Contents

Ann Lindstrand   Staffan Bergström   Hans Rosling
Birgitta Rubenson   Bo Stenson   Thorkild Tylleskär

Global Health

– an introductory textbook

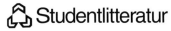
Studentlitteratur

Cover photo:
Water: Giacomo Pirozzi (UNICEF)
Vaccination: Shehzad Noorani (UNICEF)
Operation: Brian Kelly (BigStockPhoto.com)
Food: Simon van der Berg (BigStockPhoto.com)

Art. No 8012
ISBN 978-91-44-02198-0
Edition 1:9

© Ann Lindstrand, Staffan Bergström, Hans Rosling, Birgitta Rubenson,
Bo Stenson, Thorkild Tylleskär and Studentlitteratur 2006
www.studentlitteratur.se
Studentlitteratur AB, Lund

Illustrator: Niklas Hofvander
Cover design: Georg Götmark & David Herdies

Printed by Elanders Poland, Poland 2014

Preface

The enthusiasm of the students in our global health course gave us the courage to write this book. In the past the training of medical doctors and other health professionals allocated little time to the global health situation. But student demand and new government policy have recently yielded global health courses at Swedish Universities. The same is happening in many other countries. This book is intended for 5–10 weeks courses at undergraduate level in medicine, nursing, public health and pharmacy, in the training of other health professionals and in courses in the social sciences. It will hopefully also be useful in postgraduate training and as an update for those working with international health issues.

Why do health professionals need knowledge about the world outside national borders? Because the daily work in any health service today includes care for people originating from far away countries. It also includes care for local residents travelling as tourists or for work to distant parts of the world. Health staff must grasp the health variations in the whole world. Some may themselves be working in international organisations, as volunteers for Médecins Sans Frontières, as advisers for WHO or as researchers or managers in multinational pharmaceutical companies. Others will treat infections originating from the other side of the globe. Medical researchers all need to understand the global variations of the disease they spend time studying. Especially those that take part in debates and give advice on global aspects of their professional knowledge. A few will become political leaders, advisers to politicians, writers or activists for a better world.

How can global health be taught? At the University of Bergen in Norway all medical students get one week of training in global health. At Karolinska Institutet, the medical university in Stockholm, Global Health is jointly taught to medical, nursing and other students during five weeks in the elective period. The first three weeks cover the theoretical content of this textbook, with group assignments on the health development of selected countries. During the last two weeks, the students are taught in groups of 20 at medical scools in India, Iran, Tanzania or Cuba. Students study community health and follow patients at each level of health care, from the village to university hospitals. They gain an 'experience-based understanding' of what is possible at each level, and are taught by much appreciated national teachers (www.phs.ki.se/ihcar/globalhealth). Over the coming years other course formats will emerge according to the context at each university.

The aim of this textbook is to provide an overview of the global health situation for students taking such courses. It starts with a critical review of the concept of human development (Chapter 1) and of the factors that determine the health of the population in different countries (Chapter 2). Thereafter, the limitations and merits of the most used indicators of health are discussed and the sources of global health statistics and demographic data are presented (Chapter 3). Past, present and future changes in the disease panorama are explained within the concept of 'health transition' in Chapter 4.

In Chapters 5 to 9, we describe the diseases that cause most human suffering. The grouping of diseases into five chapters is mainly based on the classification used in the global burden of disease study by Christopher Murray and Allan Lopez: communicable diseases, nutritional disorders, non-communicable diseases, injuries and reproductive health. How changes in health and fertility affect world population is discussed in Chapter 10. This includes the best answers we can give to the repeatedly asked questions: "Will AIDS stop population growth?" and "Is family planning effective?" Chapter 11, on health policy and health systems, answers equally burning questions, such as: "How can world health be improved?". The chapter also explains past and current thinking on how health service should be organised and financed.

The growing number of international organisations promoting global health are briefly reviewed in Chapter 12.

The overall aim of the book is to help readers acquire an evidenced-based understanding of global health. Comments from a number of Nordic colleagues have helped us in this impossible task. The authors' own beliefs and preconceived ideas will of course have biased the selection of evidence and the conclusions presented. Several factual details may be incorrect or omitted. So please read critically. We invite all readers to provide critical comments to: hans.rosling@ki.se. Comments will be made available at www.phs.ki.se/ihcar/globalhealth/, and at the same Web site we will in due course publish revisions of selected chapters. Also check for updated animations of World Health Development at: www.gapminder.org.

Authors

All authors are attached to the division of international health at the Department of Public Health Sciences at Karolinska Institutet, the medical university in Stockholm, Sweden.

Ann Lindstrand is a medical doctor specialising in paediatrics, with a Master of Public Health from Harvard University. She has experience of working with MSF in Angola, Mozambique and Guinea-Conacry, and was the President of the Board of MSF Sweden between 1999 and 2002. She teaches international health. She is currently working in French Guiana, responsible for all Maternal and Child Health (MCH) activities.

Staffan Bergström is a gynaecologist and professor of international health. His research concerns reproductive health in low- and middle-income countries. He has worked for many years in Mozambique and other African countries. He currently coordinates extensive research and teaching collaboration with several Asian and African countries.

Hans Rosling is a medical doctor and professor of international health. His research concerns food security and nutrition in Sub-Saharan Africa, where he has served as district medical officer in Mozambique. He has developed several courses in international health, and the website gapminder.org presenting world health statistics in an understandable way.

Birgitta Rubenson is a nurse tutor with a Master of Public Health from Harvard University and a PhD in International Health from Karolinska Institutet. She has worked with primary health care, staff development and HIV/AIDS in low-income countries, both at the grass-root level and as a consultant to Sida, the World Council of Churches and Save the Children/Sweden. She also has a long experience as a teacher and course leader in International Health. She is currently working as the course-leader for the course in Global Health at Karolinska Institutet.

Bo Stenson is a political scientist with a Master of Public Health from Harvard University. He has been head of the Health division of the Swedish International Development Cooperation Agency (Sida) and has had several assignments in Africa. Currently he is principal officer in the secretariat of the Global Alliance for Vaccines and Immunization in Geneva.

Thorkild Tylleskär is a paediatrician and professor of international health at Bergen University, Norway. His focus is on nutritional disorders in low-income countries. He has a degree in African linguistics from Sorbonne and a thesis on the phonology of the kisakata language, spoken in Congo. He subsequently took a medical degree in Uppsala, where he also defended his PhD thesis on the aetiology of the paralytic disease, konzo.

Acknowledgements

Thanks to the Swedish international development co-operation Agency, (Sida) for support.

Thanks to our almost 100 colleagues in institutions abroad and in Sweden and to the many hundred students who have given valuable comments during the development of the manuscript. Through their comments many weaknesses and inconsistencies have been avoided – the remaining mistakes are the responsibility of the authors.

1 What is development?

> *Poverty means working for more than 18 hours a day, but still not earning enough to feed myself, my husband and two children.*
>
> A poor woman, Cambodia 1998

Is world health improving? Our answer is "Yes!" But all aspects of world health are not going in the right direction! The general health situation is deteriorating in several countries. Despite this, we find that the positive health trends dominate in an increasingly complex world.

Health is a good indicator of human life conditions, and the general development of a country determines the health of its population. Data of sufficient reliability is available to confirm that the average health status of the world population has improved considerably during the last 50 years. Since 1950 life expectancy at birth in the world population is estimated to have increased from less than 50 to more than 65 years (WHO 2003). On average 15 years have been added to each human life in the last two generations. This improvement is a result of both better welfare and improved health services. Literacy is an important health determinant that has increased continuously in almost all countries. Vaccines and antibiotics have in the last decades become available to most of the world population.

In spite of the overall improvement, global health variations remain very unfair by any standards of morals and justice. The differences in health reflect wide differences not only between nations but also within nations. Poverty remains the main underlying cause of disease in the world. Three major setbacks for world health slowed down the global health improvement in the last decades. The three setbacks are firstly the HIV epidemic, secondly wars, and thirdly the social consequences of the sudden transition to market economy in former communist countries. It can therefore be said that world health is getting better and worse at the same time, but the improvement dominates. With the present slow rate of overall improvement world health will remain unacceptably bad and unfair for many decades to come.

The unfairness of the world is a colossal political and moral challenge. How large is the unfairness in the world?

The consumption of an average person in the poorest country only corresponds to an expenditure of USD 500 per year, while an average person in the richest country has an annual income of USD 50 000 – *100 times more*!

Three children per thousand live births die in the healthiest country, compared to 300 child deaths per 1 000 live births in the country with most sickness – once again *100 times more*!

The World Health Chart (inside the cover) displays these income and health variations between countries. The huge difference makes it necessary to use inverse logarithmic scales to show the disparities of the world. In the "new world map" on the inside of the cover 'healthy' & 'sick' replace 'north' & 'south', while 'poor' & 'rich' replace 'west' & 'east'. The chart shows that *our world is unfair*.

This means that the world disparity in resources per health need (USD per child death) is $100 \times 100 = 10\,000$ times. That is the size of the unfairness, tenthousand times more resources are available to avoid a

Table 1.1 United Nations Millennium Development Goals and Targets for the period 1990–2015.

	Development Goals	Targets
1	Eradicate extreme poverty and hunger	1. Reduce by half the proportion of people living on less than a dollar a day 2. Reduce by half the proportion of people suffering from hunger
2	Achieve universal primary education	3. Ensure that all boys and girls complete a full course of primary schooling
3	Promote gender equality and empower women	4. Eliminate gender disparity in primary and secondary education preferably by 2005, and at all levels by 2015
4	Reduce child mortality	5. Reduce by two thirds the mortality rate among children under five
5	Improve maternal health	6. Reduce by three quarters the maternal mortality ratio
6	Combat HIV/AIDS, malaria and other diseases	7. Halt and begin to reverse the spread of HIV/AIDS 8. Halt and begin to reverse the incidence of malaria and other major diseases
7	Ensure environmental sustainability	9. Integrate the principles of sustainable development into country policies and programmes; reverse loss of environmental resources 10. Reduce by half the proportion of people without sustainable access to safe drinking water 11. Achieve significant improvement in lives of at least 100 million slum dwellers by 2020
8	Develop a global partnership for development	12. Develop further an open trading and financial system that is rule-based, predictable and non-discriminatory. Includes a commitment to good governance, development and poverty reduction — nationally and internationally 13. Address the least developed countries' special needs. This includes tariff- and quota-free access for their exports; enhanced debt relief for heavily indebted poor countries; cancellation of official bilateral debt; and more generous official development assistance for countries committed to poverty reduction 14. Address the special needs of landlocked and small island developing States 15. Deal comprehensively with developing countries' debt problems through national and international measures to make debt sustainable in the long term 16. In co-operation with the developing countries, develop decent and productive work for youth 17. In co-operation with pharmaceutical companies, provide access to affordable essential drugs in developing countries 18. In co-operation with the private sector, make available the benefits of new technologies — especially information and communication technologies

child death in Sweden compared to what is at hand to save a child in Sierra Leone.

Note that ethnic, geographic, gender and income disparities within nations are not shown in the World Health Chart.

Understanding the character and size of global disparities is also a major intellectual challenge, as is the scientific analysis of how, why and for whom life conditions are changing for the better and for the worse. The global disparities in health and wealth have probably never been wider then they are today. Yet there is no longer one single big gap between countries with healthy and sick populations. Instead there are rather many health gaps between different groups of nations, as well as between different population groups within nations. The health status of different nations currently lie at all levels between the extremes. World health is not only unfair in spite of improvements, it is also an increasingly complex continuity.

It is in the interest of all countries and persons that the global health situation improves at a faster rate. Almost half of UN's Millennium Development Goals relate to health (Table 1.1). The unjust global health disparities are incompatible with global security. Better global health will also contribute to a stable world population, which is crucial for the sustainable use of environmental resources. The improvement of world health is largely a political issue, but it also requires an understanding of which actions will be most effective in improving health in different contexts. This book is a modest summary of present understanding of global health and how it can be improved.

This chapter starts by reviewing when and why the present injustice of the world emerged? The historic injustices inflicted on the rest of the world during centuries of European colonialism and North American dominance are one important factor in explaining the present unfairness. However, our review in this chapter indicates that the injustice also has deeper historical causes that can be traced back through thousands of years. The historical causes of today's disparities of the world interact in a complex web with contemporary political, social, cultural and economic causes. We will briefly review both the historical roots and the contemporary determinants of human development. Two particular difficulties arise, however, when attempting to summarise our present understanding of the broad pattern of human development.

The first difficulty is scientific. Global development is determined by a combination of many interacting factors. The analysis, therefore, requires the involvement of many academic disciplines and the use of a wide variety of data, information and theories. You can obtain evidence on which to base your worldview from the latest developmental statistics. You can visualise these descriptive statistics using animated graphics by installing the *World Health Chart* and other software that can be downloaded free of charge.[1] The software enables you to view

a long-term perspective on global health development. This perspective may lead you to share our view that there is hope for a better world. However, the descriptive statistics provides no information about the causal relationship between the various dimensions of development, such as health and economics. Nor can world development be understood solely on the basis of numerical information; understanding also requires knowledge of cultural, social and political structures, mechanisms and contexts. In other words: it is necessary to study and consult a number of academic disciplines to obtain an evidence-based worldview. The authors of this book only know part of what is necessary, so be critical throughout your reading!

The second difficulty is political. Any conclusion about human development, even the graphic display of descriptive statistics, will conflict with a number of ideological, cultural or moral views. No review of the world situation is based exclusively on objective evidence. Some readers may even find it irrelevant to make global health development an area of academic study, pointing out that urgent action is what is needed to improve the world. However, actions for a better world will have a greater chance of success if they are based on the best possible understanding of the present situation and if they are based on knowledge of actions that have worked in similar contexts.

The analysis of global development easily lends itself to the promotion of one's own favourite political ideas or moral views concerning, for example, free trade, environmental conservation, gender equality, social justice, war on terrorism and nationalism. Writing on global health, is often dominated by skewed arguments for the importance of more resources for the health sector. The environmentalist will likewise argue for the importance of environmental protection, the economist for free trade, etc. Few specialists are in a position to provide

[1]   www.gapminder.org

an evidence-based review of the relative importance of all major aspects of global development (Sen 1999).

We hope that our attempt will stimulate health professionals to study economics, archaeology, history, demography, geography, political sciences, sociology, anthropology and all other subjects that offer explanations for the variation in health conditions between and within different countries.

Following a discussion of the concept of development, we present the cases of four contemporary young women who live at very different levels of 'development'. We then review different explanations for the historical origins of the current disparities in world health. We briefly discuss national developmental strategies of the last 50 years, and the issue of globalisation that has arisen during the preceding few decades. We conclude the chapter by providing a more evidence-based taxonomy of countries that avoids the old fashioned classification of all countries into only two groups; "*developing countries*" and "*industrialised countries*". An evidence-based view of world health today requires a classification of countries into more than two groups. We suggest the classification of countries into four groups: "*high-income*", "*middle-income*", "*low-income*" and "*collapsed*" countries.

1.1 Definitions of development

The meaning of human 'development' is straightforward, when seen in the light of the changes in daily life that took place during the Stone Age. The invention of stone tools and the discovery of how to use fire for domestic purposes were major positive developments for humanity. The same is true of the invention of baskets for collecting food, and the making of nets for catching fish. The invention of pottery led to major improvements in food preparation and storage. Despite these technologies life was rough and mortality high during Stone Age. The first 100 000 years after the origin of the human species saw the human population rise to only 10 million. Based on the slow growth of the human population we must conclude that the hunters and gatherers that lived during Stone Age had a miserable health and a short life.

Since the development of human language, no innovation has had such a great impact on human development as the introduction of agriculture. This took place less than 10 000 years ago. Most readers will agree that domestication of the major food crops (wheat, rice, maize, potatoes and cassava) and the domestication of the main domestic animals (sheep, goats, horses and cattle) were major achievements for human societies. Another important step was the domestication of dogs and cats. These animals improved security and reduced the plague of rats. The spread and adoption of all these advancements improved human welfare. The improved food supply that agriculture secured improved health: more children survived and adults lived longer. The longer life that resulted from the development of agriculture allowed the number of humans to increase gradually from 10 million during the Stone Age to many hundreds of millions before industrialisation. The sequence of improvements in human living conditions that increased health and in this way led to population growth during thousands of years of agriculture is widely accepted as 'development' of human societies and civilisations. The closer we come to the present, however, the more controversial the concept of development becomes.

To some, 'development' today means a more or less linear continuation of the historical development of human societies in the direction of better technologies, increased consumption, continued economic growth and greater human choice. To others, 'development' is interpreted as negative changes in human life imposed by 'western culture' upon ethnic groups living a 'harmonic life' in remote rainforests and high mountains. The populations of such traditional societies are considered to live a 'better' life, which may be destroyed by 'development'. In contrast to these polarised views, international debate has seen a convergence in our understanding of development during the past decade. This convergence towards "a multidimensional view" of development is largely the result of the work of Amartya Sen (1999), who won the Nobel Prize in Economics in 1999 for his studies of human development. The present consensus is that 'development' may be defined as follows:

> "Development is the desired change from a life with many sufferings and few choices to a life with satisfied basic needs and many choices, made available through the sustainable use of natural resources."

The major basic needs for development are provision of food, water, housing and other forms of basic material welfare. Others dimensions are health service, education, human rights and gender equality, freedom and democracy, and a fair distribution of economic growth combined with a sustainable use of natural resources. Most of these dimensions of development are both an end in themselves, and a means of progress. Health, for example, is a major end in itself, but also a means to accomplish education, which in turn will contribute to economic growth. Economic growth is perhaps the most important means of progress in most of the other dimensions. However, in contrast to most other dimensions, economic growth is not an end in itself. Some regard the sustainable use of natural resources as an end in itself, whereas others regard environmental protection as a matter of equity in resource utilisation between those living today and future generations.

The multidimensional understanding of development can be expressed in many ways. In his textbook on economic development, Todaro (2002) states that develop-

ment is a combined social, economic and institutional process with three objectives:

> 'to increase the availability of basic life-sustaining goods, to generate greater individual and national self-esteem, to expand the range of economic and social choices.'

A shorter definition of development is provided by the United Nations Development Programme (UNDP 1997):

> "Development is the process of enlarging people's choices."

Economic growth is central to the provision of choices in the lives of humans. But even for the very poor there is much more to development than money (Narayan 2000). Many argue that human development relates as much to the fulfilment of spiritual needs and improved self-esteem as it does to economic growth. Prominent non-economic dimensions of development are freedom, dignity, self-esteem and protection from violence and abuse. Amartya Sen (1999) emphasises that money is a means to achieve greater values, rather than an end in itself. The distribution of income is as important as the average income per capita of a country, if greater human values are to be achieved in a population.

The emerging common focus for global development is the reduction and eventual eradication of poverty. Income poverty is only one component of poverty: others include lack of self-esteem, violations of human rights, ignorance, and disease. The alleviation of poverty, both in its narrow economic sense and in its broader human definition, is both an end in itself, and a means to increase economic growth. The increased focus on the alleviation of poverty by international development agencies may also be seen as a move away from a focus on nations, towards a focus on individuals. This increased focus on poverty alleviation in the international debate may be seen as part of a globalisation trend that decreases the role of nations.

The understanding of human development and the alleviation of poverty converged gradually during the 1990s, following the end of the Cold War. The eradication of poverty, freedom from hunger, access to safe water, basic education for all children, equal human rights for women and men, a healthy life and the sustainable use of natural resources are now regarded as core aspects of human development by all concerned international agencies. The World Bank, the World Health Organization and most other UN organisations now express similar views about development. A peculiar sign of this convergence of international views of development was the awarding by the World Bank (2001) of credit to the socialist government in Cuba for progress in education and health in that country. As early as 1993, the World Bank stated in its yearbook that a better life involves more than simply higher income:

> "Development encompasses as ends in themselves better education, higher standards of health and nutrition, less poverty, a cleaner environment, more equality of opportunity, greater individual freedom, and a richer cultural life."

Two decades ago, the World Health Organization argued that good health could be achieved if the primary health care policy was followed, without mentioning how much this policy would cost to implement. Health was mainly expressed as a goal in itself. The World Bank had little, if any, interest in health at that time. Representatives of the Bank would have argued, if asked, that health improvements would come as a secondary effect of economic growth. Today, the World Bank (2004) and the World Health Organization argue jointly that public investment in improved health for the poor of the world is not only a prerequisite for broadly defined human development, but also a prerequisite for narrowly defined economic growth. Readers should critically

assess whether the broad definition of development is a valid concept; and whether the World Bank, the World Health Organization, other international organisations and national governments manage to follow the new development policy in practice.

Non-governmental organisations, united in networks such as the People's Health Movement[1], argue that the involvement of local communities in development is a prerequisite for sustainability, effectiveness and the achievement of self-esteem and freedom, as well as for the other broader objectives of development. The non-governmental organisations claim that sustainable multidimensional development is a political grassroots process, rather than a change in budget allocations between different sectors of society. As we will see, many researchers in economic history and political sciences draw similar conclusions when arguing for the important role of public institutions and civil society in successful multidimensional development.

1.2 Four levels of development

We present here four short stories about the lives of 20-year-old daughters in average families in countries at four different levels of development. These four women have four different degrees of human choice open to them. The first example is the daughter in a Swedish family living in a high-income country. The yearly income of a person in this group of countries is around USD 20 000, i.e. about USD 50 per day. One billion out of the six billion people in the world live in high-income countries. The second example is the daughter in a Brazilian family living in a middle-income country, where the average yearly income per person is between USD 1 000 and 10 000. The middle-income countries have a com-

---

[1] http://phmovement.org/

Box 1.1

Family in a high-income country (daily income about USD 50 per person)

The Swedish family gathers after the evening meal to discuss the 20-year-old daughter's holiday plans. Anna has just finished upper secondary school and has not yet decided whether she wants to start university studies after the summer holiday. But just in case she has applied for the favourable public loans that enable young people from all socio-economic backgrounds to study at universities. Her main concern is not about her future, but that she is leaving home in less than one week for her first holiday trip without her parents. She is going to travel by train through Germany, France, Spain and Portugal together with her cousin. She had planned to do this trip with her ex-boyfriend, but he left her for another girlfriend two months ago. Her mother is not happy about Anna's holiday plans. She worries that her daughter may lose the medicines she needs to take daily to treat her asthma. It may be difficult to find the same brands of tablets and inhalation sprays in foreign countries. Anna comforts her mother by telling her that she will take enough medicine with her, medicine that she buys at highly subsidised prices in Sweden. Her mother also worries that her daughter will not eat enough. In her early teens, Anna suffered a mild form of anorexia nervosa. The daughter knows about her mother's secret worries, and to comfort her further she promises to call home daily on her mobile telephone, which she will take with her. Her father suggests that it will be cheaper for her to send SMS messages. He reluctantly allows Anna to borrow his digital camera. The father reminds Anna to send postcards to her grandmother. The 80-year-old lady has been admitted to a public nursing home due to advanced Alzheimer's disease. Anna cannot see the point of sending postcards to her grandmother, as the old lady does not remember anything. However, Anna knows her father has a bad conscience for not visiting his mother every week, so she promises to send postcards to the nursing home. After all, her father has agreed to lend her his new digital camera! The daughter is finally reminded by her mother to take enough disposable contact lenses. For cosmetic reasons, she uses lenses instead of glasses to correct for her short-sightedness. Anna is happy that she can leave her parents just to enjoy travelling to foreign countries. Anna has earned part of the money needed for the travel by working in the holidays, but most of the money is a gift from her grandfather, who said that his pension was high enough to share some of it with his beloved granddaughter.

---

bined population of almost three billion people, – nearly half of the world's population. The third example is from Uttar Pradesh in India, a state in which the average income is lower than the average of all India. The average income per person and year is estimated to be less than USD 1 000. Almost 2 billion people in the world live in this reality. The fourth example is a family in Liberia at the time when the rule of government was replaced by the terror of fighting warlords. This example presents the situation in a few 'collapsed' low-income countries. Only about 50 million people live in countries or parts of countries with collapsed civil administration. They represent less than 1 % of the world's population. Consider the four fictive conversations after the evening meal in these four different families (Boxes 1.1 to 1.4).

The very different health situations of these four families show that the world health situation can no longer be described as being that of either a rich country or a poor country. The contemporary world health situation is best understood as an extremely wide but continuous spectrum of health statuses. The life situations of the

---

Box 1.2

Family in a middle-income country (daily income about USD 10 per person)

The Brazilian family in a small town in central Brazil gathers for the evening meal. The 20-year-old daughter, Ana, is upset because her father has said that he is unable to pay for her planned university studies. She was involved in a traffic accident last year, and her father explains the lack of money by reference to the high cost of her treatment. She was operated for fractures of both legs. Her father took her to a private hospital, which he believed would provide better care than the cheaper government hospital. Since childhood Ana wears glasses to correct her short-sightedness. She hates the glasses for cosmetic reasons, but the family cannot afford to buy her contact lenses. Ana often takes her glasses off so that she will look better when she is walking around town. Her father claims that the accident occurred because she was not using her glasses that day. Ana says the car hit her because the driver was drunk. Anyhow, glasses, the treatment of her fractures, and

installation of a new bathroom in the house was what this family's economy could afford, says the father. Ana must now start earning her own money.

In order for her to find a job, she has been offered the opportunity to stay with her cousin's family in Rio de Janeiro. This is on the understanding that she helps to care for their sick grandmother, who lives with the cousin's family. The 66-year-old lady had one leg amputated last year due to complications from diabetes, and since then she has had to take regular medication against depression. Ana is told that it is a good offer to go to Rio. The cousin's family has a new DVD-player, something that her own family has not yet been able to afford to buy. Ana is reluctant to leave her hometown because of her new boyfriend, whom she has not yet introduced to her parents. She would really like to study at the university in her hometown instead of working and caring for her sick and sad grandmother.

---

first two women, indeed – all of the first three women – can today be found within the same country, or even in the same town or village. Fortunately, the tragic life of the fourth young woman remains relatively rare. Such horror is found in only a handful of collapsed nations in Asia and Africa. The United Nations has taken wise actions during the previous decade, and these actions have assisted countries, such as Mozambique and Cambodia, to turn prolonged civil wars into stable peace.

The lives of the four young women exemplify the situation for the average citizen in each of four groups of countries. The classification into high-income, middle-income and low-income countries, with the fourth group of collapsed countries, is useful but very far from perfect. The statement that high-income countries are more developed than the countries in the other groups does

not mean that all aspects of life are better in the richest countries. Undoubtedly, many cultural, social and spiritual aspects of life are better for the young women in Brazil, India and perhaps even in war-torn Liberia than they are for large parts of the populations in high-income countries.

One useful overall indicator of where life is, on average, better than in other contexts is the direction of human migration in the contemporary world. Very few young persons from rich countries migrate to middle-income or low-income countries. In contrast, people migrate overwhelmingly in the direction away from poverty, disease, and lack of human rights towards material wealth, education, a good health service and human rights. Many foreigners immigrate to Sweden in spite of the cold weather, the strange language and the reserved social attitudes in this northern country. The very

16

Box 1.3

Family in a low-income country (daily income about USD 2 per person)

The Indian family gathers for the evening meal on the veranda outside their small house in rural India. Ana's family lives in a village in the state of Uttar Pradesh.

The 20-year-old daughter, Ana, is today visiting her parents to show them her second child, a baby who was born the year before. Ana says she wants to listen to her father's radio. Her husband's family has a radio, but has been unable to afford batteries for the radio for several months now. The reason is that her last delivery was costly for her and her husband. She is still weak following the delivery, and has developed a cough in recent months. The cough syrup she was prescribed at the public health centre did not cure her. The 8-kilometre walk today from the village where she lives with her husband's family has tired her. The hidden aim of her visit to her parents is to discuss whether they can help to pay for medicines to treat her cough and her weakness. She and her husband hope that her parents will help to pay for good medicines. She looks at her small family and thinks: "Well, at least I still have two healthy children and a kind husband, although we are so poor that we only get enough food to eat every second day." She thinks that it is a shame that she should be a burden to them. How long will her husband put up with her if she remains sick?

She cannot read, as she had to leave primary school after only one year. Her father said there was no point in continuing, since she could not see what the teacher wrote on the blackboard. The family could never afford to buy glasses for her short-sightedness. The teacher had told her father that glasses were the only thing the clever little girl needed to learn to read and write. Her younger brother, went to school long enough to learn to read. He is now reading the text on the bottle of cough syrup that she has been taking every day for a week, without any effect. Her parents are very concerned about her health, but no one realises that, in addition to anaemia, she has pulmonary tuberculosis. The latter diagnosis was missed due to the limited diagnostic resources at the health centre where she was very briefly examined.

Her grandmother died some years ago, after coughing blood for many months. The family thinks she died from tuberculosis, but she was never taken to the clinic for diagnosis. She was instead given traditional medicines at home. Tuberculosis is considered to be a shameful sign of poverty. Consequently, the word 'tuberculosis' is never mentioned in the family discussion. The family knows the possible significance of chronic coughing, but use an old Hindi word for chronic cough when talking about Ana's disease. Her mother says she should be taken to a private doctor. Her father says it is too expensive; it would be cheaper to take her to a traditional Ayurvedic clinic. The herbal treatment given at that clinic cured his back pain last year, and he thinks it also may cure his daughter's cough. He is willing to pay for traditional treatment, but not for consultation with a private doctor. The reason for his reluctance is that doctors always prescribe very expensive medicines. Ana knows precisely what she would do if she had her own money and the right to decide for herself. But this is not the case, and she does not want to embarrass her husband by begging her father for more money. She will try the herbal medicine, but the tuberculosis bacteria will continue to destroy her lungs and infect her children. Ana does not have any other choice, not even to cry. But she has a secret determination: "I must survive this disease, to make it possible for my daughter to go to school!"

Box 1.4

Family in a collapsed country (daily income less than USD 1 per person)

The family in Liberia lived in a rural village not far from the capital Monrovia during the recent period when the political and administrative functions of this West African country collapsed during a prolonged armed conflict. Liberia is presently in the process of regaining peace and basic public functions.

The young Liberian woman Ana had never been to school. This had always saddened her. This story begins when her parents returned to what used to be their home before the war. Ana's father had been in hospital close to the capital for two months. He suffered severe injuries during the fighting that took place between two armed gangs in their village two months ago. After the fight, the victorious armed gang started to burn down all the houses in the village. While trying to stop them from burning the family house down, her father was badly cut with a big knife. His right elbow joint was cut open, but he managed to escape to his family, who were already hiding in the forest. The mother told Ana to remain with her small brothers in the hiding place in the forest while she tried to help her husband to get to a hospital. They knew of a hospital supported by a humanitarian relief organisation. It was situated a few day's walk away. Ana's mother had heard that this hospital also treated poor people who could not pay. Her father reached the hospital in time and recovered, following amputation of his right arm above the elbow. He now thanks God that he is alive and still has his left hand.

Ana lived in the forest with her brothers while their parents were at the hospital. They ate from the family's cassava field. This productive root crop protected them from starvation. During the second week of hiding, her youngest brother suddenly developed a high fever, and she had to return to their village with her sick brother on her back, to look for treatment. The older brothers had to follow. On the path, they met a passing gang of armed teenagers, who raped Ana in front of her brothers. She had not recognised the kind of people who were approaching in time to be able to hide. Once, the imam in their village had said that her problem in recognising people was due to

the fact that she was short-sighted. The family could never afford to buy her the glasses that the imam said she needed.

Following the rape, she managed to get back to their village with her sick brother. However, the man who owned a bicycle and used to bring and sell modern tablets against malaria had left the village, as had the traditional healer who sold herbal medicine against fever. The sun set and in the darkness of the night she could do nothing but sit beside her young brother and try to comfort him. His fever became worse, he got convulsions and died in the middle of the night. The next morning, some old women who had remained in the village helped her to bury the little body. She now shows her parents the grave, where they all pray together.

Ana is relieved that her parents do not blame her for her brother's death. Although her parents are kind, she does not want to tell them that she was raped. In spite of all the tragedies that have affected them, Ana and her mother are comforted by the reunion of the family, and they cook a full meal for everyone. They have not eaten much in recent weeks, because one night someone stole almost all the cassava plants in their field. The children have been extremely hungry, but tonight they will be able to eat well. The parents have brought back a sack of maize flour that they were given when leaving the hospital. Ana's two surviving brothers have managed to catch two small birds. Ana fries the birds over the fire, while her mother prepares the maize porridge. She and her brothers are allowed to eat as much as they want. In silence, they watch their father learning to eat with his left hand. The father thinks: "Had we fled in time to the neighbouring country, we would have avoided all these sufferings." Ana thinks that she is pregnant, as she has not had any bleedings since the rape. It saddens her immensely that this is not the child of the man she loved. He was killed in the war last year. What she will not know until several years later when peace has returned to her country is that she was infected with HIV during the rape. She and her only child will only have a few years to live together.

fact that people from all continents are willing to settle in Sweden shows clearly that wealth, health, education, peace, and human rights are highly valued by humans from all over the world.

But how and why did human health and welfare become so unevenly distributed in the world? As far as we know, there were no major differences in human health between the continents during the Stone Age. So why and at what point in time during the last 10 000 years did the present differences in human health and development emerge? An old hypothesis is that the differences can be explained by differences in climate (Landes 1999).

1.3 Climate

None of the early agricultural civilisations developed in a cold climate, and it was people living under a hot sun who invented writing and mathematics. The first advanced civilisations were developed by the people living in hot climates along the Indus River in what is now Pakistan, by the Maya Indians in tropical Guatemala and Mexico, and by the Nile valley populations of what is now Egypt and Sudan. Even though advanced civilisations arose first in the tropics, one explanation of the global disparities in human health and welfare that is frequently advanced is that a cold climate favours planning and development. A hot climate, in contrast, is perceived to hamper activity and to enable people to live with less planning (since there is no winter that must be lived through). The populations that now live in the areas of ancient civilisations have inherited the hot climate from their ancestors. Paradoxically, many of the offspring of the great civilisations now live under more modest socio-economic conditions than the descendants of the barbarian tribes in the cold climates of northern Europe. This suggests that if cold climate has been a positive determinant for human development, the climatic effect on develop-

ment must have differed tremendously between different historic periods.

A humid, tropical climate is believed to hamper development because it favours the spread of many parasitic and viral diseases that are transmitted by insects that only live in the tropics. The most important of such diseases is malaria. Humans originated in the tropics, but it is assumed that the migration to sub-tropical climates improved health and facilitated the growth of the human population due to a lower incidence of the parasitic diseases of the tropics (McNeill 1976). Studies of the contemporary impact of climate on development also suggest that the burden of malaria is a major reason for the slow economic growth in many lowland tropical countries. It is also possible that malaria contributed to the decline of ancient civilisations in the humid tropics. It is remarkable that an emerging human civilisation was successful in the hot and dry climate of northern Sudan and Egypt along the Nile. However, this civilisation stopped north of the hot and humid climate of southern Sudan. The much heavier burden of malaria in the humid tropics is one plausible explanation of this early developmental demarcation. Today, Egypt has completely eradicated malaria, but the disease remains a major health problem in southern Sudan.

It should be noted that what is commonly called 'malaria' is actually several different diseases, all caused by different species of the malaria parasite. Falciparum malaria is the most severe form, because it affects the brain. This form only exists in humid, tropical countries; whereas a malaria parasite that gives a milder form of the disease, *Plasmodium vivax*, existed as far north as Sweden less than a century ago. The malaria parasites that were common in colder countries, when the countries at these latitudes were poor, survived the winter in a dormant form in the human liver. Malaria disappeared from Sweden following the draining of the marshlands where the mosquitoes that acted as hosts for the parasites bred. Better housing also greatly reduced the number of mosquito bites. The use of quinine, a herbal drug from South America, for the treatment of malaria also contributed to the disappearance of the disease. The *Anopheles* mosquito, which is capable of transmitting malaria parasites, is still common in Sweden, but it is only a nuisance for humans now, inflicting itchy bites during the summer months. The mosquitoes in Sweden no longer carry malaria parasites, since nobody in the population is infected. The climate did not change, but poverty disappeared.

In lowland tropical areas, malaria mosquitoes can transmit the parasite from human to human all year round. Falciparum malaria requires transmission between mosquitoes and humans in order to continue uninterrupted all year around. Hence, this severe form of malaria only constitutes an obstacle to human development in lowland tropical regions. An increase in population density in such areas will inevitably increase the occurrence of malaria, if no special measures are taken to control the disease. However, even in the most tropical countries all forms of malaria can be overcome with knowledge, resources and political determination. Singapore, Cuba and some other highly developed tropical countries have eradicated malaria. The reason that malaria remains a problem in other tropical countries is the poverty of these countries, which leads to poor human life conditions and insufficient malaria control. But it is fair to conclude that malaria contributes to the poverty remaining in these countries. The relationship between poverty and malaria is reciprocal: poverty causes malaria and malaria causes poverty. The alleviation of poverty in countries with hot, humid climates requires extra resources for the control of malaria (McMichael 2001).

Another example of a disease that hampers development in tropical areas is yellow fever, which is a viral disease. The virus is transmitted by a number of mosquito species, most readily by *Aedes aegypti*, which is common in tropical areas. Epidemic outbreaks of yellow fever halted the first attempt to construct the Panama Canal between 1881 and 1889. The French company that tried to build the canal housed thousands of workers under miserable conditions. The workers were constantly bitten by mosquitoes, and the resulting epidemics of yellow fever killed a large proportion of the workers. It was the Cuban researcher, Carlos Juan Finlay that in 1881 suggested that mosquitoes transmitted yellow fever. Experiments on humans carried out by Walter Reed in 1901 proved that the mosquito hypothesis was correct. Reed was at the time a physician in the US Army during the US occupation of Cuba. He showed, long before a vaccine became available, that mosquito control could prevent yellow fever. Based on Reed's findings, an American company started the second attempt to build the Panama Canal in 1907. A substantial investment was made in sanitary control by qualified public health staff throughout the entire period of work. The company started by draining the swamps. They built mosquito-free living quarters for the workers, in this way also contributing to preventing malaria. The construction of the Panama Canal was successfully completed in 1914. A memorial at the Pacific end of the canal honours Finlay for the discovery that made this major economic investment possible (Desowitz 1998). The US Army has named its main medical research institute after Reed, and the Cuban government has named its vaccine institute after Finlay. Both governments honour their heroes of public health. This shows the enormous importance of medical advances for development in tropical regions. The climate hampers economic development in tropical regions by facilitating the spread of some infectious diseases, but with extra investments these infectious diseases can now be controlled, and this will promote economic development in the tropics.

A cold climate has also been an obstacle to development, by favouring the transmission of infectious diseases that thrive when poor people live under cramped conditions in frosty and miserable houses. Prominent examples are tuberculosis and leprosy. Leprosy is also known as Hansen's disease, after the Norwegian researcher Armauer Hansen, who identified the leprosy bacterium in 1874. His studies were conducted among poor patients in the leprosy hospital in the town of Bergen in western Norway. At that time, leprosy was common among the poor in Norway. Leprosy was transmitted when many persons survived the cold winter packed into cold and miserable cottages. The Center of International Health at Bergen University is situated in "Armauer Hansen Building". In this way the country with cold climate also honors its conqueror of the poverty diseases that were specifically prevalent in the cold climate.

Climate has undoubtedly affected the development of societies. Some scholars attribute a major role to climate (Landes 1999) when explaining the present lower level of human development in tropical climates. Others mention that tropical climate also has favoured economic development, as a number of very valuable crops, such as spices, sugar cane and tobacco, can only grow in warm climates. It is clear that different climates can stimulate or hamper development, but it cannot be convincingly demonstrated that climate is the main explanation for the great differences in living conditions and health status in today's world.

We will search for the major causes of contemporary developmental differences by reviewing history and identifying the period during which the great differences in development emerged. We commence where all humans originated, in Africa. We shall briefly review human society from a time when all our ancestors were hunter-gatherers in Africa until they had eventually spread to all corners of the world. What determined the spread of agriculture among our stone-age ancestors, and what determined the formation of the great empires and civilisations with written languages and

advancing technologies? We shall ask why European colonialism, followed by North American dominance, has ruled the world for the last 500 years. If we can identify the period at which the developmental and health differences emerged and increased, we may identify the major causes of these differences.

1.4 Hunters and gatherers (up to 10 000 years ago)

Different academic disciplines study the development of human living conditions over very different time scales. Evolutionary biology covers many millions of years. Archaeology studies the human development that has taken place during the last one million years. Historians are only concerned about written history, approximately the last 5 000 years since the art of writing was invented in present Iraq. Economists study the last few hundred years. Political science focuses mainly on the last 200 years, and its sub-discipline 'development studies' focuses on world development during the last 50 years.

Historical documentation of human diseases exists already in ancient Chinese, Persian, Indian, Arabic, and Greek texts. However, reasonable quantitative documentation of disease occurrence and mortality are limited to the last two centuries. We must therefore depend on research in demography, history and archaeology to assess indirectly human health in earlier historical periods. An estimate of the health of pre-historical and historical populations can be obtained from the population growth. People must have been healthier where more of them survived and the number of people increased. From this follows that there must have been long periods when people were healthier in India and China than anywhere else in the world.

But let us start from the beginning. Present scientific consensus is that humans originated from Africa (Kaessmann & Paabo 2002). Human ancestors started to spread from Africa more than 100 000 years ago. Several waves of early human ancestors managed to adopt to the environment in the Middle East and on the Eurasian continent. The evolutionary origin of modern *Homo sapiens* has not been resolved. According to the "multiregional hypothesis", modern human populations inherited their genes from different waves of human ancestors that came out of Africa at widely different periods. A different hypothesis proposes that one isolated population of early humans evolved into modern *Homo sapiens*. This population succeeded in spreading across Africa, Middle East, Europe, Asia, Australia, and eventually to the Americas. They displaced, killed and eventually replaced all early human populations as they spread. Support for this hypothesis comes from molecular biology, especially studies of DNA. These methods date the time of divergence from the common ancestor of all modern human populations to less than 200 000 years ago. This date is incompatible with the "multiregional hypothesis", since it gives a human species that is too young for the waves of migration to have occurred. Whichever model (if either) is correct, the oldest fossil evidence for anatomically modern humans is about 130 000 years old in Africa, and 90 000 years old outside Africa. The present differences in external traits in humans from different geographic regions, sometimes referred to as human races, have thus existed for less than 100 000 years. The genetic variation that lies behind these differences constitutes less than 1 % of the evolutionary history that all people have in common (Boyd & Silk 2000).

Humans advanced to using stone tools and the creation of art about 40 000 years ago. This marked the start of the older Stone Age, which ranged from 40 000 to 10 000 years BC. During this period all our ancestors lived from gathering edible plants and hunting animals. Humans slowly increased in number, filled new areas, and parts of the population migrated to new locations. As long as there was enough plants to gather

for food and sufficient animals to hunt, humans remained in one place and their numbers grew in the newly occupied areas. When food supplies became insufficient, some migrated to new places. The main driving force was probably the gradual increase in the number of people. The average number of children born to each woman in the hunter-gather populations is estimated to have been at least six. If four of these died during childhood, the population would not grow. If less than four children died, the population would grow. Human populations are capable of a more than two-fold increase in their numbers in one generation and a more than 16-fold increase in a century. In periods of good availability of food, the health of our ancestors may have been relatively good during some generations. They ate a variety of foods. The population density was low, which minimised the transmission of infectious diseases. In spite of this, the human population increased very slowly following the exodus from Africa. This means that the good periods were few and the harsh periods many. Our Stone Age ancestors suffered many injuries and lived a risky and hazardous life. During long periods they had a very low life expectancy due to frequent early deaths.

The increase in numbers that occurred as soon as most children survived made the local life of hunter-gatherers unsustainable. That is why they had to move on, gradually and in stages, until they filled the world. During good periods, their numbers doubled in a generation. When humans crossed from Asia into the Americas and arrived at the prairies of North America, they found many wild animals to hunt. This probably led to a period of plenty, and the number of hunters multiplied. The humans caused in this way the extinction of many of the animal species in North America. The same happened in all areas where humans found an excess of easily-hunted animals.

By the end of the last Ice Age, about 10 000 years ago, human populations had reached every continent. Following Europe,

Asia and Australia, they moved on *via* Alaska to North, Central and South America. Archaeological evidence indicates that the present genetic variations between human groups had already been formed. The human population of the world 10 000 years ago is estimated to have been less than 10 million people, approximately the same as the present population of Sweden. All groups on all continents still lived from gathering edible wild plants, catching fish and hunting wild animals and birds. No major differences in 'development' or health emerged in the period during which humans spread to all continents.

Why was the world population so small 10 000 years ago? Why did the human population not exceed 10 million people in the course of the first 90 000 years of human life, equal to about 4 000 generations? The growth rate of the human population was less than 0.02 % per year during the older Stone Age, which corresponds to adding less than one person to a group of 1 000 during one generation.

Very few human groups that live primarily from hunting and gathering remain today. These few remaining groups are integrated into the world economy in several ways. However, before such integration takes place the capacity of the ecological system in each area to provide edible wild plants for the gatherer and game for the hunter determines the size of the hunting-gathering populations. Research among these groups reveals their harsh living conditions, with high mortality among both children and adults. Each woman on average gives birth to six to eight children during her life. Pre-agricultural societies were able to regulate their birth rate through prolonged breastfeeding, abstinence and the expulsion of young adults from the community. Many also used infanticide, the intentional killing of a newborn, to maintain ecological balance. However, the main explanation for the slow growth of the human population before agriculture is that the death rate was very high (Livi-Bacci 1995).

All human populations lived in similar ways 10 000 years ago, but why did human societies develop differently during the last 10 000 years? Why and when did the present large differences in levels of development and health emerge?

1.5 Agriculture (10 000 to 5 000 years ago)

The introduction of agriculture was undoubtedly the first major reason for the differences in health and living conditions between different human societies that we find today. Agriculture improved health through its more efficient ways of producing food and clothing. But due to new social organisations agriculture also gave rise to health differences between groups in the same society.

Agriculture enabled the size of the human population to multiply by a factor of 100, from ten million at the end of the Stone Age to about one billion at the start of the industrial revolution (1820). However, agriculture did not improve human health in a straightforward way. More food improved health but by increasing population density, agriculture also resulted in many cases to the spread of new and lethal infectious diseases, such as measles and smallpox. Agriculture often resulted in a more monotonous diet, resulting in iron deficiencies and other nutritional deficiencies. However, the overall effect of agriculture on health and survival was favourable, as indicated by the steady increase in the global population. This increase in population was, of course, interrupted by many catastrophic events, such as famine, war and epidemics, but agriculture provided much better chances for survival for more people in the world.

There is clear evidence that agriculture emerged independently in a few areas of the world between 9 000 BC and 2 000 BC (Figure 1.1). The cultivation of food crops was independently invented by the ancestors of today's Indians in South and Central

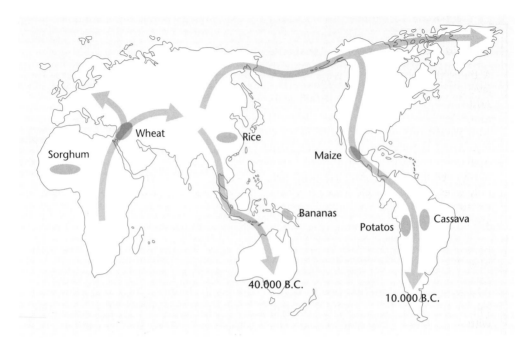

Figure 1.1 The spread of humans to all continents and the areas of domestication of the main staple crops.

America, by the ancestors of Africans and Arabs, and by the ancestors of populations in India and China. The crucial events of this agricultural revolution were the domestication of the ten plants that have remained the major staple crops of humans until this day. The first of these events was the cultivation of wheat. It was probably a Turkish, Kurdish and/or Arabian female ancestor in what is now Syria, Turkey or Iraq who started the cultivation of cereals about 10 000 years ago. She used seeds from a wild grass that grew in the region. The farmers that followed gradually selected better and better varieties of what became wheat. The domestication of rice took place in China, maize in Mexico, the potato in Peru, and cassava in what is now Brazil. These are now the five most important staple crops in the world. Sorghum, millet, sweet potato, yams and plantains (cooking banana) are the other major staple crops. These ten plant species were all domesticated more than 4 000 years ago. In combination with the domestication of ten animal species this

changed forever human life in this world. The ten animals were the cow, horse, sheep, goat, pig, camel, lama, chicken, duck and turkey.

But why did agriculture emerge and develop in particular locations? Was it because the humans living in these places were smarter than those living elsewhere? Were the ancestors of Chinese rice growers smarter than the ancestors of the Australian aborigines? Were the Aztec Indians who domesticated maize in what now is Mexico smarter than the Indians on the colder plains of North America, who never domesticated any major crop? Were the ancestors of people living at the sources of Euphrates and Tigris rivers smarter than the ancestors of the Swedes?

Jared Diamond (1997) has published a general hypothesis about the major trends in human development. His hypothesis is that the major determinant of the global development of the human societies on different continents was access to plants and animals that could be domesticated, and how

24

Box 1.5

Why did the Aborigines of Australia not colonise England?

A thought-provoking question is why the level of development of the Aborigines of Australia in the 18th century differed so much from that of the British occupiers, who arrived in 1788. In other words: why did the Aborigines remain hunters and gatherers, and thus succumb to cruel colonisation by the British, and why were there only an estimated 300 000 Aborigines living in Australia when the British occupation started?

The Aborigines arrived in Australia long before any humans settled in the British Isles. Australia lost its land connection with Asia due to geological events after their arrival 40 000 years ago. The Aborigines subsequently lived in Australia without contact with the rest of the world. In many parts of Australia, the soil is fertile and the rainfall is suitable for agriculture. Why did the Aborigines not develop agriculture during these 40 000 years? There must have been many Aborigine families who were very, very hungry many times during those 40 000 years. If we can understand why they did not start agriculture, we will also understand why they did not develop an alphabet, mathematics, shipbuilding and weapons to protect themselves against the British.

The reason is that the Aborigines did not find any plant to cultivate. The natural flora and fauna of Australia do not contain any wild plant or animal that can be domesticated. European immigrants to Australia have also failed to find any plant suitable for

domestication in the flora of Australia. The inhabitants of the British Isles were originally hunters and gatherers, living a life similar to that of the Aborigines in Australia. In the course of history, those who lived in the British Isles acquired wheat from the Middle East. It was the wheat from the Middle East that the British eventually took across the oceans and that eventually made agriculture such a success in Australia. Australia's isolation from the rest of the world meant that wheat did not reach Australia until the arrival of the Europeans. The simple explanation for the society of the Aborigines remaining pre-agricultural is thus that there was nothing to domesticate in Australia.

It should be noted that the only important domestication that took place in Europe was that of the olive tree. Europe got agriculture from the Middle East and Asia. The Europeans had land connections at similar latitudes, while the unfortunate Aborigines were isolated from all plant domestications that occurred in the rest of the world. Their hunting and gathering could only sustain about 300 000 people. The decimation that took place during the British occupation decreased the Aborigine population to about 60 000 people in 1930. Thereafter the size of the Aborigine population has increased. Today there are more than 400 000 Aborigine people, probably a higher number than ever before during their 40 000-year-long history.

these plants and animals could be spread across the globe. There is no convinsing evidence that differences in intelligence determined where agriculture started and where it was later adopted. The current belief is that hunter-gatherer populations must have tried desperately many times to find new ways to feed their starving children in times of unsuccessful hunting and gathering of wild plants. *Where nature provided suitable*

plants and animals for domestication, people developed agriculture!

The main support for this theory is that all the major domestic crops and animals were already in use 4 000 years ago. Since then an increasing number of people have passed through every part of every forest during the last 4 000 years, but no-one has found one single additional plant or animal that became an important new crop or domestic animal. Many have tried. One example is the attempts to domesticate the zebra. This has repeatedly proven impossible, as zebras bite anybody who tries to treat them as domesticated animals.

The Swedish botanist, Carl Linné, classified all plants and animals in a scientific manner. Yet neither he nor any of the thousands of botanists and zoologists that followed have found any additional plant or animal that could become a major staple crop or domestic animal. The only explanation for the failure to find new plants and animals for domestic use is that our human ancestors as early as 4 000 years ago had attempted to domesticate all existing plants and animals in the world in their struggle to survive (Box 1.5).

Jared Diamond suggests on the basis of several pieces of evidence that the subsequent development of human history was determined by how agriculture and animal husbandry spread from the few sites of domestication. Domesticated plants and animals were adapted to a specific climate. For this reason, populations living at the same latitudes east or west of a site of domestication, and thus having similar climate, could rapidly adopt the domesticated plants and raise the domesticated animals. Due to the east-west direction of the longest geographical axis of their continent the peoples on the Eurasian continent were very successful in exchanging the fruits of domestication. There are similar agro-ecological zones extending from what is now Portugal in Europe to Eastern China. The highlands of Central Asia constituted less of a barrier to the transfer of domesticated crops and animals than the hot, dry Sahara of Africa, and the tropical Panama peninsula in the Americas. In Eurasia, the domesticated crops and animals could relatively easily be spread and adapted to areas outside their sites of domestication. Wheat spread relatively rapidly to both Asia and Europe following its domestication around 8,500 BC.

Agriculture and the ability to store carbohydrates in the form of cereals, were the basis for the development of urban life. The ability to create a storable food surplus was essential in allowing human societies to form cities. The storage of food surplus and the foundation of urban life are believed to be the basis for major inventions, such as mathematics and alphabets. No human society developed an alphabet before adopting agriculture as their main form of food supply. At the time of the arrival of Europeans in the Americas, the agricultural empires of the Incas, Mayas and Aztecs had developed cities, and some had developed a basic sign alphabet. The Native Americans on the northern plains had no cities and none could read or write. Most of the disparities in development that were created by the adoption of agriculture persist to this day. This is a consequence of the population of agricultural societies obtaining more food, better health and lower mortality. Their numbers increased, and eventually the farmers became a hundred times more numerous than neighbouring hunters and gatherers. The farming populations developed new cultures, institutions and technologies; whereas the societies of the hunters and gatherers remained relativety similar over the centuries, as did their high mortality rates and the small populations that resulted from this. On all continents, societies based on agriculture and cattle-herding have come to dominate over neighbouring hunters and gatherers. This domination has often resulted in cruel and catastrophic reductions through genocide and diseases of the already small populations of hunter-gatherers.

1.6 Empires (5 000 to 1 000 years ago)

One process by which agriculture expanded was the spread of domesticated plants and animals to populations that had not previously practised agriculture. However, agricultural expansion probably occurred mainly through the occupation of the lands of gatherers and hunters by rapidly growing farming populations from other areas. The last major example of this was the occupation by northern European farmers of the fertile lands of the hunting native Americans, as described in a series of well-known Swedish novels, first published in 1949 (Moberg 1995).

Agriculture gradually resulted in larger populations and larger kingdoms, and eventually in several major civilisations and empires. China, India, Iran, Egypt and Mexico are examples of modern nations that approximately correspond to the areas of ancient empires that emerged thousands of years ago. The major civilisations and empires that developed on the Eurasian continent gradually came into more frequent contact with each other. The size of a particular population and the wealth of a particular empire changed as a result of wars, which were numerous. However, contacts between the empires and kingdoms also included trade. The agricultural civilisations improved agricultural methods, transport systems and other technologies in a stepwise fashion. These civilisations exchanged goods, technology, institutional organisations, knowledge and culture through trade contact. The kingdoms of Sub-Saharan Africa were involved in this exchange to a limited degree. East-west contacts were always easier than north-south contacts. The ancient civilisations on the American continent: the Incas, the Mayas and the Aztecs, were not only isolated from those in Europe, Asia and North Africa; they were also isolated from each other.

One explanation for the later domination of the world by the populations of Eurasia are the waves of epidemic infectious diseases that spread through the contact between European and Asian populations. Trade within and between the major agricultural regions of the Eurasian continent allowed viral diseases such as smallpox and measles to spread in epidemics across the continent. Exposure to these diseases probably resulted in the surviving Eurasian population devel-

oping partial resistance to most of them. The populations of the Americas, who met these viruses for the first time during the European colonisation, remained susceptible. The viruses became as deadly to the people of the Americas as were the weapons of the European invaders (Diamond 1997).

Agriculture, trade and the rise of an urban lifestyle had major impact on human health. New infectious diseases emerged due to the higher population density at which people lived and closer contacts between humans and domesticated animals. The cultural aversion to living with and eating pigs that is observed in many parts of the world is based on rational considerations. The pig is the domestic animal that is physiologically most similar to humans. It is therefore more likely than other domestic animals to transmit diseases to humans. The pig tapeworm, which can cause neurological damage and epilepsy in humans, is a prominent example. The origin of several major epidemic infectious diseases, such as smallpox, measles and influenza, is genetically traced to diseases among domestic animals (cows, pigs and ducks). The increase in food supply that agriculture made possible resulted in denser human settlements and much closer contacts between animals and humans. The exchange of infectious diseases between humans also increased considerably through the introduction of agriculture. Human society responded by developing sanitary rules, hygienic practices and water supply technology.

The provision of safe drinking water, the disposal of urine and faeces, and improvements in personal hygiene became major determinants for the success of urban societies. The storage of food also made rat-control a major task of ancient public health. Bacterial diseases spread across the Eurasian continent. The Plague, a bacterial disease that uses the rat louse as a vector, reached Europe in 1347. The first epidemic of this plague had a devastating effect on the European population. The effects of plague were less severe when the disease returned in smaller epidemics in subsequent centuries. This was probably partially due to greater resistance among the surviving population, and to the use of more rational actions to stop the epidemics. Cholera, a bacterial disease that causes the most severe form of acute diarrhoea, has occurred for thousands of years in Bengal. The cholera bacteria are transmitted directly from human faeces to the human mouth, and have a very short incubation time. Therefore cholera reached Europe as late as 1832, as a result of the increased speed of transport brought by the industrial revolution.

The agricultural revolution and the cultural and technological developments in the great empires had both positive and negative effects on human health. These societies had striking health differences between the ruling classes and slaves, but the net effect must have been improved health as the size of the populations grew. Population growth was fastest in China and India, since these two countries for long periods had slightly better health than the rest of the world. The successful development of their agricultural civilisations many thousands of years ago thus explains why these countries today are the most populous in the world (Table 1.2). Agricultural civilisations, and the accompanying improved health that resulted in population growth, also developed in South-East Asia, Persia, the Middle East,

Africa and the Americas. The Roman Empire was the principal example in Europe. The Romans built impressive aqueducts to provide cities with fresh water. The major diseases were kept under control and the population grew. Two thousand years ago, the Roman Empire had a population of 50 million. This was more than one fifth of the estimated world population of 230 million. The majority of the population of the Roman Empire lived in the Middle East and North Africa (McMichael 2001).

How did human development differ in the world 1 000 years ago, when the Roman Empire had split and largely collapsed? Agriculture, and the institutional and technological improvements that followed, had yielded a slight improvement in health that had increased the world population to more than 250 million. Differences in human living conditions had emerged. However, the greatest disparities in health were found within the empires, rather than between them. The most significant determinant for a person's health was whether he or she belonged to the ruling class or was a slave. The ability to read and to make decisions about one's own life was still a privilege of a few male members of the ruling classes. Ethnic differences remained throughout the world between agricultural societies and hunter-gatherer societies. It is difficult to assess how gender differences in living condition

Table 1.2 Estimated population (in millions) of the main world regions.

Year	0	1000	1500	1600	1700	1820	1870	1913	1950	1973	1998
Asia (excl. Japan)	171	175	268	360	375	680	731	926	1 298	2 139	3 390
Japan	3	8	15	19	27	31	34	52	84	109	126
Western Europe	25	25	57	74	81	133	188	261	305	358	388
Eastern Europe*	9	14	31	38	46	91	141	236	267	360	412
North America**	1	2	3	2	2	11	46	111	176	251	323
Latin America	6	11	18	9	12	21	21	40	81	166	508
Africa	17	33	46	55	61	74	90	125	228	388	760
World	230	268	438	556	603	1 041	1 270	1 791	2 525	3 913	5 907

* Includes former Soviet Union.   ** Includes Australia & New Zealand.

Source: Maddison 2001.

changed with the transition to an agricultural society and later to a feudal agricultural society. We have reasons to assume that the life situation for the majority of the human population in the empires on the Eurasian continent was relatively similar 1 000 years ago. Europe had no clear developmental advantage in comparison with other empires at that time. Estimates of economic development 1 000 years ago (Table 1.3) indicate that Asia lay slightly ahead of the rest of the world. China was also ahead of Japan at that time. Knowledge, technology and social institutions were more advanced in the Arabian and Islamic cultures of the Middle East than they were in Europe.

Our brief search for the origin of contemporary developmental differences between the 'western countries' and Japan, on the one hand, and the rest of the world on the other hand shows that these differences must have emerged during the last 1 000 years. However, development on the Eurasian continent lay ahead of that of the rest of the world 1 000 years ago. The people of America, Africa and Australia were already destined to succumb to the cruel occupation of people from Eurasia. However, Western Europe was by no means ahead of the rest of the Eurasian continent. The origin of the global dominance of Western Europe from 1500 to 1950 must be found between the years 1000 to 1500.

1.7 European dominance (1 000 to 50 years ago)

It is difficult to explain why the economic, social and military development of Western Europe surpassed that of Asia and the Middle East in the last Millenium. It is easier to explain why the populations of Western Europe, and their offspring in North America, became much healthier than most of the people in the rest of the world. This was a consequence of the socio-economic advantages that followed the Western European world dominance.

The last 1000 years of European colonialism and world dominance has seen a twenty-fold increase in world population, with most of this increase taking place during the last 500 years (Table 1.2). The last 500 years have seen a ten-fold increase in the average per capita GDP in the world (Table 1.3). This undoubtedly reflects an improvement in the average living conditions for the world population. This improvement has taken place despite the numerous wars and genocides and other cruelties that European dominance has inflicted on the peoples of other continents. However, the health improvements for the majority of the populations of the colonial powers and their allies only came gradually, being in fact concentrated in the last one or two centuries. The related improvements in North

Table 1.3 Gross domestic product per capita in international US dollars (i.e. purchasing power parity).

Year	1000	1500	1820	1870	1913	1950	1973	1998
Asia (excl. Japan)	500	600	600	500	600	600	1 200	2 900
Japan	400	500	700	800	1 400	2 000	11 400	20 400
Western Europe	400	800	1 200	2 000	3 500	4 600	11 500	17 900
Eastern Europe*	400	500	700	900	1 500	2 600	5 700	4 400
North America**	400	400	1 200	2 400	5 300	9 300	16 200	26 100
Latin America	400	400	700	700	1 500	2 600	4 500	5 800
Africa	400	400	400	400	600	900	1 400	1 400
World	435	600	700	900	1 500	2,100	4 100	5 700

* Includes former Soviet Union.   ** Includes Australia & New Zealand.

Source: Maddison 2001.

America and Japan have taken place even later. It is the health improvements for the general population of the richest countries during the last century that have caused health to be so extremely unevenly distributed throughout the world. The wide health disparities as measured by life expectancy are only to a minor extent due to a deterioration of the health status of the population in the rest of the world.

During the first eight centuries of the previous millennium, until industrial development started to make an impact around 1820, most people living in rural or urban societies in the world experienced approximately the same miserable level of health. Most citizens of the colonial powers did not have significantly longer lives than the inhabitants of the colonies, at least not during the first few hundred years of European colonialism. There are, of course, many exceptions. Europeans inflicted severe horrors onto the Native American population. The Native Americans were either annihilated or greatly reduced in number following the European invasion (Table 1.2). Another exception is the impact of the slave trade on the health of Africans. Severe oppression was a constant aspect of European dominance of the world. However, the majority of the population of Western Europe also continued to live in misery and illiteracy, until the last two centuries. This was largely due to the effects of frequent wars within Europe. Life expectancy in England, France and the Netherlands was less than 40 years at the start of the industrial revolution in 1800. One century and an industrial revolution later life expectancy in these countries had only increased to 50 years in 1900. Further economic growth and the establishment of democracy and welfare policy led to an increase in life expectancy to 70 years in 1950. Public investment in education and sanitation, in parallel with popular movements for social justice, gradually led to the creation of the European welfare states. It was these social changes, which followed the industrial revolution, in combination with direct public health actions that improved health in Western Europe.

In his long-term study of the history of the world economy, Angus Maddison (2001) estimates that the total size of the world economy has increased nearly 300-fold during the last 1 000 years. This means that the value of all goods and services produced in the world has increased by a factor of 300. However, most of this increase is due to a 20-fold increase in the world population from 0.3 billion in 1000 AD to 6 billion today (Table 1.2). The economic increase per capita is thus 15-fold. An improved economy means that humans work more efficiently, but its effect on health depends on how the economic resources are distributed and used. Maddison (2001) identifies three main reasons for strong economic growth, which benefited the populations of Western Europe, North America and Japan. It is clear that the increased survival and improved health of the populations in these regions during the last 200 years are partly explained by economic growth, and partly by the social changes that both preceded and followed this economic growth.

1.7.1 Trade and capital

The principal reason for world economic growth was increased international trade and the movement of capital. The start of Western European international trade on a large scale can be dated to 992 AD. In this year the Republic of Venice signed its first trade agreement with the Byzantine Emperor in Constantinople (now Istanbul). The Republic of Venice, and the other major North Italian city-states of Milan, Florence and Genoa, established and maintained a very profitable Mediterranean trade with the Middle East. These city-states also established overland trade between Northern Italy and several towns in Flanders, in what is now Belgium. The economic importance of Flanders gradually increased. The 'trading houses' of Northern Italy developed the capitalist system that emerged as the driving force of economic development in Western Europe. Portugal and Spain replaced Northern Italy as the dominant economic region around 1500, following successful transoceanic voyages by Columbus and Vasco da Gama. In the following centuries, the Netherlands, followed by France and Britain, took over most of the transoceanic world trade. This world trade was based on the superiority of the European warships. The Europeans frequently used armed attacks on other countries to support their trade, and in this way favoured the economic growth of Western Europe. The countries that were attacked, and later colonised, often suffered devastating effects from the same trade that gave economic growth in Europe. The most dramatic example is the transatlantic slave trade by which 13 million Africans were forcibly transported to the Americas, to work mainly on sugar and coffee plantations (Thomas 1998). Undoubtedly, European colonial dominance of the rest of the world was a prerequisite for what was to come, but it was only after the industrial revolution that the wide economic, social and health disparities emerged between the populations of the world.

1.7.2 Agriculture and crops

The second reason for world economic growth during the last thousand years was the introduction of agriculture into new fertile areas, and the introduction of new crops into areas where agriculture was already practised. Both of these processes took place mainly by the migration of agriculture from northern to southern China, and from Europe to North America and Australia. Many important crops were transferred between continents in the "agricultural globalisation" that took place from 500 to 200 years ago, as a result of European colonisation. Maize and cassava were transferred from the Americas to Africa, wheat from Europe to Australia and North America, and the potato from the Americas to Europe. In Sweden the

consumption of potatoe grew from negligible levels in the year 1800 to almost 300 kg per person per year in 1850. Potatoes were more productive than any crop previously grown in Sweden. The potato put an end to famine in Sweden. The last major famine occurred in 1863. Sweden, indeed all of Europe, owes a debt of gratitude to the natives of the Andes who had domesticated the potato thousands of years earlier, and to the sailors who brought the potato to Europe. One of the first and most noticeable positive effects of the globalisation of agriculture that followed transoceanic European colonialism was the spread of all major staple crops from the agricultural revolution to all continents where they could be grown. This spread occurred between 1500 and 1800, before the start of the industrial revolution. It should be noted that the benefits of growing maize and cassava also spread across Africa many centuries before the European colonists penetrated the continent.

1.7.3 Technology and institutions

The third reason for the world economic growth of the last 1 000 years was technological and institutional innovation. Until 500 years ago, Europe advanced mainly by importing technology that had been developed in China, India or the Middle East. Only during the last 500 years was Europe the world centre for technological and scientific development, a status that has now been taken over by North America and Japan.

The explanation of Western Europe's world dominance lies in the period between the years 1000 and 1500. The gradual development of Western European agriculture resulted in a steady population growth during these medieval centuries. Agricultural development was accompanied by gradual development in culture, architecture and knowledge. This development was largely related to the spread of the institutions of the Catholic Church, and universities associated with the Church, and to a gradual improvement in the system of trade and its financing. Western European development was severely retarded by the Plague epidemic around 1350, but the effects of this epidemic were eventually overcome. Centres of development grew in a crescent from Northern Italy *via* France to the Netherlands, and later crossed the sea to Britain. The establishment of social institutions, such as universities and banks, was as important as technological advances in shipbuilding and book printing.

In the centuries before 1500, Western Europe had developed a slight technological lead over Asia in weapons technology and in shipbuilding technology. The European lead in maritime technology was largely due to wide differences in political and economic priorities in Europe and Asia. Chinese ships did sail to East Africa before 1500, but China made a political decision not to invest further in transoceanic dominance. A simplistic explanation for this is that the wealthy of Europe were keener to obtain silk from China than the wealthy of China were to obtain woollen cloth from Europe. Similarly, Europe was keener to obtain spices from India than India was to obtain salted herring from Europe. European trade with Asia after 1500 was combined with repeated armed attacks and, whenever possible, the use of military and political dominance to improve European trade conditions. The European powers skilfully used political conflicts in Asia to gain dominance in trade. Only Japan managed to maintain fully its independence from Europe, which it first achieved by isolating itself! However, Japan entirely changed its policy towards Europe around 1830. A very active process started to obtain European technology and knowledge for the industrialisation of Japan. Japan also invested early in general primary education for both boys and girls. This multidimensional Japanese strategy was successful. Education, health and wealth improved in Japan. In 1905 Japan won the war against Russia. Thereafter Japan also copied European colonial ambitions and started its own ag-

gressive colonial policy towards Korea and China, and later towards other parts of South East Asia.

1.7.4 The industrial revolution

The industrial revolution started in Europe around 1820. The economic level of Europe, North America and Japan were at the time approximately only twice that of the rest of the world. This difference has now increased to its current level of seven to one. Asian countries have started to close the gap in recent decades, but the total economic disparity between the richest and the poorest nations of the world continues to grow. Major technological and socio-economic advances occurred in Western Europe following the industrial revolution. These advances continued for more than a century. Advances were driven as much by institutional development as by technological innovation. Core elements were the mechanisation of production, the use of new raw materials, and the replacement of human energy by mechanised energy from steam engines and improved hydroelectric energy. The mechanisms of the industrial revolution are well-documented (Landes 1999). Table 1.3 shows the effects of the industrial revolution on the economic growth of Europe and other parts of the world. The economic benefits of the industrial revolution were extremely unevenly distributed, and thus it was during industrialisation that European dominance of the world created the present economic disparity in the world. This resulted from the direct control that Western European countries exerted over colonized countries, and from the strong indirect control that they exerted over countries such as China, whose foreign trade lay completely under Western European control. European colonisation expanded during the industrial revolution into Africa and Asia. The European colonisation of Africa was relatively late, and the territorial partition and domination of African societies took place largely after the Berlin conference of 1885. Due to strong resistance it took several decades for Europeans to gain control of the occupied territories in Africa.

Mozambique was dominated by Portugal for more than four centuries. However, the Mozambican territory was not effectively controlled by Portugal until after the First World War. The period of colonial administration of the territory of Mozambique, and of many other African countries, lasted only 60 to 80 years. The developmental challenges for the newly independent African countries thus relate both to the structure and institutional systems of the pre-colonial societies and to the effects of less than a century of colonial administration.

The European colonialism and North American dominance that followed the industrial revolution gave the impression of a homogeneous situation for the majority of the world population, who lived under this dominance. However, the differences in health development that have arisen during recent decades suggest that the precolonial situation is an important determinant for the present developmental situation in many countries.

1.7.5 The end of colonialism

The colonial period started to come to an end in 1776 with the independence from Britain of the United States of America. Decolonisation continued with countries of Latin America becoming independent during the next century, and most countries in the Middle East, Asia and Africa becoming independent after the Second World War. Most African nations became independent between 1960 and 1980. Following the fall of the apartheid regime in South Africa the county received its true independence from colonialism. With the return of Hong Kong to China, and the independence of East Timor, the world today consists almost entirely of independent nations. The newly independent states were initially seen as a homogenous group referred to as 'developing countries' or 'the Third World', but their eco-

nomical, social and institutional development varied greatly. Due to very different developments in these countries in recent decades, the variations are even greater today.

The communist revolutions in Russia in 1917 and in China in 1949 were important developments in the 20th century. All the nations with communist regimes and centrally planned economies developed initially in similar ways. The similarities were seen in social advances, slow economic growth and limitations of human rights. The rapid transition from centrally planned economies to market economies in the countries that emerged from the former Soviet Union during the 1990s gave rise to different socio-economic developments than those that emerged from the transition to market economies by the ruling communist parties in China and Vietnam. These different changes combined with the maintenance of centrally planned economies in Cuba and North Korea has further contributed to the widely differing socio-economic situations in the former group of communist countries.

The transformation of almost all countries and territories into national states with widely different development, and the diversity of the transformations of communist regimes, have given rise to a world with tremendous variations in development. The health disparities between and within the countries of the world are today related to these enormous disparities, as shown by the World Health Chart on the back cover of this book. The wide differences in the progress of former colonies are linked both to the prerequisites that were available for development at independence and to the chosen developmental strategy. The progress of each former colony does, in fact, depend on how the chosen strategy suits the situation in each country. We summarise in subsequent sections ideas about the determinants of the development of nations during the last 50 years, and opinions about the ongoing globalisation of the world.

1.8 Development strategies (the last 50 years)

The debate about what determines the development of nations is as old as social science and economics. Adam Smith's classic work published in 1776, *An Inquiry into the Nature and Causes of the Wealth of Nations*, may be regarded as the start of the modern debate. Smith argued that wealth came from the accumulation of capital for investment through savings, the division of labour and free trade. Another classic work that discussed the development of human societies, a work that constituted the foundation of communism, was Karl Marx's *Capital*, published in 1867.

Most analysis of economic and social development before 1950 was focused on the driving forces in the richest and most industrialised countries. Following the independence of the former colonies, an increasing amount of research has been focused on the development situations of the newly independent countries. This change of focus has generated a number of development theories and new research areas, such as 'development economics' and 'development studies'. These theories are based on the observation that the situations for the newly independent developing countries differ from the historic situations of the contemporary high-income countries. The new nations have had to develop under the continued dominance of a world economy controled by richer countries. Therefore it may still be relevant to divide the world into two types of countries when considering solely economic and military power. Theories for the development of the newly independent countries have differed considerably during the last half-century. We will review the strategies for development that emerged from the different development theories by describing some major trends in the process that have dominated the strategy of governments and international organisations. References to further information on the determinants of development are given in the reference list (de Vylder 2002, Todaro 2002, Middleton 2001, Allan & Thomas 2000, Gunnarsson 1995).

1.8.1 Import substitution (1950 to 1985)

Most newly independent countries embarked on rapid industrialisation based on a strategy of 'import substitution'. They chose this strategy based on a number of development theories known collectively as 'structuralism'. The goal of import substitution was to improve the terms of trade for the newly independent countries. Prices of exported raw materials kept falling, and this meant that such countries could never afford to improve welfare by paying for imported industrial goods with the earnings from the export of raw materials. The decision to focus on government planning and protection from the international market was based on the premise that free trade would only benefit the rich countries. Instead, the newly independent countries founded industries that were supported by government subsidies or directly owned by the state. High customs duties on imported goods protected the new domestic industries. In contrast, the domestic industries could import machinery without customs duties.

Many economists criticised this strategy, but many new national governments favoured it. The governments gained a central role in the national economy through the import substitution strategy. All new governments also, to different degrees, invested in public education, health services and infrastructure, such as roads. However, the subsidised industry did not become sufficiently profitable. The heavy public investment and subsidies to industry soon eroded the economy of many newly independent countries. A large part of the national investment was made with borrowed money. Countries for which the import substitution strategy did not pay off were caught in a debt crisis.

A striking example of the import substitution strategy is provided by the investment made in pharmaceutical industries by many

African countries. This investment was based on the observation that the costs of drug imports were increasing rapidly, due to both population growth and improved coverage of the health service. The solution was to make this import unnecessary by the rapid development of a national pharmaceutical industry. The Ministry of Health was expected to buy cheaper drugs from the national industry in the future. However, the pharmaceutical industry proved to be technologically complex to operate, and productivity was low. It was also found that the making of tablets and ampoules for injection was a very minor part of the cost of drugs. The main cost was the purchase of active substances, and these substances still had to be imported from countries with more advanced chemical industries. It then turned out that sometimes tablets made in the country were even more costly than imported tablets. Import substitution contributed to fewer drugs being available in the health service and to an increased debt that could not be repaid. The increasingly competitive world market in generic drugs from middle-income countries provided tablets at lower price, and the national industry could not compete. A West African pharmaceutical consultant summarised the plans for a pharmaceutical industry in Angola in the 1980s as follows: "The government wants to construct a pharmaceutical temple, on the altar of which it will burn large amounts of dollars in honour of the young nation." A rational economic analysis showed that an effective means of reducing the cost of drugs for low-income countries was to buy annual drug requirements through a competitive and non-corrupt international tender system. The import substitution strategy was often based on a mixture of insufficient economic analysis and excessive political prestige.

When many of the attempts at rapid industrialisation failed, the poor countries became unable to pay back their loans. Indeed, many countries became unable to pay even the interest on their loans. Their recent in-dependence was replaced by total dependence on international banks and economic organisations. Economic failure meant that governments could no longer maintain the quality of public schools and health service systems. The low salaries of teachers and health staff prohibited them from working full-time, and health centres and hospitals often lacked the drugs and equipment needed to treat the patients. The currency of an indebted country lost most of its value. It can be said, somewhat simplified, that the import substitution policy ended in the debt crisis of the 1980s. More and more countries were forced to renegotiate their debts with the International Monetary Fund and the World Bank, at annual meetings known as the 'Paris Club'. The debt crisis was particularly severe in Sub-Saharan Africa and in Latin America, but it also affected several Asian countries. Consequently, international economic institutions soon dictated the development policies of the indebted countries. They correctly diagnosed that something was wrong, but the treatment they prescribed, known as 'structural adjustment programmes', often caused more problems than it solved.

1.8.2 Structural adjustment programmes (1985–1997)

The International Monetary Fund (IMF) and the World Bank reacted at the end of the 1980s to the increasing debts and frequent failures of government intervention in most low-income and many middle-income countries. The standardised reactions of these international organisations, however, did not take differences in local contexts in each country into consideration. The IMF and the World Bank enforced similar neo-liberal so-called 'structural adjustment programmes (SAPs)' in all countries. In brief, SAP meant more market economy and a smaller public sector. This new policy was largely supported by the international development agencies in the high-income countries. The governments of the indebted

**Purchasing Power Parity (PPP)
(= International Dollars)**

The domestic currency is converted to US dollar by an exchange rate at which all the goods and services that comprise the gross domestic product will cost the same to buy in the country as in United States. As PPP conversion reflects the services and goods that inhabitants can buy in their own country, the GDP/capita expressed in international dollars (= PPP) is the best estimates of the economic differences between the countries in the world.

countries were obliged to apply SAP if they were to have their debts renegotiated.

The philosophy of SAP was that the state should do less, but do it better. The impoverished nations were to achieve macroeconomic balance by cutting public expenditure. They had to privatise formerly state-owned industry and they had to open their countries to free trade. However, the economic growth that was expected as a result of these measures did not materialise in many countries. In those countries in which economic growth was achieved, the new wealth did not benefit the majority of the population, at least not in the short term. How was it that the treatment prescribed by the main economic institutions of the world did not achieve what was promised?

The diagnosis on which the launch of the SAP was based was to a large degree correct. Most of the indebted countries were in macroeconomic chaos. They could no longer pay for public health services by printing more banknotes. SAP brought inflation under better control, and the reforms re-established reasonable stability of the exchange rate of the national currencies. The macroeconomic balance was a positive result of the SAP policy in several countries. Yet the treatment that was prescribed cured only a small part of the problem, and it had

several severe side-effects. SAP did not achieve rapid economic growth, particularly not in the low-income countries of Sub-Saharan Africa, where economic growth was and is most desperately needed. The education systems and health services that had been weakened by economic chaos were not improved by SAP. It is, however, simplistic to blame the whole crisis in the economy and public health services on SAP.

Printing more banknotes in an economy with severe inflation and increasing international debt could no longer finance a growing government health service. This became obvious to many African governments during the 1980s, and the problem was unofficially noted long before SAP was introduced. The value of staff salaries had fallen to negligible levels and the supply of drugs and consumables was insufficient to maintain even a minimum quality of the service. In many low-income countries in Africa, patients only received treatment in a government hospital if informal 'fees' were paid directly to the staff, and if the relatives bought the drugs, gloves and other equipment that was needed for the treatment from private pharmacies. Relatives even had to bring water for the surgeons to wash before surgery in some hospitals, since the hospital was incapable of maintaining a water supply. The structural adjustment programmes did not destroy functional economies, but neither did the programmes improve the faltering economies in the way that was intended. This neo-liberal policy did not restore the basic functions of the health and education sectors.

The movement in high-income countries for debt relief in poor countries failed to recognise fully the catastrophic economic situation that had caused the debts and the introduction of SAP. It has now been acknowledged in most countries that it was the combination of imposed "blue print" type of SAP and poor national governance that resulted in the crises for the public sector (Bhutta 2001). In many low-income and middle-income countries in Africa, Asia and the Middle East, opposition to the neo-liberal policy of the 1980s was not dominated by the traditional political left, but by other movements. A movement known as the "People's Health Assembly" effectively voiced health-focused opposition. The People's Health Assembly is an international grassroots network of organisations and individuals with thousands of participants. It arose spontaneously in 2000 at a meeting in Bangladesh. The participants defend public investment in the health service and debt relief for poor countries.[1]

Improved macroeconomic stability remains a favourable effect of the SAP programmes. The dominance of the neo-liberal strategy ten years ago is now being replaced by a more multidimensional development strategy, of which the macroeconomic reforms are only one component. The SAP erred in trying to achieve development by isolated economic reforms. Its failures led to a general recognition of the multi-dimensional character of development and a deeper understanding of the complex links between the economic, social and institutional aspects of development, as well as of the crucial role of good governance in achieving an optimal balance between the different development dimensions.

1.8.3 Prerequisites for economic growth (1998–)

Several non-economic dimensions of development are now recognised as being crucial for economic progress and human develop-

[1] http://phmovement.org

ment. While sound economic policies are necessary, economic policies are far from sufficient to achieve socio-economic development in poor countries. The 1993 Nobel Laureate in Economics, Douglass North, eloquently summarised that *neo-classical economic theory is simply an inappropriate tool to analyze and prescribe policies that will induce development. The reason for this is that classical and neo-liberal economists have been concerned with the operation of markets, not with how functioning markets are developed.*

A simplified analogy is that neo-liberal economists are excellent Formula 1 drivers that can drive established market economies well. However, the same economists do not know how to construct the cars that they love to drive (some times so fast that they cause crashes). The question arises concerning what it takes to construct a market that can be driven by economists with sufficient safety? Four principal non-economic dimensions of development are today widely recognized as being necessary for a functioning and safe market economy. A summary is given in Box 1.6.

The first dimension is public investment in improved health and basic education, termed "investment in human capital" in economic jargon. When the structural adjustment programmes reduced government investment in human capital, construction of the foundation for a functioning modern market economy – a healthy and educated population – stopped.

The second dimension is the creation and maintenance of well-functioning public institutions. This requires public funding, human capital and good governance.

> **Box 1.6**
>
> **Non-economic requirements for economic growth**
>
> 1 Human capital   = A healthy and educated population
> 2 Public institutions = Police, courts, tax authority, legal property register, etc.
> 3 Civil society   = Trades unions, religious organisations etc, with strong values.
> 4 Good governance   = Ruling in the interest of the majority without corruption

The third dimension has been termed 'civil society'. This term refers to the range of social organizations, of varying degrees of formality that are autonomous from the state, market and family, and are formed through voluntary association. Prominent examples are trades unions, sports associations, development NGOs, human rights groups, women's groups, religious and other faith-based organizations, social movements, advocacy networks, etc. Many specific values, norms and cultural patterns are transferred through these organizations. Current research attributes a considerable role to such organizations in the development of nations. Much of the successful development of the market economy in Western Europe is attributed to the social environment created by the combination of a strong civil society and well-functioning public institutions.

The fourth dimension has been termed 'good governance'. Good governance describes a government that is doing the right things in the right way. Leaders make optimal decisions for the benefit of the majority with due respect to the interests of minorities. Human rights are protected, gender equality is advanced and the mass media are free to inform and debate national and international issues. A government ruling with good governance rules in the interest of the majority, not in the interests of a wealthy minority.

The continued unfair trade conditions imposed by the richer countries continue to hamper development in the world. However, researchers also increasingly emphasize important internal reasons for the slow socio-economic development in many low-income and middle-income countries. The Peruvian economist Hernando de Soto has analysed the failure of a market economy to generate rapid economic growth and welfare improvements in so many countries in Africa, Middle East, Asia and Latin America. His book *"The Mystery of Capital: Why Capitalism Triumphs in the West but Fails Everywhere Else"* (2001) starts as follows:

"The fall of the Berlin Wall ended more than a century of political competition between capitalism and communism. Capitalism stands alone as the only feasible way to rationally organize a modern economy. At this moment in history, no responsible nation has a choice. As a result, with varying degrees of enthusiasm, Third World and former communist nations have balanced their budgets, cut subsidies, welcomed foreign investment, and dropped their tariff barriers. Their efforts have been repaid with bitter disappointment."

De Soto's hypothesis is that the informal economic sector is much larger and more important in most middle-income and low-income countries than has been realised. This informal sector is sometimes referred to as "the black market", but it includes all economic activities that occur outside of the control of tax authorities and without legal protection and documented property rights. Investments in the informal sector by small entrepreneurs, such as fishermen and tailors, are not protected by the legal system of the state. Small entrepreneurs are unable to mobilize capital for further investment by using their property as security for needed loans. De Soto claims that a market economy will not function until the state serves the interests of the whole population. The correct enforcement of laws and property rights is needed for a free market to create prosperity. To put it simply, governments must fight corruption, permit a free flow of information, and defend the rights of small-scale enterprises instead of acting as the guardians of a small traditional elite. Studies of the successful Asian 'tiger economies', such as Taiwan and South Korea, have shown that it is the ability of a government to provide these public functions that gives rapid economic growth. De Soto criticises the form of globalisation that is currently being developed because it interconnects only the elite groups of the different countries. His recommendation to the governments in low-income and middle-income countries is to make capitalism function for all citizens by creating functioning public institutions. His underlying argument is that capitalism is "the only game in town" that can create the massive surplus value that is needed to eradicate poverty.

Consensus about the prerequisites for a functioning market economy is emerging from economic research. Gunnarsson and Rojas (1995) identify three main reasons for the success of the Asian 'tiger economies'. These reasons are (1) an egalitarian social structure; (2) an autonomous state; and (3) socio-cultural coherence in the civil society. The egalitarian social structure means that all parties are treated equally in the courts and by public authorities. Both South Korea and Taiwan gave everyone access to land for farming, and achieved a reasonably fair distribution of income. The differences in income between rich and poor in these successful Asian economies are smaller than they are in Sweden, and many times smaller than they are in Africa and Latin America. Income equality seems to be good for economic growth. The autonomy of the state means that the government acts in the interests of the whole nation, and does not focus on the protection of the wealth of a small elite. Socio-cultural coherence refers to the shared values in the civil society. Economic growth is greatly facilitated in countries in which citizens enjoy not only the protection offered by law, but also trust each other, due to shared values originating from different social networks.

Development in eastern Asia is also related to the interplay between economic and demographic factors. A rapid fall in fertility in eastern Asia has created a favourable 'dependency ratio' in the population. The decline in family size and in mortality rates, will cause a distinctive sequence of effects on the population composition. The number of adults relative to the number of children and old people in the population will be very high during the initial decades.

Later, a rapid aging of the population will take place. The population composition during the decades between a population with many children and that with many old people has a low 'dependency ratio'. There are many people who produce goods and services, relative to the number who need to be supported. This favourable age distribution has been found to provide a *"demographic gift"* that facilitates economic growth. The former communist countries in Eastern Europe did not receive a demographic gift when they converted from a planned economy to a market economy. Economic growth is a major factor pushing the demographic transition, but the demographic transition can also help to push economic growth during a period of a few decades. This period has already passed in Eastern Europe.

Contemporary development policy corresponds to Amartya Sen's broad definition of development (see Section 1.2). Development policy takes into consideration that development is driven by a number of mutually reinforcing dimensions, of which economic growth is just one. Other major dimensions are education, health and freedom. Increased gender and economic equality are also widely recognised as being crucial for socio-economic and health development (Sen, 1999). The social conflict in Bolivia that in 2003 stopped planned gas exports provides a dramatic example of how economic inequalities and social distrust can stop economic growth.

There is now a clear agreement among international agencies that public investment in the health service and wise government health policies are crucial to human development and to economic development. The 1993 yearbook of the World Bank was entitled "Investing in Health". The World Bank announced in 1993 for the first time that expenditure on public health services was an investment. The World Health Organization has recently reinforced this view with a report from its Commission for Macroeconomics and Health published in

2001.[1] This report is based on commissioned research that shows that investment by the international community in improved health in low-income countries will increase economic growth in these countries. It predicts that health investment in the poorest countries will produce an economic return that is to the benefit of the global world economy. The report estimates that public funding at a level of the exchange rate of USD 35 per person per year is needed to provide essential health services. Low-income countries in Africa currently allocate only USD 5 to 10 per person, and these countries receive only about USD 2 in development aid per person for the health sector. The WHO now states that if governments double their investment, the international donor agencies must increase their support, in order to achieve the improvements in health that are needed to enable economic growth where it is most needed. (The cost estimates given above are quoted in current US dollars, i.e. at the 2004 exchange rates of the national currency.)

It has been recognised for many years that debt relief is a prerequisite for development of the poorest countries. It remains to be decided, however, under what conditions debt relief should be provided. Low-income countries must present to the World Bank and the International Monetary Fund 'Poverty Reduction Strategy Papers (PRSP)'.[2] This "PRSP process" implies that debt relief is offered in exchange for a description of how

the government plans to use the money made available when it is no longer obliged to pay the debts. The rich countries are willing to write off the loans if the money is to be spent in ways that will relieve poverty. Furthermore, the General Secretary of the United Nations, Kofi Annan, has convinced the rich countries to contribute to a global fund to fight AIDS, tuberculosis and malaria. This fund would make drugs and vaccines cheaper for low-income countries.[3]

A particularly striking development failure can be seen in Sub-Saharan Africa, which is also the region of the world that has been worst hit by HIV/AIDS. Most countries in this region have lagged behind world development throughout the last 20 years (Table 1.4). This is considered to be mainly due to the failure to provide the institutional structures and governance that are needed for positive national development. During the last two decades, most Sub-Saharan African countries have become marginalised in the world economy. Africa is yet to benefit from the "demographic gift". Analysis of this failure with a longer development perspective and placing more emphasis on the civil society and institutional factors reveal clearly why post-colonial development has been less successful in Sub-Saharan Africa than it has in Latin America, the Middle East and most parts of Asia.

The Latin American countries are offspring of Western Europe, and the relative failure of their socio-economic development

[1] www.cmhealth.org
[2] www.imf.org/external/np/prsp/prsp.asp

[3] www.theglobalfund.org

Table 1.4 General economic development in groups of countries.

Countries	1960s	1970s	1980s	1990s
High-income countries	Good	Relatively bad	Good	Relatively good*
Africa	Good	Fair	*Very bad*	*Bad*
Latin America	Good	Fair	*Very bad*	Fair
China & South East Asia	Fair	Good	Very Good	Good
India & South Asia	Fair	Fair	Good	Good

* With great variations: very good in USA, reasonable in Europe and bad in Japan.
Source: Adapted from de Vylder (2002).

when compared to offspring of Britain such as Australia and New Zealand is surprising. This is especially so as Argentina, Uruguay and Cuba in many ways were on a par with large parts of Western Europe during the first part of the past century.

The Middle East and most of Asia are descendents of ancient civilisations that knew how to read and write long before the Europeans learnt these skills. These countries have a stronger coherence in their civil societies and a much better institutional base for the modern state than is the case in Sub-Saharan Africa. The recent successful socio-economic development in Asia and the Middle East may be seen as a reversion to the more homogenous development level of the Eurasian continent that existed before the European colonial expansion during the last centuries.

At the beginning of the European territorial occupation, the present nations in Sub-Saharan Africa were mainly small political units of subsistence farmers and cattle-herders. These small units had advanced and ancient social organisations and cultures, but there were few large civilisations that used an alphabet. Ethiopia was an exception. Contemporary Sub-Saharan African nations have much less of civil society coherence and weaker social institutions on which to build the present nations than is generally the case for the countries of Asia and the Middle East.

The farming systems in much of Sub-Saharan Africa are still based on rain-fed agriculture using shifting cultivation. This involves cultivating land for three to four years and then leaving it fallow for a generation. Women largely carry out the agriculture labour in these systems. This is quite different from the system of irrigated rice cultivation that was used for thousands of years and that formed the basis of many Asian civilisations. The kingdom of Thailand thus had a much better chance of succeeding in the modern world than the republic of Tanzania had when it became an independent country in 1960.

Although national leadership and governance is crucial for positive development, it may be an error to attribute the development crisis in many Africa countries to the occurrence of less capable leaders. Post-colonial nation-building may rather be regarded as a much greater challenge in Sub-Saharan Africa than elsewhere in the world. It seems that the immense challenge in Africa has yielded both the best and the worst of leaders. The best leaders include persons like Mandela, Annan and Nyerere; while Amin, Bokassa and Mobutu form a stark contrast.

The labelling of most of the world as "colonies" gave the impression that the potential and difficulties facing development was similar when the new nations rather suddenly became known as "developing countries" or "the third world". The importance of the widely different historical and cultural backgrounds of these "developing countries" was not sufficiently appreciated during the last decades. Labels such as "the third world" gave the impression that the development challenges were similar in Argentina and Mozambique. Both countries had the same unfair trade barriers of the high income countries, but Argentina had without doubt a much higher socio-economic development than Mozambique. However, given the situation in these countries 50 years ago, it is more surprising that Argentina has not achieved the same level of development as Western Europe than it is that Mozambique is still struggling with severe poverty and ill health. In contrast, one can admire the leaders of Mozambique for having achieved independence, and for bringing a peaceful end to the brutal civil war that followed. Mozambique now faces enormous challenges with widespread poverty, weak public institutions, prevalent corruption and increasing HIV prevalence, but given the history of the country this is not surprising. Good governance thus involves making the best out of a country's situation at any given moment. Although there is agreement on the main components of a good national development policy, a country still needs excellent politicians who are able to implement these policies in a continuously changing context.

The emerging consensus on national development policy does not include how to balance socio-economic development against environmental sustainability. This debate remains extremely polarised, and will be reviewed below.

1.8.4 Sustainable development

The term 'sustainable development' is the established term for the concern that development must maintain natural resources for coming generations. The human species has had a tremendous impact on the ecology of the whole world. Hunters have driven animals to extinction, and farmers have changed vegetation and caused erosion. Industrialisation and the increased energy consumption that followed have changed the chemical composition of the atmosphere. The enormous increase in the number of humans that these revolutions gave rise to has also had profound environmental effects. The way in which human societies use and protect the natural resources while they improve their livelihood is one criteria for "good development". Paul Harrison (1993) argues that contemporary human development is compelling us to stage a third revolution, the sustainable use of natural resources. The Rio Conference in 1992 converted environmental concern into global and national policies known as "Agenda 21". The need for the sustainable use of natural resources makes it necessary to include a biological dimension in the definition and analysis of development. The understanding of global development involves a progressively more complex system analysis. Peace & conflict research and meteorology play a more central role than health sciences, but more evidence about the relationship between climate change and health is one component of the global system analysis that is now required.

The debate about the relationship between human development and the environment has been highly polarised (Sarre & Blunden 2000). The biologists fear that humanity is irreversibly changing the biological basis for its own survival. This is now supported by clear scientific evidence that global warming is taking place. Recent research has shown that the climate of the world has warmed by about 0.6 °C compared to earlier average, and that this change corresponds to observed changes in the natural ecology (Gian *et al.* 2002). It has been predicted that a number of health effects will result from this warming (Patz & Kovatz 2002). The diseases that are expected to increase range from an increase in malaria due to more favourable conditions for the mosquitoes to an increase in skin cancer in populations with deficient skin pigmentation.

It is also possible to interpret the links between human activity and environmental change by assuming that humanity will be able to adapt to changing conditions through a series of mechanisms. This view finds support in the fact that earlier catastrophe scenarios have not come true. Three decades ago, Paul Ehrlich published a book entitled *The Population Bomb.* He forecast that human population growth would result in lack of raw materials and food (Ehrlich 1968). He was wrong. Six billion people are today being fed by increased agricultural output, and population growth is slowing. The prices of many raw materials have fallen. There is firm evidence that agricultural development will be able to feed an expected stable world population of about 10 billion, 50 to 100 years from now (Evans 2000).

The very definition of global environmental problems is controversial. Many argue that a lack of latrines, poor hygiene and unsafe water remain the main environmental problems of mankind. Many families cannot avoid drinking water that contains their neighbours' faeces, and this is responsible for millions of child deaths each year. The most important contribution that health sciences have made to the discourse on global ecology is demonstrating that basic sanitation and health services result in a decline in child mortality. This decline, in turn, leads to lower birth rates, giving a stable population. This corresponds to "the invention of the two-child family", which will yield stable human populations. It is noteworthy that 30 years ago the growth of the human population was regarded as the major threat to sustainable development. Fertility reduction is today not included when the United Nations defined in 2000 its Millennium Development Goals (Table 1.1) to be achieved by 2015. The reason is that the number of children born per woman has already fallen to three or less in most parts of the world, with the exception of the countries in Sub-Saharan Africa and a few other countries. The average number of children born per woman in India has decreased from 6.5 to 2.9 during the last four decades. This huge nation has thus in a few decades achieved more than 75 % of the requirement for changing unsustainable family sizes with six children to sustainable two-child families. This is a neglected success in human development! "World opinion", instead of celebrating a problem solved, rapidly changed its focus to a new alarm. This is probably unavoidable, but for those in despair it is good to know that the global problems of past decades have been largely solved.

It is impossible to reach scientific consensus about how to handle the links between human development and the global environment. The book *The Skeptical Environmentalist*, by the Danish statistician Bjørn Lomborg is a prominent example of the controversy regarding sustainable development. Lomborg (2001) reviewed the available data underlying not only the assessment of environmental change but also other aspects of world development. He concluded that most of the debate in high-income countries concerning global development constitutes of "a litany" of pessimistic forecasts, despite many measurements of development showing favourable trends. His conclusion is that the common image of the state of the world is a mix of prejudice and deficient analysis. His book has been met with attacks from both scientists and cake-throwing environmentalists.[1] The Danish Committee on Scientific Dishonesty stated in January 2003 that Lomborg had been "systematically one-sided", while Lomborg has replied that the Committee had failed to give one single example of this.[2] We find the review of data and the conclusions of his short chapter on global health development to be accurate. Interested readers may engage in the debate about *The Skeptical Environmentalist* through the websites mentioned below. It remains difficult to draw a line between scientific reviews and advocacy statements in the debate about global environmental change and human development. It is also difficult to draw such a line in the intense debate on how global political governance should be organised in the present period of economic globalisation.

We conclude that global warming now should be regarded as a fact, but that the degree and the future distribution and character of impacts of this warming remain unknown, as well as to what degree it is wise to invest in halting the warming or in adapting to the consequences, respectively.

1.9 Globalisation (the present)

The term 'globalisation' is much used but rarely defined. To some, it designates the *goal* of world development. Globalisation, they argue, has been around for a long time. The current phase is just an intensification that will strengthen market economy and bring more wealth to the world. To others, globalisation designates the *evil forces* that increase the unfairness of the contemporary world, leading to further dominance by the

[1] www.anti-lomborg.com
[2] www.lomborg.com

United States and its closest allies. To a third group, the term globalisation is a *descriptive term* for the present state of world affairs: an increasingly neo-liberal world economy with increasing movement of capital across national borders, and with decreasing power of local communities and nations to regulate these economic activities. As a descriptive term, globalisation, however, also includes a growing global commitment for the environment and for joint human values. The future may bring a free trade that in the end benefits the poor in both low-income and middle-income countries, or it may bring just a continuation of the neo-liberal merging of global elites, with increased suffering for the poor. The descriptive interpretation refers to globalisation as an open-ended and contradictory process that generates forces that act in both good and bad directions.

We use the term 'globalisation' as a description of a number of changes in the world that have accelerated in the last decade following the end of the Cold War. The term 'globalisation' refers to more than the dominance of neo-liberal policy in the global economy. The present process of change in the world is both wider and deeper than an expansion of western economic dominance. From an Asian perspective globalisation may even be seen as the beginning of the end of European and North American dominance.

In short, the descriptive term 'globalisation' refers to an increased interconnectivity of remotely living populations. The life situation of people in one part of the world has an increasing direct significance for the well-being of populations in very distant parts of the world. A dramatic example of this was the terrorist attack on World Trade Centre on 11 September 2001. This attack was originally planned in a remote part of rural Afghanistan and killed thousands people in downtown Manhattan in New York. The reciprocal attack on Afghanistan that followed probably killed even more civilians.

The increased interconnectivity not only between remote parts of the world but also between local communities within a nation is blurring the distinction between domestic and foreign politics. Globalisation has been described as a process of denationalisation following a century in which the nation-state had considerably more importance than the local and global communities (Cooper 2003). The Nobel Prize winner Joseph Stiglitz (2003) argues that globalisation can be a positive force for the poor around the world, but only if the IMF, World Bank, and WTO dramatically alter the way they operate. After having worked in these organizations he has become their main critic, but remains positive to economic globalisation. Another leading economist and UN adviser (Bhagwati 2004) claims that globalisation has reduced poverty in China from 28 % of the population in 1978 to only 9 % in 1998. Nevertheless, he recommends that continued globalisation should be better managed. He suggests taxing of skilled workers who leave poor countries for jobs abroad, using non-governmental organisations as corporate watchdogs, slowing financial liberalisation and loosening intellectual property safeguards.

The globalisation process may be seen as comprised of at least eight components:

1 *The economic forces of transnational capitalism* have induced a process of economic investment with progressively fewer links to nationally owned companies. Nations are today adapting to companies, rather than companies adapting to nations. There is an increasing deficit of global democratic governance that can match the global capital movements. Capitalism has become global at a much faster rate than democracy.

2 *New communication technologies* for satellite-meditated TV, the Internet, e-mail and cheap telephone connections have revolutionised communications between remote parts of the world. Through the application of new technologies and

commercial mechanisms that require only limited involvement of state-owned telephone networks, connections are being established to remote parts of rural Africa in ways that were impossible only a few years ago.

3 *National governments increasingly share power*, not only with transnational companies but also with other types of organisations, such as agencies of the United Nations, international voluntary organisations such as Greenpeace, and mass media, such as CNN, which are becoming increasingly international.

4 *A growing global cultural identification* of the national elites in most countries, i.e. a cultural identification by rich, well-educated and powerful social groups. With this comes an increasing global cultural conformity, especially in youth culture. The habit of eating hamburgers and listening to MTV music is rapidly spreading across most national borders. But a global culture is also promoted by an expanding non-commercial global civil society. This has resulted in world music, a global environmental movement and a growing integration of cultures and ethnic groups from other continents into local cultures. Another aspect is the growing importance of diasporas, i.e. people of the same origin and culture who live in a large number of local communities across the globe.

5 *Global environmental changes*, such as global warming, know no borders. This compels nations to negotiate about global regulations to protect a shared global environment. The world must also deal more efficiently with the common global microbiological environment, as exemplified by infectious diseases such as HIV and SARS, and by resistant strains of older microbes (WHO 2003).

6 *Patents are questioned on global level.* An example of the uncertainty with respect to patenting can be found in pharmaceutical drugs, which have become a central issue for the World Trade Organization (WTO). It was agreed at the last WTO meeting that poorer countries with public health emergencies should be given the right to obtain drugs at the lowest possible production cost. A major reason for this change in policy was that the United States broke the patent rules with respect to the best antibiotic needed to control a minor anthrax epidemic in 2001. This is a prominent example of a case in which global health interests are attempting to limit the negative health effects of a neo-liberal trade policy. The outcome remains unclear.

7 *Intellectual property rights go beyond nations* when scientific advances in molecular genetics have made plant genes the property of transnational companies. An intense struggle about the right to patent genes is currently raging between national institutions and transnational companies.

8 *Global ethical values and human rights* are further issues confronting the principles of sovereign national states. An organisation such as Médicines Sans Frontière (MSF) bears the principle of denationalisation in its name, and hence constitute a prominent feature of globalisation. The humanitarian organisation MSF was founded during the civil war in Nigeria, when the International Red Cross was not allowed by its national Nigerian counterpart to assist the population in the breakaway territory of Biafra in 1968. Assistance from the International Red Cross was refused because one of the fighting fractions did not have a recognised national Red Cross organisation. The Red Cross was formed in 1863 to act in armed conflicts between recognised nations. A number of relief workers did not accept that national borders should stop them from relieving the suffering of people. These workers founded MSF. This is a clear example of global ethical values being awarded greater significance than national integrity.

Globalisation is thus characterised by simultaneous changes in several social, economic, technological, political and cultural dimensions. The effects that globalisation has had and will have on health are a topic of heated debate at the time of writing this textbook, and opinions differ as much as the definitions of globalisation do. The nation state is beneficial for health by providing the public investment that is needed for health promotion, the provision of primary health care, and public hospital services. Many claim that globalisation threatens the health service that is provided by the welfare states, and prevents poorer nations from building welfare states. Commercial globalisation is catastrophic for health by facilitating the free promotion of tobacco, alcohol and other health-threatening goods. Others conclude that globalisation increases economic growth and in this way mainly benefits the global health situation (Feachem 2001). One line of thinking also suggests that globalisation may apply pressure on the richest countries to support the alleviation of poverty for the sake of joint security and global stability.

The agricultural subsidies in high-income countries correspond to a "lack of globalisation", i.e. the national governments use tax revenues to subsidise national agricultural products that could be purchased at lower prices on the world market. The agricultural policies of the European Union and US do not allow free trade. This was the reason the meeting of the World Trade Organisation in Mexico in 2003 did not reach an agreement on the conditions for world trade. China, India and Brazil lead a united front against the high-income countries. They demanded trade that was truly free – trade that included agricultural products. Looked upon in this way, fair globalisation may open new opportunities for low-income and middle-income countries to receive foreign investment and to sell their products on the world market. Good governments will thus gain greater tax revenues, which they can invest in the health sector.

A contrasting prediction is that nations will lose power, and that health services in poor countries will be organised to serve a rich minority in a neo-liberal economy with private health care. There are several examples of this happening (WHO 2003). It may confuse some readers that the communist parties currently in power in China and Vietnam are leading the international transition of health service to "out-of-pocket payment" and "private-for-profit" provision. A strong voice in the global health debate for free primary health care is the People's Health Movement, which in 2000 presented the People's Health Charter (Box 1.7). The charter argues strongly for a publicly financed health service and for development policies that favour health. The charter ad-

---

Box 1.7

The People's Health Assembly and the Charter

The idea of a People's Health Assembly (PHA) has been discussed for more than a decade. A number of organisations launched the PHA process in 1998 and started to plan a large international Assembly meeting, which was subsequently held in Bangladesh at the end of 2000. A range of pre-Assembly and post-Assembly activities were initiated, including regional workshops, the collection of people's health-related stories and the drafting of a *People's Charter for Health*.

The present Charter builds upon the views of citizens and people's organisations from around the world, and was first approved and opened for endorsement at the Assembly meeting in Savar, Bangladesh, in December 2000.

The Charter is an expression of a vision of a better and healthier world, and calls for radical action. It is a tool for advocacy and a rallying point for a global health movement. http://phmovement. org

vocates strongly against the commercial aspects of globalisation. This network, presently led from Bangalore in India, is a leading representative for NGOs in the global health debate. This global network is in itself a new aspect of globalisation.

1.10 A taxonomy of nations

There is a strong association between socio-economic development and the health status of the population in each country of the world. There is also a strong association between the socio-economic situation of different population groups within countries and the health status of each of these groups. The old division of countries into two groups, 'industrialised' and 'developing', or 'north' and 'south', may remain relevant with respect to political, economic and military considerations. However, we find that the old division into two groups of countries today constitutes an irrelevant taxonomy for an evidence-based view of the contemporary global health situation. This is because there is today a continuous spectrum of health status across the populations of the more than 200 nations of the world. There are countries with all levels of child mortality. The worst child health situation corresponds to countries with several hundreds of children dying per one thousand born; while the best child health situation corresponds to countries with only three young children dying per one thousand born. Countries are found that have all different levels of economic development. There is no longer one single big gap between two types of countries (see World Health Chart on back cover).

A division of countries into more than two groups is therefore long overdue when analysing the global health situation. This new pattern of social and health situations favours the division of nations into three, four or more groups, based on their levels of socio-economic development. This does not imply that clear dividing lines can be easily found between such groups. On the con-

trary, such lines must be arbitrarily chosen, as the world health situation constitutes a continuum between two extremes that are wider apart than ever.

Most authors who review global health and social development no longer use the previous concept of two types of countries (Cooper 2003; Allen 2000). This is not a trendy change of terminology, but rather a delayed reflection of a major change in the pattern of global health and social development. We suggest that the use of terms such as 'industrialised' and 'developing' countries, or 'north' and 'south', should be avoided when discussing global health. The most used alternative taxonomy is a division based on economic level into high-income, middle-income, and low-income countries. A group of 'collapsed' nations, with prolonged complex emergencies due to armed conflicts, may be added to these three groups. Most previous taxonomies of nations have grouped countries into two groups. This has been true ever since the ancient empires conceived the world as being composed of the empires and the barbarian territories. Both the Chinese and the Roman Empire saw the borders between the two groups as a line, often in the form of a wall cutting across continents to divide mankind (Table 1.5). Humanity seems very prone to divide itself into a "we" group and a "them" group. Understanding of the modern world requires higher ambitions.

The dichotomisation of mankind was prominent during the European colonisation of the world. It was expressed linguistically in terms of 'civilised' and 'primitive' cultures. Many concepts of world health remain influenced by this colonial division of countries into two groups. During decolonisation, colonial powers and former colonies became 'industrialised' and 'developing' countries. The frequent use of the term 'developing country' is surprising, as this category lacks definition. The limitation of the term is notable in many ways, especially within the UN system and in various agencies for international development co-oper-

Table 1.5 Taxonomy of nations based on their level of "development".

Time period	Taxonomy of countries into named groups			
Early Historic	Empires	Barbarians		
Colonial	Colonial Powers	Colonies		
1946–1960	Developed	Underdeveloped		
1960–1990	Industrialised	Developing		
1975–	North	South		
1946–	First	Second	Third World	
1983–	Industrialised	Newly industrialised	Developing	Least developed
1990–	High-income countries	Middle-income Countries	Low-income countries	*

* Collapsed or war-torn nations.

ation. It seems that these organisations do not want to recognize progress in formerly developing countries. In UNICEF's Yearbook, State of the World's Children 2004, Singapore is still labelled a developing country (UNICEF 2004, page 136.). Yet Singapore in the same book is ranked as having the second lowest child mortality in the world, and Singapore's gross national product per capita is also on a par with that of the richest countries in the world. The use of country labels without definitions is a result of subconscious prejudice when trying to make sense of the world situation. The use of the terms 'north' and 'south' also suffers from the problem that there is no definition regarding which country should belong to which group. The terms 'first world', 'second world' and 'third world' reflected a first attempt to construct a new form of categorisation, namely one in which countries may belong to more than one group. However, only the term 'third world' became widely used, and it remains unclear whether South Korea, Turkey, Russia, Saudi Arabia, Poland, Mexico and Singapore, for example, are third world countries today.

Taxonomies with more than two groups of countries were first devised by the United Nations. The UN introduced a new taxonomy in the 1980s that grouped countries into 'industrialised countries', 'newly industrialised countries', and 'developing coun-

tries' with a subgroup called 'least developed countries'. The 'human development index' (HDI), which is composed of measures of national economy, life expectancy and literacy rate of a country, offers an alternative division of countries. The HDI for all countries is published annually in the 'Human Development Report' by the United Nations Development Programme, UNDP.[1] The human development index has become used mainly for ranking countries, rather than for dividing them into groups. This provides further evidence that the development of all of the countries in the world today are found on a continuum.

The World Bank launched in the 1990s a classification into 'high-income', 'middle-income' and 'low-income' countries, based on well-defined cut-off values of the gross national product expressed in current US dollars (this measure thus considered the exchange rate of the currency against the dollar, and not its purchasing power) (Box 2.2). We have added to these three categories a distinct, small group of war-torn, low-income countries, which in the last decade have been designated as 'collapsed countries' or 'failed states'. It should be noted that the cut-off levels used to classify countries are arbitrary, but they are at least well-defined values, and this taxonomy al-

[1]   www.undp.org

lows for countries to change group from one year to the next. The World Bank adds a caveat to their income taxonomy:

> The use of these three terms is not intended to imply that all countries in one group are experiencing similar development, or that other economies have reached a preferred stage of development. Classification by income does not represent development status.

This taxonomy is, of course, far from perfect, but we have found it to be a convenient description of the present variations in demographic patterns, disease panoramas and health statuses of the countries of the world.

The World Bank[1] provides the latest cut-off values. Countries divided according to their 2002 gross national income (previously known as 'gross national product', see Box 2.2) per capita in current US dollars at levels calculated by the World Bank *Atlas method* form the following groups: *low-income*, 735 USD or less; *lower middle-income*, 736–2 935 USD; *upper middle-income*, 2 936–9 075 USD; and *high-income*, 9 076 USD or more. This classification gives Indonesia as the richest low-income country and Ukraine as the poorest middle-income country. Saudi Arabia is the richest middle-income country and Slovenia is the poorest high-income country. Until a better taxonomy is proposed and widely used, the classification of countries into three groups based on economic performance remains useful, because this classification departs from the previous worldview with only two types of countries. A display of countries according to both economic and social performance is available in the World Health Chart on the back cover.

1.11 The hopeful future

The Secretary General of the United Nations outlines the challenge to the world in the UN Millennium Declaration.[2] It is impor-

tant to note how he summarises the multi-dimensional development consensus into diplomatic language. Later he lays down the concrete Millennium Development goals that are to be used for monitoring. Kofi Annan spoke as follows to the gathered national leaders:

"We recognise that, in addition to our separate responsibilities to our individual societies, we have a collective responsibility to uphold the principles of human dignity, equality and equity at the global level. As leaders we have a duty therefore to all the world's people, especially the most vulnerable and, in particular, the children of the world, to whom the future belongs.

We reaffirm our commitment to the purposes and principles of the Charter of the United Nations, which have proved timeless and universal. Indeed, their relevance and capacity to inspire have increased, as nations and peoples have become increasingly interconnected and interdependent. We are determined to establish a just and lasting peace all over the world in accordance with the purposes and principles of the Charter.

We rededicate ourselves to support all efforts to uphold the sovereign equality of all States, respect for their territorial integrity and political independence, resolution of disputes by peaceful means and, in conformity with the principles of justice and international law, the right to self-determination of peoples which remain under colonial domination and foreign occupation, non-interference in the internal affairs of States, respect for human rights and fundamental freedoms, respect for the equal rights of all without distinction as to race, sex, language or religion and international co-operation in solving international problems of an economic, social, cultural or humanitarian character.

We believe that the central challenge we face today is to ensure that globalisation becomes a positive force for all the world's people. For while globalisation offers great opportunities, at present its benefits are very unevenly shared, while its costs are une-

---

[1]   www.worldbank.org/data/countryclass/
      countryclass.html
[2]   www.un.org/millennium

venly distributed. We recognise that developing countries and countries with economies in transition face special difficulties in responding to this central challenge. Thus, only through broad and sustained efforts to create a shared future, based upon our common humanity in all its diversity, can globalisation be made fully inclusive and equitable. These efforts must include policies and measures, at the global level, which correspond to the needs of developing countries and economies in transition and are formulated and implemented with their effective participation.

We consider certain fundamental values to be essential to international relations in the twenty-first century. These include:

- *Freedom*
  Men and women have the right to live their lives and raise their children in dignity, free from hunger and from the fear of violence, oppression or injustice. Democratic and participatory governance based on the will of the people best assures these rights.

- *Equality*
  No individual and no nation must be denied the opportunity to benefit from development. The equal rights and opportunities of women and men must be assured.

- *Solidarity*
  Global challenges must be managed in a way that distributes the costs and burdens fairly in accordance with basic principles of equity and social justice. Those who suffer or who benefit least deserve help from those who benefit most.

- *Tolerance*
  Human beings must respect one other, in all their diversity of belief, culture and language. Differences within and between societies should be neither feared nor repressed, but cherished as a precious asset of humanity. A culture of peace and dialogue among all civilisations should be actively promoted.

- *Respect for nature*
  Prudence must be shown in the management of all living species and natural resources, in accordance with the precepts of sustainable development. Only in this way can the immeasurable riches provided to us by nature be preserved and passed on to our descendants. The current unsustainable patterns of production and consumption must be changed in the interest of our future welfare and that of our descendants.

- *Shared responsibility*
  Responsibility for managing worldwide economic and social development, as well as threats to international peace and security, must be shared among the nations of the world and should be exercised multilaterally. As the most universal and most representative organisation in the world, the United Nations must play the central role."

1.11.1 Millennium Developme nt Goals (MDGs)

The United Nations Millennium Summit in 2000 agreed on a set of time-bound and measurable goals and targets for combating poverty, hunger, disease, illiteracy, environmental degradation and discrimination against women.[1] These 8 goals and the corresponding 18 targets and 48 monitoring indicators concern the main advances to be made in the major development dimensions between 1990 and 2015. In other words the MDG tells how much to do during one generation of 25 years.

The statistical data for the 48 indicators is available at the web page of the UN Statistical Division.[2] The goals, targets and indicators have been selected such that they make global policy concrete to national governments and in people's lives by showing what can and must be achieved within one gener-

[1]   www.un.org/millenniumgoals
[2]   http://millenniumindicators.un.org/unsd/mi/mi_goals.asp

ation. The definition of 'development' in the millennium declaration is also a confirmation of a global acceptance of the multidimensional view of development. The goals show the ambitions of the Secretary General of UN, Kofi Annan, to improve co-ordination within the UN organisation, both in action and in monitoring the impact of the actions taken. Three of the eight UN Millennium Development Goals (MDGs) to be achieved by 2015 directly concern health (Table 1.1).

The goals make the general aims of the global community operational. However, there are obviously no binding agreements in this area, and no agency has been given ultimate responsibility for reaching the targets. The UN emphasises that countries should monitor their own development goals. This process is being co-ordinated by the UN development group.[1] The MDGs constitute an ambition to reach shared responsibility between national governments, international organisations and other partners in development. Some of the goals and targets are impossible to monitor for several countries because the 1990 value is too uncertain. However, the way in which the targets have been defined involves rates of development, rather than absolute levels. The rates of development set down in these targets are not impossible. The goal to reduce child mortality by two thirds in 25 years has already been achieved during the past 25 years in several countries, including Egypt, South Korea, Mauritius, Malaysia, Chile and Iran. Many other countries have reached the rates of development specified by other targets. An animation on Human Development Trends and MDGs is available at the gapminder site.[2]

The world and the countries are advised to simultaneously keep track of several dimensions of development. The MDG approach does actually not set a fixed goal, but rather a rate for development in each dimension. These goals can be criticised for including indicators for which no reliable data is available. They can also be criticised for not taking into consideration the possibility that a country in 1990 may have had an uneven development profile, while all countries are assumed to advance at an equal rate in all dimensions. Thus, a country that was doing very badly in 1990 may show the best progress in fulfilling each goal. For example, China already had low child mortality in 1990, while that of Egypt was high. Egypt is, therefore, in a better position to fulfil goal number four, since this goal is expressed as a relative improvement. However, these are technical issues that need to be addressed without calling the MDG concept as such into question.

Kofi Annan's basic approach in the Millennium Declaration and in the Millennium Development Goals is firmly based on the best current understanding of how multidimensional development can be achieved. The fact that the United Nations development policy is evidence-based and will be monitored brings hope for a better global future! You may be surprised that the World Bank has done advanced analyses on how to improve global health.

References and suggested further reading

Allen T, Thomas A. (Eds.) Poverty and development into the 21st century. Oxford University Press; 2000.

Bhagwati J. In Defense of Globalization. Oxford University Press; 2004.

Bhutta ZA. Structural adjustments and their impact on health and society: a perspective from Pakistan. Int J of Epidemiology 2001;30:712–16.

Boserup E. Population and Technology Change, a study of long-term trends. The University of Chicago Press; 1981.

Boyd R, Silk JB. How humans evolved. Norton; 2000.

Cohan JE. How many people can the world support? Norton; 1995.

---

[1]   www.undg.org
[2]   www.gapminder.org

Cooper R. The Breaking of Nations: Order and Chaos in the Twenty-first Century. London: Atlantic Books; 2003.

de Soto H. The Mystery of Capital: Why Capitalism Triumphs in the West and Fails Everywhere Else. Times Books; 2001.

Desowitz, R. Tropical diseases from 50 000 BC to 2500 AD. Flamingo; 1998.

de Vylder S. The driving forces of development (in Swedish). Forum Syd; 2002.

Diamond J. Guns, Germs and Steel. A short history of everybody for the last 13 000 years. London: Vintage; 1997.

Ehrlich PR. The Population Bomb. New York: Ballentine Books; 1968.

Evans LT. Feeding the 10 billion – plant and population growth. Cambridge University Press; 2000.

Feachem RG. Globalisation is good for your health, mostly. BMJ. 2001;323:504–6.

Gian R, et al. Ecological responses to recent climatic change. Nature 2002;416:389–95.

Gunnarsson C, Rojas M. Growth, stagnation, chaos (in Swedish). SNS; 1995.

Harrison P. The Third revolution – population, environment and a sustainable world. Penguin Press; 1993.

Kaessmann H, Paabo S. The genetic history of humans and the great apes. J Intern Med 2002;251:1–18.

Landes DS. The Wealth and Poverty of Nations: Why Some Are So Rich and Some So Poor. Norton; 1999.

Livi-Bacci MA. Concise History of World Population. Blackwell; 1995.

Lomborg B. The sceptical environmentalist. Cambridge University Press; 2001.

Lutz W. The future population of the earth: what can we assume today? Earthscan; 1996.

Maddison A. The World Economy: A Millennial Perspective. OECD; 2001.

McMichael T. Human Frontiers, environments and disease. Cambridge University Press; 2001.

McNeill W. Plagues and People. Anchor Press; 1976.

Middleton N, O'Keefe P, Visser R. (Eds.) Negotiating Poverty. London: Pluto Press; 2001.

Moberg W. The Emigrants. Penguin Books; 1995.

Narayan D. Voices of the poor – Can anyone hear us? Oxford University Press; 2000.

Patz JA, Kovats RS. Hotspots in climate change and human health. BMJ 2002; 325:1094–8.

Roberts JM. The Penguin History of the World. Penguin Books; 1995.

Sarre P, Blunden J. An Overcrowded World? Oxford University Press; 2000.

Sen A. Development as Freedom. Oxford University Press; 1999.

Sen G, George A, Östlin P. Engendering International Health – the Challenge of Equity. MIT Press; 2002.

Stiglitz JE. Globalization and its discontents. W.W. Norton & Company; 2003.

Thomas H. The Slave Trade. The History of the Atlantic Slave Trade 1440–1870. Papermac; 1998.

Todaro M, Smith SC. Economic development, 8th edition. Addison Wesley; 2002.

UNDP, Human Development Report 1997.

UNDP, Human Development Report 2003.

UNICEF, State of the world's children 2004.

WHO, World Health Report 2003.

World Bank, World Development Report 1993.

World Bank, World Development Report 2001.

World Bank, Responsible Growth for the New Millennium: Integrating Society, Ecology, and the Economy; 2004.

2 Health determinants

> *Poverty is pain; it feels like a disease. It attacks a person not only materially but also morally. It eats away one's dignity and drives one into total despair."*
>
> A poor woman, Moldavia 1997

The basic requirements for good health in human populations are not so many, but they interact in a very complex way. Since the degree of fulfilment of these requirements determines health status, they are jointly designated *health determinants*. The determinants can be grouped and labelled in various ways. We group the determinants under seven headings:

1 *socio-economic*
2 *food*
3 *water*
4 *sanitation*
5 *other environmental determinants*
6 *behaviour*
7 *health services*

Any grouping of health determinants is a simplification of the complex web of factors that jointly determine the health status of human populations. This web is composed of many mutually interacting socio-economic, cultural and environmental factors, which, through various links with individual behavioural and genetic factors, determine the health of a human being. Public health is about understanding the role of each factor in this web and about how to modify factors or to intervene with new factors in ways that improve the health status of a population.

The cause of each of the main diseases in the world can also be regarded as a long chain of causative factors within a wider web of interlinking factors. The causative chain behind a specific disease may start in underlying poverty or ignorance. Interventions like primary schooling for all children will affect one of these underlying causative factors, which is far away from the actual disease at the other end of the web of determining factors. Primary schooling for all will reduce the occurrence of many diseases. In fact primary schooling for all children appears to be the most effective health intervention of all, but it will take half a century before it has full effect.

Poverty and ignorance are underlying causative factors that act upon many intermediate causative factors, such as insufficient food supply and unsafe water supply. Each causative chain is ultimately linked to the direct biological cause of a specific disease. One example is how a polluted water supply results in poliovirus infection, as virus particles from the faeces of one infected person are transmitted via drinking water to the gut of a previously healthy child. If the child has been vaccinated, she will manage to resist the virus and remain healthy. But if the health service has been inadequate, the unvaccinated child who drinks water that has been contaminated with poliovirus may be at risk. This child can thus acquire an acute infection with the poliovirus, which causes high fever and may lead to permanent paralysis in one or both legs. In poverty-related diseases such as polio, the effect of one determinant is strongly dependent on the other determinants.

The provision of vaccination services in poor communities, where few mothers have attended school, will not have the same effect as if the same service is provided in communities where all women are literate and conversant with how infectious diseases may be prevented by an injection at an early age. In many communities, a high proportion of children will remain unvaccinated although the health service provides safe vaccinations, because of reluctance by many illiterate mothers to have their children vaccinated. Many factors may thus be regarded as the cause of the paralysis of one of the legs of the little girl mentioned previously: the poverty of her family and community; the unsafe water supply in that community; the poorly functioning health system that failed to vaccinate her; or the virus itself. Hypothetically speaking, the individual child's genetic susceptibility to developing paralysis when exposed to poliovirus infection may also be put forward as the cause of the paralysis, as paralysis only occurs in a few percent of those infected with this virus. All of these factors can intellectually be regarded as causes, although some may, in certain circumstances, be easier and less costly to prevent than others.

We may go even deeper in analysing the cause of paralysis in the child. This requires a study of how the global political and economic situation relates to the occurrence of the underlying determinants of diseases within the poor community of the victim. Global economic and health policy may alleviate or aggravate the poverty of the family and thus affect their access to safe water and health service.

The satisfying message in relation to polio infection is that the international community has taken up its responsibility. Technical and financial resources have been made available for polio vaccination of all children throughout the world. The disease has already been eradicated from Latin America. The eradication of the poliovirus from the world is now within our grasp through concerted international action and funding. It is interesting to note that the contemporary global health governance is successful in dealing with health problems that can be solved by highly technical interventions such as vaccination. In sharp contrast to such technical achievements stands the fact that the world is still far from providing primary schooling for all its children. This is in spite of free elementary schooling being declared a human right in 1948[1].

Another example of interactions between different health determinants can be found in contemporary Sweden. An increasing proportion of highly educated parents abstain from vaccinating their children against infectious diseases, e.g. measles, due to the influence of new cultural values originating from anthroposophy and related philosophical trends. There are two main reasons as to why the unvaccinated Swedish children are very rarely infected with the measles virus. A minor reason is that good housing standards decrease the risk of measles transmission in Sweden. However, the main reason is that the vast majority of Swedish parents do continue to have their children vaccinated. The vaccination of most of the children provides 'herd immunity', meaning that an infectious disease will not spread in a population in which the vast majority are vaccinated. Acting in combination, these two factors reduce the risk of measles epidemics in Sweden to almost zero among vaccinated and unvaccinated alike. The advice from parts of the anthroposophy movement that vaccination is unnecessary will continue to be supported by empirical evidence only as long as it is not followed by too many. If an unvaccinated Swedish child travels to a low-income country where measles occur, she will be at great risk of acquiring the disease and hence to transmit it to other children. This demonstrates the fact that the health effect of one and the same determinant may be different in different contexts.

The scientific evidence for the relative importance of each determinant in a web of causation is surprisingly limited. The reason is that the strong interdependence between the different factors makes it very difficult to separately quantify the effect of each factor in observational studies. Many factors would also only exert their positive effects if another factor changed at the same time.

[1]   www.un.org/Overview/rights

Table 2.1 Major preventable risk factors for disease in the world in 2000.

Risk factors	% of total disease burden[*]
Under nutrition[**]	15
Over nutrition[***]	13
Unsafe sex	6
Tobacco	4
Alcohol	4
Unsafe water, sanitation and hygiene	4
Indoor smoke from solid fuels	3
Occupation[****]	2

[*] (attributable DALYs see chapter 3 for definition)
[**] including: underweight, iron-VitA-and Zinc deficiency
[***] including: hypertension, high cholesterol, overweight, low fruit and vegetable intake and physical inactivity
[****] including: risk factors of injury, carcinogens, airborne particles, ergonomic stressors, noise
Source: World Health Report 2002. WHO.

Provision of safe tap water in a village will only reduce the occurrence of diarrhoea if health education is simultaneously provided and if poor households have the means to maintain the water clean when storing and drinking it in their homes. In addition many causative factors, such as literacy, are not possible to study in randomised controlled trails. It is therefore difficult to answer questions such as: "How much healthier would country X be if every household gained access to clean, safe water?" "How much would child survival improve in country Y if malnutrition was eradicated among children?"

The World Health Report 2002 presents the first coherent attempt (Table 2.1) to estimate at a global level the relative importance of each major preventable risk factor responsible for the loss of disability adjusted life years (DALY, see chapter 3). It is estimated that the world at the beginning of the new millennium has reached the point where the degree of ill health due to being overweight, eating foods with a high dietary fat content and lack of physical activity is almost as great as the ill health resulting from lack of food. Too much food accounts for 13 % and too little food 15 %, of lost healthy years in the world today. Table 2.1 also shows the estimates of how much of the global burden of disease is caused by each preventable risk factor. The eight most common risk factors are together responsible for half of the healthy life years lost in the world.

The difficulty in defining causes and best preventive actions against ill health also relates to difficulties in defining health. A discussion of health determinants must include an attempt to define health (Box 2.1). The

---

Box 2.1

Definitions of health

The definition of health agreed upon in 1948 at the foundation of the World Health Organization:

Health is a state of complete physical, mental, and social well-being and not merely the absence of disease or infirmity.

This eloquent holistic definition encompasses a broad psychosocial view on the health of humans. However, it is useless for monitoring the effect of health promotion and disease prevention. When WHO in 1977 reformulated its overall goal a more practical health definition was included.

Health permits a socially and economically productive life.

---

health aspirations of the poorest people in the world remain a matter of survival and a hope of living without disability. The promotion of world health in the last 50 years has also focused on improving survival. Mortality statistics have thus been the main means of monitoring the result of health promotion, as will be discussed further in chapter 3.

At the start of the new millennium, global health problems are still dominated by high mortality among the poor in low-income countries. In low-income countries, most premature deaths, diseases and disabilities are caused by varying combinations of the seven types of determinants described in this chapter. We fully recognise that individual genetic factors also are important in all human populations, but the genetic disease determinants are not dealt with in this book. Many behavioural and social health determinants that are not mentioned in this book are also of great importance for health in high-income countries and in some middle-income countries. Many contemporary health issues of populations in the most affluent countries are not related to survival. A very low or non-existent pregnancy-related mortality is now taken for granted in Sweden. The health impact of birth delivery services in contemporary Sweden is very much a question of the direct psychosocial outcome of the experiences of the delivery. Most psychosocial health determinants in high-income countries are not covered in this text. The chapter focuses on determinants of worldwide importance for survival.

The main determinant of disease in the world is poverty. Gender is another health determinant that transcends all societies and modifies the effect of other determinants mentioned in this chapter. Ethnicity and other cultural dimensions are also overarching factors that modify other health determinants.

2.1 Socio-economic determinants

It is agreed that the poverty of households and individuals, as a result of the level and distribution of economic resources of each nation, is the most important determinant of health. There is less agreement on how to define and measure poverty (Öyen 1996). Two different definitions of poverty are currently used. The first is the conventional economic understanding, which is known as 'income poverty'. The second is a wider concept of poverty that includes income, ignorance, ill health, disempowerment, gender issues and vulnerability[1]. There is even greater disagreement about the relative importance of each of these components. In the past, the debate has related to the relative importance of pure economic factors such as household income in relation to social factors such as literacy. Some have argued that, if a country had strong economic growth, this would almost automatically lead to all of the changes that result in improved health status. Others have stated that health is marginally or even negatively associated with economic growth, and that improvements in health result from improved education, human rights, gender equity and general access to health services, rather than from any economic change. Today, social and economic changes are regarded as intensely interlinked. The understanding of the complex interactions between different socio-economic factors has been advanced by the Bengali Nobel Prize Laureate in Economics in 1998, Amartya Sen (1999), as described in chapter 1.

Amartya Sen simultaneously emphasises the close relationship between economic progress and health improvement, and the fact that health improvements also are strongly related to non-economic development dimensions, such as education. There are two influences in particular that weaken the relationship between the economic level

[1] www.worldbank.org/poverty/voices

of a country and the health status of its population.

The first influence is how the economic resources are distributed between communities, households and individuals. One striking example of this is that the child mortality of countries with a very uneven distribution of economic wealth, such as South Africa, Brazil and Turkey, is several times higher than in countries with the same income per capita but with a more even distribution of economic wealth, such as the Czech Republic, Costa Rica and Malaysia (See the World Health Chart on the back cover).

The second influence is how public and household resources are spent with regard to their effect on health. Diseases induced by severe poverty can be largely prevented or alleviated at a relatively low cost. The past 50 years provide many examples of countries that, despite limited economic resources, have managed to provide primary education for all children and a general primary health care service that greatly reduced the burden of disease. Prominent examples are China, Vietnam, Costa Rica and Sri Lanka. Other countries with well-developed social services and general access to health services have had periods of severe economic decline without a deterioration of the general health status. The reason was that the social and health services were maintained and that prior investment in human capabilities helped the population during the economic crisis.

An interesting comparison can be made between Cuba and Iraq (See the World Health Chart on the back cover). These two countries are estimated to have had about the same per capita income during the last decade. During this period both countries experienced international trade boycotts, and political isolation that contributed to an economic decline. In spite of the economic and political similarities between the two countries, the health status varied widely. Iraq's child mortality rate before the 2003 war was estimated to have been 15 times greater than that of Cuba. This enormous difference in child health was mainly explained by differences in domestic health policies between the two governments. The extensive development of the Cuban social and health systems secured the good health of the population through long periods of economic hardship, while the Saddam Hussein regime failed to make optimal priorities during the period of economic hardship. Economic growth will have little health impact if money is wrongly or unfairly spent.

What has been said about economic progress and health at national levels can also be applied to this relationship at the household and individual level. Increased income within a family may be spent exclusively on the alcohol consumption of a cigarette-smoking father. Such an application of economic progress will obviously only result in a deterioration in the health status of the family. In contrast, a family that spends an increase in income well will be able to gain daily access to safe water, improved hygienic sanitation, a more nutritious diet, and better access to health information through media.

The World Health Organization has recently taken the discussion about the relationship between economic growth and health development one further step forward. The Director-General of WHO in 1998 to 2003, Gro Harlem Brundtland, argued that improved health is a necessary prerequisite for economic growth. The basis for this argument is that recent decades of rapid economic growth in many Asian 'tiger economies' was preceded by extensive public investments in improved health. These investments in South Korea, mainland China and Taiwan concerned both preventive programmes and the equitable provision of basic curative health services. These countries provide good examples of economic growth being preceded by improved health. There is in fact no good example of a country that has had a rapid, stable and diversified economic progress over several decades without preceding or simultaneous improvements in the health status of its population occurring. The exceptions are so-called 'mineral countries'. However, these countries did not have a diversified economic growth. In Saudi Arabia and Botswana the sudden economic progress was due to the onset of the exploitation of oil and diamonds, respectively. In the 'mineral countries' health improvements only followed after more than a decade of economic growth.

The World Health Organization's *Commission for Macroeconomics and Health* delivered its report in December 2001 (Sachs 2001). This research programme led by Jeffery Sachs commissioned 87 studies, which reviewed aspects of the relationship between economic growth and health investments. The conclusion is that increased investments in health in the world's poorest countries will save millions of human lives and also contribute to economic growth in these countries (see chapter 11).

2.1.1 Income, poverty and equity

The level and distribution of economic resources is today the main determinant of health throughout the world. One reason for income poverty emerging as the most important determinant of the health of nations is that the disparity in average income within and between the nations of the world is so very wide. Calculated as the income per capita in US dollars using the exchange rate between national currency and dollar, the differences range from a little more than USD 100 to USD 40 000 per inhabitant, i.e. more than a 100-fold difference.

There are several problems related to the comparison of economic indicators between countries. The main problem is that the cost of living varies between countries in a way that is not expressed when using the exchange rate to convert national currencies into US dollars. This has been partly overcome by using the *Purchasing Power Parity (PPP)* of the national currency when con-

verting GDP per capita to US dollars as an estimate of the economic development of a country (Box 2.2). This conversion factor for GDP takes into account the number of units of a country's currency required to buy the same quantities of goods and services in the domestic market as one dollar would buy in the United States. In other words, how many US dollars' worth of goods and services can be bought for a unit of the country's currency? This has also been called the 'international dollar'. If we use the value of the purchasing power of the national currency, the difference in GNP per capita or GDP per capita decreases a little, but a 100-fold difference remains between the economic level in the richest and the poorest country. Counted as purchasing power, the average income per capita in the poorest countries increases from USD 100 to USD 300–500 per person. The Indian rupee, for instance, is worth about five times more if used for purchases in India than if it is changed into US dollars at existing exchange rate and used to make purchases in the United States. In contrast, the Japanese yen is worth less if used in Japan than if it is exchanged into dollars and used in the United States. The difference between the exchange-rate dollar and the purchasing-power dollar is more important when comparing economic level in the countries of the world than if the level is measured by GNP per capita or GDP per capita. As a rule of thumb, the poorest countries have a purchasing power that is 3–5 times stronger than the exchange rate of their currency, and for most countries GNP is almost the same as GDP.

However, it is not mainly the relative differences in income per capita in the world that makes money such an important determinant of global health. What makes money so important is that daily incomes are so very low among the poorest two billion people. They live on the purchasing power of less than USD 2 per day. This implies that they spend the major part of their economic resources on buying the staple food needed to survive. There is today almost unanimous

---

Box 2.2

The two main measurements of economic level of nations

GDP (Gross Domestic Product)/capita	The value of all goods and services produced in a country by nationals and foreign residents during one year divided by the mid year resident population of that year.
GNP (Gross National Product)/capita = GNI (Gross National Income)/capita	The value of all goods and services produced during one year by the nationals in a country plus the income of nationals earned abroad divided by the mid-year national population of that year.

GDP and GNP can be expressed in US dollars in two ways:

Current U.S. dollars by 'Atlas method'
The domestic currency is converted to US dollar by a factor that averages the exchange rate for a given year and the two preceding years, adjusted for differences in rates of inflation between the country and the rate of inflation of France, Germany, Japan, UK and USA. If the official exchange rate does not reflect the rate effectively applied to actual foreign exchange transactions or if the exchange rate fluctuates considerably alternative conversion factors may be used.

Purchasing Power Parity (PPP) (= International Dollars)
The domestic currency is converted to US dollar by an exchange rate at which all the goods and services that comprise the gross domestic product will cost the same to buy in the country as in United States. As PPP conversion reflects the services and goods that inhabitants can buy in their own country, the GDP/capita expressed in international dollars (= PPP) is the best estimates of the economic differences between the countries in the world.

---

agreement among international organisations, national governments and researchers that poverty is the main obstacle to human development. The majority of the two billion poor people in the world live in the western part of China, India, Bangladesh, Pakistan and Sub Saharan Africa.

There is agreement that the world has improved in social development areas such as schooling, health, lowering of fertility rates and improvement of human rights in recent decades. The improvements in these 'softer' dimensions of development have, however, only partly been matched by economic growth in the less affluent countries. The proportion of people living in poverty has started to decrease, but the total number has not decreased.

The total income of a country can be measured in different ways (Todaro 1997). The average income measurements listed in Box 2.2 do not tell us anything about how the income is distributed within each national population. To understand the health impact of national economics, it is therefore crucial to simultaneously measure both the average income level and the distribution of income within a country. This can be done in several ways, but each method has a number of limitations.

One way to measure income inequality is by calculation of the Gini-coefficient. This measure is named after the Italian statistician who formulated it in 1912. The Gini-coefficient is based on the much-used Lorenz curve. This curve shows the relative

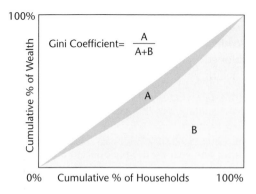

Figure 2.1 How the Gini-coefficient is calculated based on the Lorenz curve.

distribution of income in a population, with the percentage of population on the x-axis and the percentage of income on the y-axis. A perfectly equal distribution of income yields a straight line, and the more unequal the distribution, the more bent the curve will be. The Gini-coefficient is the proportion obtained by dividing the area between the straight line and the curve by the area of the half square under the straight line (Figure 2.1). A small Gini-coefficient means an equal distribution, while a large value of the coefficient means more inequality. A value of 0.0 means perfect equality, while a value of 1.0 means that one person earns the entire national income. Recently, the Gini-coefficient of Brazil and South Africa was estimated at 0.57; of United States and Thailand 0.39; and of Sweden and Japan 0.27.

Another way to express income distribution is to calculate the percentage of national income earned by the richest 20 %, the next 20 %, the middle 20 %, the second lowest 20 % and finally the poorest 20 % of the population. This calculation may also be used to express the income ratio of the 20 % richest (the upper income quintile) to the 20 % poorest (the lower income quintile). The World Bank used the indicator 'percentage share of income or consumption by the richest and poorest 10 %' in their World Development Report 2003. In Brazil, for example, the richest 10 % earned

48 % of the total income and the poorest 10 % only earned 0.7 % of the total income in 2002.

A third way to measure income distribution is to calculate the proportion of the population living in absolute poverty, defined as being unable to satisfy basic needs. A household is classified as living in absolute poverty when found to have a daily income of less than the purchasing power of one US dollar per person. This line is defined as purchasing power in dollars and is intended to be the same cut-off point throughout the world. Some countries may define poverty in relative terms, but relative income poverty just means that someone has low income in relation to the majority in the country. The most widely used definition of absolute poverty is an average income of a purchasing power parity of less than USD 1 per day. For a nation, poverty is expressed as the proportion of households that live either in poverty, with less than USD 2 in PPP/day, or in absolute poverty, with less than USD 1 in PPP/ day. Brazil has about 12 % of its population living on less than 1 USD/day and 26 % living on less than 2 USD/day. Mozambique is estimated to have 38 % of its population living on less than 1 USD/day and 78 % living on less than 2 USD/ day (World Bank 2003).

Almost all data from low and middle-income countries are based on surveys of household income that are being carried out several years apart. It must be emphasised that this data will not show the distribution of the economic resources within the household. Gender differences further exacerbate a very unequal distribution of income in countries with a low general economic level. In practice, this means that, even if the gross national product of Guatemala is measured together with the proportion of income between the richest 20 % and the poorest 20 % of households, this does not tell us how much of the country's resources are available for women and children in the poorest households. Unfortunately, gender differences often disfavour women most in the poorest households in the poorest countries (Sen 2002).

Unequal distribution of health exists in every country in the world. Health inequalities constitute unfair and avoidable gaps in health status within populations. These inequalities are due to differences in socio-economic status, effects of gender roles and ethnicity, and effects from combinations of these factors and other contextual factors determined by the geographical location. The inequity in health is partly explained by differences in access, utilisation and quality of health care. This has been summarised by the Indian scholar, K. Park (1997), in his textbook on public health:

> *Health is not mainly a matter of doctors, social services and hospitals, but an issue of social justice.*

A surprising finding has been that many inequalities in health remain very pronounced even in high-income countries with a well-developed social security system and general access to health services. It has been shown that cardiovascular disease in Northern Europe is much more common among less educated people with low income than among people with more education and a greater income. This difference remains after controlling for differences in tobacco smoking, diet, degree of physical activity and all other known individual risk factors. In high-income countries, the unequal distribution of major diseases is much more pronounced among adults, while child morbidity and mortality do not differ as much between income groups (Evans 2001).

2.1.2 Gender

Gender is the social construct and interpretation of the biological sex difference between men and women. Gender differences are determined by how female and male roles are perceived on the basis of social values, on cultural norms and on how societies are organised. Gender inequity in health

emerges when an unequal distribution of resources, responsibilities and rights of access to health exists between the sexes. As mentioned before, gender is a socio-economic health determinant that modifies all the other determinants, as do poverty and ethnicity. Gender determines access to and use of resources, be they financial or educational; it determines the type and quality of social support a person receives; it determines access to food and water, as well as individual behaviour such as alcohol and tobacco use. Finally, gender determines accessibility and use of health services.

One biological reason for health differences between the sexes relates, for example, to the biological difference of the reproductive organs e.g. pregnancy complications and breast cancer in women, or prostate cancer in men. However, besides the biological differences there may be a low and unfair coverage and quality of health services for pregnant women. There may also, due to cultural norms, be a greater tendency by men to drink more alcohol. The consequence will be inequity in health due to gender differences, not due to biological differences. Striking examples are that maternal mortality is exceedingly high in countries such as Yemen. The performance of harmful traditional practices such as female genital mutilation is another striking example of gender differences in health. The higher rate of death in men due to substance abuse is yet another gender difference.

Inequity in disease occurrence between men and women may thus depend on varying underlying and interacting biological, social and political causes. The fact that women and men work in different jobs or have different tasks in agriculture is one example. The gender role may vary between different regions and ethnic groups within a country. In parts of many African countries, women are the main farmers, and this places a very heavy physical burden on them and decreases their opportunities to offer optimal care to young children. Back pain in nursing employment has a high incidence in women in high-income countries. Women in low-income countries are more prone to infection from water-borne parasites, because they are exposed to infection when they fetch water for the family. Studies in high-income countries show that, even if women work and earn money, which increases their economic independence, they still have a higher burden of household work. On the other hand, in societies where men are responsible for the greater part of the family economy, the psychological burden on men may be harder in times of economic recession and unemployment. One example is Russia where, during the last decade, the suicide rates and high-risk behaviour such as drinking alcohol and taking narcotic drugs increased much more in men than in women. Today the Russian female life expectancy is 23 % longer than the male whereas in Sweden women only live 6 % longer than men. A study in Central America revealed an interesting relation between parental gender differences and child survival. Children with two illiterate parents had a better chance of survival than the child of the family where only the father could read (Aleman 1997).

The high degree of domestic abuse of women relates to the powerlessness of the woman in relation to the man she lives with. In South Africa domestic violence against women has recently been recognised as a major health problem. The background to this violence is the social norm that accepts male dominance in society and at home. The weaker social and economic position of young women makes it difficult for them to refuse to have sex with a dominant man; they are therefore at greater risk of acquiring HIV infection than men in the same age group.

Knowing the level of discrimination against women in the world, it is surprising that women live longer than men in almost all societies, except for those societies unusually oppressive towards women. There is a considerable difference in life expectancy between men and women. This is probably due to interrelated biological and social factors, but it is noteworthy that the precise causes are unknown. The male lifestyle contributes to a higher injury frequency in men and partially explains the life expectancy differences (see chapter 8). The increased risk of injury for men outside the home relates to the higher exposure of males to dangerous professions and to their different social roles. It has also been explained partially by biological differences. The higher incidence of male victims of road traffic accidents, as opposed to women victims, probably reflects both a higher male presence and more risky behaviour in the traffic environment.

More male than female babies are born in societies where either sex is equally socially acceptable. The proportion of 105 boys to 100 girls is believed to be a biologically determined relationship. Where this ratio is not observed, as in China, this most probably reflects the application of selective abortion, or underreporting of female births. It may even occasionally be due to female infanticide, due to a social preference for boys and the national policy of the one-child family. After birth males have higher death rates than women at all age intervals, but social class modifies this trend. It is wrong to attribute this difference entirely to biological factors, and it may even be wrong to attribute it mostly to biological factors.

In contrast to the mortality statistics, in most countries women report a higher degree of morbidity than men. This tendency is more pronounced in mental rather than physical illness. The reason may be that men have greater difficulty in accepting that they are sick, or that the burden of disease affecting women causes greater morbidity, while that affecting men causes greater mortality. Excess female reporting of illness can also be related to more frequent illnesses in their reproductive organs i.e. a biological explanation. Higher female acceptance of reporting morbidity may be a social effect among women. Men may instead under-report morbidity due to their social roles and norms. It should be noted that most of the gender research on morbidity has to date been carried out on the populations of high-income countries and results should not be extrapolated to other contexts.

2.1.3 Social support

An individual's social support network consists of family, friends, neighbours, teams at work and relatives or members of the same clan or ethnic group. It can be defined as 're-sources provided by other persons' (Cohen 1985). A good social support network has been found to be important for sustaining good mental and physical health. It is further essential for a person's ability to deal with periods of illness. This means that a person may not have the financial resources needed for treatment and care, but through the social network money may be borrowed at a reasonable interest rate. An individual with a good network may deal with a period of disease more effectively than one in a better financial situation but with a weaker network.

It has been shown in numerous studies that married people have a lower mortality rate after myocardial infarction than single, widowed or divorced people. This is particularly true for men. Part of this differential death rate is explained by a selection effect, in that unhealthy people may remain unmarried, or that people are divorced because of unhealthy behaviour such as alcoholism. People with large social support networks have lower death rates than people with few contacts with family and friends. The size and quality of the social support depends on many factors, such as size of family, the individual's social abilities, occupation and skills. These factors in turn may all affect the ability to stay healthy. A social network thus provides a range of support from psychological counselling to fast loans of cash when most needed.

An example can be taken from Kerala, the state that has the best health status in all of India. Although there are public hospital services available to all, there is no functioning public ambulance service. If a woman has a life-threatening haemorrhage in the last month of pregnancy, the family has to find money for emergency transport to the hospital. Among poor people, it is common that the husband or the relatives have to borrow money from neighbours to pay for a taxi to the hospital. They become indebted to their neighbours and will eventually repay the loan. If they can borrow from friends at a low interest rate, they will not be as severely impoverished as if they have to borrow at an exploitative interest rate from the local commercial moneylender.

The very special social bond between mother and child is essential for child survival in every society. This is most needed in societies with high risks for children. In low-income countries if the mother dies at or following delivery, up to 95 % of their new-born children will die before the age of five. An infant is usually dependent on the mother for both breastmilk and care. Of course the father or another responsible adult may replace the mother, but they can not fulfil all aspects of childcare, breastfeeding being the most important one. Breastfeeding is one of the most important determinants of survival from infectious diseases and of prevention from malnutrition in the young child. The mother's basic care, along with her knowledge of how to treat common diseases and when to take the child for health care are also necessary for survival. If the mother is continuously able to stay close to the child, she can prevent accidents. A woman's status in society and social support network largely determines what care she can offer her child. This also depends on her education, workload and decision-making power.

2.1.4 Education

After income education is one of the most important determinants of health. Female education in particular has proved to be of

Table 2.2 Adult literacy rate[*] by region in 2000 for male and female.

Region	Male	Female
East Asia and Pacific	93	81
CEE/CIS and the Baltic states	99	96
Latin America and Caribbean	90	88
Middle East and North Africa	74	52
South Asia	66	42
Sub-Saharan Africa	69	53
High income countries	99	97

* Adult literacy = % of persons >15 years old who can read and write.

Source: State of the world's children 2004. UNICEF.

Table 2.3 Percent[*] of relevant age group (male and female) attending primary,[**] secondary and tertiary education in different regions in 1997–2000*.

Region	Primary school male	Primary school female	Secondary school male	Secondary school female	University total
East Asia & Pacific	106	106	65	61	17
CEE/CIS and the Baltic states	99	95	81	78	47
Latin America & Caribbean	126	123	82	87	26
Middle East & North Africa	95	86	68	62	23
South Asia	107	87	53	39	10
Sub-Saharan Africa	89	78	29	23	5
High income countries	102	102	105	108	67

* Ratio of total enrolment regardless of age to the population of the age group that officially corresponds to the level of education, which is why it may be >100 %.
** Primary = elementary or primary school, Secondary = high school, Tertiary = university.

Source: State of the world's children 2004, UNICEF and World development indicators 2004, The World Bank.

great significance for child survival. It is therefore most promising that the worldwide adult literacy rate has increased from 70 % in 1980 to 80 % in 2000. The adult literacy rate is expected to continue to rise to 83 % by the year 2010 (UNESCO 2002). However, due to population growth, the absolute number of illiterate adults remains almost the same as 20 years ago. There are between 600 and 700 million adults in the world who cannot read or write. Of these one-third live in India and another one-third in China, Pakistan and Bangladesh. Despite the fact that Africa has the greatest proportion of illiterate adults, more than half of the illiterate population of the world live in the four big Asian nations. Gender disparities in primary education have not changed much in the last 20 years; 400 million of the illiterate are women. In South Asia a total of 66 % of adult males are literate, but only 42 % of adult females are literate (Table 2.2).

Large gender disparities in literacy rates also appear in Sub-Saharan Africa, the Middle East and North Africa. Within each region, the disparities in national literacy rates are wide. In the year 2000, Ethiopia had a male adult literacy rate of 47 % and a female rate of 31 %, while the rates in Botswana were 75 % and 80 %, respectively. In Bangladesh, the male literacy was 49 % and the female 30%, while in Sri Lanka the rates were 94% and 89%, respectively (UNICEF 2004).

School enrolment at the primary school level is depicted in table 2.3. The disparities between geographical regions increase at higher levels of education. Sub-Saharan Africa is lagging particularly far behind when it comes to university education.

The state of Kerala in South India is known for its high literacy rates, 94% in men and 86% in women. This is high compared to India as a whole, where male literacy is 68% and female 45%. The high literacy is regarded as the main reason why Kerala has achieved an under-five mortality rate of less than 20 per 1 000 live births, while India as a whole had an under five mortality rate of 96 per 1 000 births in 2002. If all of India had the same literacy rate and social development as the state of Kerala, in the tropical southern tip of this vast nation, the lives of more than one million children would be saved each year.

Kerala is the rule, not the exception. High parental, particularly maternal, literacy is linked to low child mortality rates almost everywhere in the world where this relationship has been studied. Using data from the 41 countries covered by the World Fertility Survey (ISI 1984) it was shown that the association between mother's education and survival of children is stronger for children aged 1–4 years than in infants. This study also showed that more maternal years in school were associated with better child survival. Latin American mothers with 4–6 years in school had a 35% lower infant mortality compared with mothers without any schooling. If the mother had 7 or more years in school, the infant mortality was half of that for children of uneducated mothers. The positive effect of female literacy on health has been shown in many studies but this finding has been notably difficult to translate into political actions.

Several factors may explain the disparity in child survival between educated and uneducated mothers. Education may be a proxy variable for higher family income, but even after controlling for socio-economic situation, maternal education remains an important health determinant. The advantages of higher income, clean water, safer sanitation and better housing account for only about half of the association between education and child survival (Cleland 1988). Education itself is thus associated with better health. Educated mothers can, of course, be expected to have more knowledge and therefore adopt new health interventions, such as immunisation, to a greater extent than illiterate women. An understanding of the causation of disease, nutrition, preventive and curative home care may be enhanced in the educated mother, leading to improved hygiene and a healthier diet. The educated mother may sense a larger personal responsibility for the child's survival than someone who has a more traditional and fatalistic view of health and disease. She may be less prone to practising dangerous forms of traditional medicine. She may be more vocal, with greater social confidence, and more persistent in demanding care for her children from health care personnel. In fact, higher education in women may also be an indicator of a stronger social position for women in the family and the community. The association between a mother's education and her child's survival may thus largely represent an association between greater empowerment of women and child survival. The educated mother may have both greater motivation and greater ability to travel promptly to seek health care for her child, and also better compliance with prescribed treatment. She may also have a greater decision-making role in health-related matters, if she is educated because of her higher status in the society (Caldwell 1996).

There are some exceptional examples of low-income societies, such as Kerala and Sri Lanka, which have achieved a very good health status for their populations. These countries' success stories have come from a conscious choice of public policy to achieve high female educational levels, coupled with a high degree of female autonomy, a radical tradition and a deep-rooted respect for education. It should also be noted that a high literacy rate in women may be associated with improved health and decreased fertility despite many limitations in women's rights. Iran, where literacy rates have improved considerably during recent decades, provides a prominent example.

In conclusion, children of educated parents, especially educated mothers, have lower death rates, because education is associated with other positive health determinants, because parents' increased knowledge helps them to make more rational decisions and because education is accompanied by higher status and more power. Access to primary school education is crucially dependent on public policy and public financial allocations. The amount and type of public spending on education is thus a central issue for health policy in low and middle-income countries.

2.1.5 Culture and ethnicity

Culture is a concept that designates the acquired behavioural pattern and conceptual views on life of a group of people. Culture is intertwined with language, the arts, social structure, laws, religion, ethics and morals. Culture profoundly affects people's attitudes, beliefs and actions. However, no culture is static. All cultures are in constant change at a faster or slower rate, depending on the pace of other changes in society. New cultural trends emerge, and some aspects of culture disappear over time. Concepts of health and disease, diet and the choice of modern evidence-based health care or traditional and complementary health practitioners are all aspects of human cultural behaviour that affect health. Cultural factors may thus affect health in both negative and positive directions, while many cultural phenomena are quite neutral in relation to their effect on the health status of populations.

In all parts of the world, the strongest cultural traditions and rituals surround the main stages in life, such as conception, birth, and passage from adolescence into adulthood, marriage, reproduction and death. Circumcision of boys is a widespread cultural practice, representing an initiation rite in several ethnic groups and countries. Circumcised men have a lower risk of developing cancer of the penis and a lower risk of transmitting sexually transmitted diseases, including HIV. In contrast, there are considerable health risks following the female genital mutilation practised mainly in Egypt, Somalia and Sudan. This is complicated by an increased risk of infections, impaired urination and complications at delivery, not to mention the psychological distress of the circumcision itself and the loss of the sexual pleasure (WHO 1996).

When a child becomes ill its survival largely depends on the family's cultural attitudes towards treatment. In some cultures, children's health is believed to be under the control of God, fate or luck (Caldwell 1989). Infanticide or differential care of female infants when boys are more valued in society is another tragic consequence of cultural beliefs. Some generations ago, some African ethnic groups had strong cultural beliefs directed against twins, who were believed to represent evil spirits. As a consequence of this belief, one of the twins used to be killed directly after birth. This is a traditional cultural practice that has disappeared due to severe legal actions taken during colonial times, as well as bold interventions by religious leaders. The number of children a family has is influenced by the preference of sex, but also by the customary age at marriage, socio-cultural preferences of number of children, concerns for security in old age, customs surrounding sexuality and family planning practices.

Dietary practices are closely related to culture. In the cultures of the Middle East, pork is not included in the diet. This naturally protects against parasites transmitted by the pork tapeworm. This tapeworm is a great health problem in other parts of the world. Breastfeeding customs also vary across cultures and over time. In Europe there has been a resurgence of breastfeeding, particularly in the Nordic countries, since the 1970s. In Islamic countries breastfeeding is practised widely, partly due to promotion on religious grounds. Presently there is a sub-cultural trend among the youth population of Northern Europe to eat vegan food, on the ethical basis of respecting the rights of animals. The influence of culture upon diet may both remain stable over thousands of years and change over short time periods.

Elderly people are regarded with different levels of respect in different cultures. In many countries in Asia and Africa, old people stay with the family and still enjoy an important role, based on the life-experience they possess. In Japan elderly women, who enjoy a high status, have the greatest life expectancy in the world. In Europe and North America most of the elderly stay by themselves or in homes for the elderly that may lead to isolation and a feeling of lowered self-esteem. These cultural changes with respect to the elderly are largely explained by changes in population composition and longevity. The matter may be summarised crudely as follows. Where old people are rare and do not survive so long, they are 'respected', but when the old are common in the population and live longer, they become 'less respected'. This change has great implications for the occurrence of depression among the elderly. Japan is facing a dramatic situation because the proportion of old people has rapidly increased in the last decade. The cultural norms still state that younger women in the family must take care of the old at home, but this cultural obligation will most probably change.

Different cultural rituals of burial surround death. Such practices may have considerable health implications. One of the most drastic examples induced the neurological disease, kuru, until fairly recently practised in New Guinea. This disease was caused by prions infecting family members

engaging in the cannibalistic practices of eating the deceased person's brain and viscera during the mourning ritual. When the practice was discontinued, the disease disappeared. Cholera is a very contagious bacterial disease that causes vomiting and diarrhoea, leading to dehydration and possibly death within 24 hours if untreated. Burial ceremonies in northern Mozambique include a practice by which family members jointly and carefully clean the dead body before the funeral, and thereafter eat a shared meal. As the body of an individual who has died from cholera remains highly contagious, this respectful practice places the whole family at risk of contracting cholera. Cholera control in such communities depends to a high degree on the early modification of this cultural ritual.

Ethnicity is a term that is used with different meanings. It is sometimes used as a synonym for race, or to refer to a specific culture, and sometimes to both at the same time. In the health context, this changing terminology relates to the old question of whether genetics or the environment is the main determinant of human behaviour and health. The most common use of the term ethnicity in social science is that it refers to a subjective understanding of common origin by a group of people. It may refer to either a national identity or the identity of a minority within a nation (Allen 2000).

The formerly common view that behavioural and health differences in the world were related to genetic differences between races is rarely advanced today. However, some people still think of ethnicity as partially a matter of genetics. They claim that population groups in the course of evolution have developed certain genetic differences in response to the environment in which they live. Few would argue that this is completely wrong. Pigmentation of the skin is one factor that has undoubtedly changed genetically with differing environmental exposure. When genetic factors determine prejudices against and social oppression of a population group, it is obvious that, through social mechanisms, these genetic factors may be health determinants for the whole group. However, the view that the health risks conveyed by ethnic identity are mainly genetic is not evidence-based. There is no reason to assume any significant genetic explanation for the wide disparity in health status between black, Hispanic and white people in the US.

As a health determinant, ethnicity is mostly used to refer to cultural and social heritage alone, as distinct from any genetic factors that may be associated to a certain ethnicity. The high prevalence of the haemoglobin mutation causing sickle cell anaemia in people of African origin is not considered to be due to the ethnicity of those African population groups. The differences between ethnicity and genetics resemble the difference between the social concept 'gender' and the biological concept 'sex'. The former refers to a social construction, the latter to differences due to molecular genetics. An illustration of the terminological issue is provided by the question of whether Swedish citizens who were adopted from other countries as young infants have a Swedish ethnicity or the ethnicity of their country of birth e.g. Korean or Bengali. These persons share Swedish norms of behaviour and are thus ethnic Swedes, but they may also be regarded as a special ethnic sub-group in Sweden that shares 'a collective sense of common origin'.

We conclude that genetic factors are very strong health determinants at an individual level, but of minute significance as determinants of the considerable differences in health status between different parts of the world population. That ethnicity is regarded as a significant factor in the web of factors that explain the health status of a population is mainly because ethnicity conveys behaviour and socio-cultural patterns that are linked to direct causes of diseases or injuries.

In conclusion, culture influences health status and health care utilisation in all stages of life. Culture is not static, but is constantly changing, and new practices develop with the arrival of new technologies and knowledge. For health services to function, the cultural context must be understood and respected. But culture should not be confused with other social and economic health determinants. Cultural factors such as a cast system, may be an obstacle to poverty alleviation, but income poverty and illiteracy should be separated from the marginalisation induced by cultural concepts when making a social analysis of contemporary India. This is especially important for the understanding of what poverty means for health. Medical sociologists and anthropologists help greatly with their research to unravel the relationships between social change and culture in the complex causational web of disease.

2.1.6 Security

The nature of armed conflicts has changed since the Second World War. In the last decades, most wars in the world were internal conflicts. The armed conflicts involved different ethnic groups in the same low-income countries. Such were the wars in Sierra-Leone, Rwanda, Bosnia and parts of the former Soviet Union. Due to the character of these conflicts the number of civilian victims has increased considerably. Civilians now far outnumber the deaths of soldiers directly involved in the fighting. It is estimated that about 85% of casualties of war are civilians and only 15% military personnel. During the First World War, these proportions were reversed. Targeted violations of human rights, such as rape, forced displacement and 'ethnic cleansing', are used as part of war strategies.

Refugees and internally displaced people are victims of armed conflicts who cannot stay within their country's borders or in their home community. The health deterioration caused by armed conflict is often severely aggravated by drought and other natural disasters. The United Nations High Commissioner for Refugees (UNHCR) estimates that there are currently about 40–50

Table 2.4 Countries with most refugees in 2002.

Country of origin	Main counties of asylum	Refugees
Afghanistan	Pakistan, Iran	2 480 000
Burundi	Tanzania	574 000
Sudan	Uganda, Democratic Republic of Congo, Ethiopia, Kenya, Central African Republic, Chad	505 000
Angola	Democratic Republic of Congo, Zambia, Namibia	432 000
Somalia	Kenya, Ethiopia, Yemen, Djibouti	429 000
Gaza	Saudi Arabia, Iraq	428 000
Democratic Republic of Congo	Tanzania, Zambia, Rwanda, Congo Brazzaville	415 000
Iraq	Iran	400 000
Bosnia-Herzegovina	Yugoslavia, Croatia, USA, Sweden, Netherlands, Denmark	371 000

Source: UNHCR 2003 (http://www.unhcr.org).

million people who have been forced to flee their homes. This means that about one percent of the world population have fled their homes! Half of these people are what is known as 'internally displaced persons', i.e. they have left their homes but not their country of origin.

The countries of origin of most refugees in 2002 are listed in table 2.4. As shown the vast majority of the world's refugees end up in a neighbouring country whose economy was strained even before the refugees arrived. The health care of refugees in the emergency stage usually depends on international aid organisations access to the refugees and the resources of the host country. Swift provision of basic needs and actions against malnutrition and epidemic diseases such as cholera and measles can dramatically reduce the mortality in these populations. The ten most significant actions at the beginning of a refugee crisis are listed in Box 2.3. The future life of the refugees will depend on the political situation in their country of origin and on how they are accepted and integrated into the society of the country that provides asylum. It is estimated that more than 170 000 people were killed in 2002 as a consequence of war and armed conflict. An estimated 2 million children and young people have been killed and 6 million have been seriously injured due to armed conflict in the last decade. Today an estimated 300 000 children serve as soldiers (Human Rights Watch 2001).

War affects health in many ways apart from direct physical or psychological war injuries. The breakdown of infrastructure e.g. water, sanitation, education and the health service systems, as well as deteriorating socio-economic and nutritional situations, all affect the health of populations. In times of war governments may be weak or absent

---

Box 2.3

Top ten priorities at the beginning of a humanitarian crisis

1. Initial assessment
2. Measles vaccination
3. Water and sanitation
4. Food and nutrition
5. Shelter and site planning
6. Basic health care in the emergency phase
7. Control of communicable diseases and epidemics
8. Public health surveillance
9. Human resource mobilisation and training
10. Co-ordination

Source: Refugee Health, MSF 1997

---

in parts of the country, and unable to prioritise the health of their population. The economies of countries and families are severely damaged by war.

Antipersonnel mines cause thousands of deaths and mutilations every year. Landmines also affect the social and economic recovery for decades after a conflict. An estimated 100 million mines remain to be removed in 64 countries of the world. A major achievement in global health was reached by the International Campaign to Ban Landmines[1]. This organisation promoted the treaty, which has been signed by 146 countries, banning the use, production, stockpiling, and transfer of antipersonnel landmines. However, landmines are still being produced and many mines remain to be removed. The worst affected countries are Afghanistan, Angola, Cambodia, Laos, Iraq, Mozambique, Somalia and the former Yugoslavia. Mine clearing is exceedingly expensive, risky and time-consuming. Clear health priorities for the populations in the worst affected countries, are firstly to reduce the incidence of injury and, even more importantly, to restore access to land for agricultural activities to recommence.

The level of socio-economic development of a country at war clearly affects the way people cope with the crisis situation. This can be seen in the greater increase in mortality in Sierra Leone compared with the Balkans during the recent periods of war. In the war-affected societies in the Balkan countries, people were able to apply innovative technological solutions to maintain a minimum of basic hygiene, safe water supply and life-saving energy supply for warming and cooking. This resilience to external crisis shows that, once people have acquired the necessary technological knowledge and skills of how to maintain health, their acquired health status is amazingly resistant to severe military conflict. In Sierra Leone the population in peace time lived very close to or under the poverty line, and when the war

broke out they were thrown into suffering of biblical proportions. The resulting infant mortality was estimated to be one of the highest in the world. Contrary to many assumptions, highly developed, technological societies seem to have better resources to maintain health during war than poorer societies with less modern technology in use.

2.2 Food

Food is required both as fuel and as building blocks for the body. The most basic requirement for food is to satisfy daily energy needs. The minimum dietary energy need for an adult is around 1500 kcal per day. This corresponds to a daily consumption of half a kilogram of rice, maize or wheat. The daily energy need may also be satisfied by the corresponding amounts of carbohydrates from root crops like potato or cassava, but due to their high water content, the daily minimum need corresponds to 1.5 kg fresh weight of these starchy root crops. Physical activity increases energy needs and heavy work may double the energy requirements. A cold climate also increases energy needs. Children need more energy per kilogram of bodyweight because they are growing. Energy is not enough for normal growth and body function; a supply of proteins, vitamins and minerals is also essential, but as a basic rule of thumb humans need half a kilo of cereals per day to survive in the short term.

2.2.1 Food supply

A family needs to have enough food for all its members every day of the year. The fulfilment of this need used to be called 'food security'. It is important to realise that when a family is food insecure, i.e. it does not have enough to eat; this may not necessarily mean that there is not enough for the small children. The reason is that small children need relatively small amounts, compared to adults. Still, food insecurity will damage the

---

[1] www.icbl.org

Box 2.4

Definition of food security

"Sustainable access to safe food of sufficient quality and quantity, including energy, protein and micronutrients, to ensure adequate dietary intake and a
healthy life for all members of the
household".

---

small child's health, because the parents
cannot fully care for them if they have to
spend much of the day in search of food. Insufficient quantities of food and the resulting hunger will affect all aspects of family
life. In the mass media malnutrition in children is often portrayed as a direct effect of
food shortages. However, pure food shortage
will have a greater direct impact on the nutritional status of the adult population.
Small children will suffer to a greater degree
from the combined effects of food shortage,
reduced care and increased susceptibility to
infectious diseases, when food insecurity
strikes a family.

World food production can sustain the
present population, even at a population
growth rate of 1.5 %, but a more equitable
distribution is necessary. Food production
has increased to match population growth,
and it is estimated that, with the technological advancements of increased yield and increased arable land, world food production
will support the estimated 7 billion or more
people who will live on earth by the year
2010, and also the billions more to be added
in the decades to come (Cohan 1995).

Diet changes as a country develops socially and economically. In low-income
countries most people eat mainly starchy
cereals and root crops. During development
this changes to a diet with a higher content
of sugar, fat and animal products. This is
presently taking place in most middle-income countries. Access to food in the world
depends on how we solve the increased de-

mand to feed animals for meat production.
Perhaps future generations will become veg-
etarians for economic reasons.

2.2.2 Breastfeeding

Children place special demands on their environment if they are to thrive. An additional set of health determinants comes into
play concerning young children. At delivery
the child leaves a highly protected life in the
mother's womb. The human child is help-
less when exposed to the outer world.
Nature's way of supporting the child in this
new environment is through the mother's
breastmilk and intensive parental care during years to come. It is possible to replace
nature's food supply artificially, but it requires time, money and special efforts and
skills. For mothers living under difficult conditions, breastmilk substitutes are inferior to
nature's supply by any criterion. For children born into poverty breastfeeding is a
matter of life or death.

Bottle-feeding is costly and implies severe
risk of contamination if optimal hygienic
conditions are not maintained in the
mother's environment. The commercial promotion of feeding bottles and breastmilk
substitutes in low-income countries in the
1970s and 1980s killed many small children.
The risk of infections and diarrhoea is particularly high when the feeding bottle is handled in a home with poor, unsanitary conditions, using un-boiled water and, as often occurs due to poverty and illiteracy, an under-
dosage of milk powder.

Breastmilk provides the child's first immunisation; the colostrums (first breastmilk) in
particular contains lymphocytes, antibodies
and vitamin A. It is tailor-made to the specific environment into which the child is
born, because the mother has met most of
the microbes in this environment and provides ready-made antibodies against the
microbes for the child through the breastmilk.

Breastmilk is also the optimal food for
the child. It is composed of all the nutrients

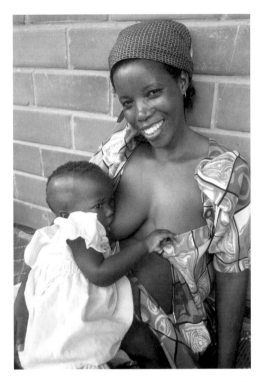

UGANDA, Masaka. Woman breastfeeding her child.
© Sean Sprague/PHOENIX.

the child needs in adequate amounts for optimal growth and development. It is probably even better than we understand. For instance over the last decade it has been established that the fatty acid composition of breastmilk is optimal for the development of the central nervous system. In fact, anything else given to the child will be inferior in composition. Adults have the ability to cope with foods of varying quality, but the infant's capacity to do this is very limited.

Breastfeeding reduces exposure to microbes. While suckling from the breast, the child avoids being contaminated with bacteria and viruses from water and unsafe food. Exclusive breastfeeding for the first six months prevents unnecessary exposure to potentially infectious foods. Infant mortality from diarrhoea decreases considerably if the child is exclusively breastfed during the

first 6 months of life. The risk of non-breast-fed babies in a low-income country dying from diarrhoea during the first months of life may be 25 times greater than that of exclusively breastfed babies. Exclusiveness of breastfeeding during the first 6 months is therefore an important determinant of child health in many parts of the world.

In many cultures breastmilk is traditionally given together with water, cow's milk or other food. This is considered a harmful traditional practice. Not until the age of six months should the infant begin to consume food products other than breastmilk. The practice of exclusive breastfeeding for the first three months varies from 1 to 90% among mothers in different countries, mainly due to different cultural traditions (Table 2.5). Breastfeeding creates a psychological bonding between mother and child that protects the child from neglect. It also protects the child from getting siblings too soon as it releases hormones in the mother that reduces fertility through what is known as 'lactation amenorrhoea'. Breastfeeding also stimulates a hormone release that helps the uterus to contract, which is helpful to stop bleeding after birth.

In almost all countries around the world the 'modernisation' in the last 50 years was associated with a decrease in breastfeeding. In the 1970s the use of a feeding bottle also

Table 2.5 Percent of babies exclusively breastfed for the first six months 1995–2002.

Country	% exclusively breastfed children < 6 months
Bangladesh	46
Pakistan	16
Egypt	57
Gabon	6
Kenya	5
Madagascar	41
Rwanda	84
Sierra Leone	4
Vietnam	31

Source: State of the world's children 2004. UNICEF.

spread to poor population groups in low and middle-income countries with disastrous effects on child health. Since then there has been a considerable change. In the last decades, WHO and UNICEF successfully promoted national regulation concerning the commercial promotion of breastmilk substitutes. The success was partly due to the advocacy campaigns carried out by the International Baby Food Action Network[1]. The health regulation concerning artificial feeding was made possible through the International Code of Marketing of Breastmilk Substitutes which was adopted by UN in 1981 as a 'minimum requirement' to protect infant health. The extensive scientific documentation of the benefits of breastfeeding was the basis for the almost unanimous acceptance of this code by all member countries of WHO. The promotion and protection of exclusive breastfeeding has in fact been one of the most successful actions for improved child health in the world over the last 20 years. This has shown that the promotion of better nutrition may be more beneficial than medical interventions such as vaccines and drugs.

Child feeding is determined by a complex set of socio-economic factors, such as the status of young mothers in society and in the family, the availability of time for care and food for preparation, but most of all by how well breastfeeding is protected and promoted. The practice of bottlefeeding has had an interesting boom and decline in the Scandinavian countries. In the 1950s it became popular, initially among the well to do, as a sign of wealth and modernisation, and with time it trickled down through all the social strata. At 1970 less than 10 % of Swedish mothers breastfed for 6 months. The decrease in breastfeeding changed due to actions of female action-groups outside the health system. Today breastfeeding rates in Sweden are lowest among less educated, young and unprivileged groups. Bottlefeeding has thus followed a similar

---

> ### Box 2.5
>
> **United Nations advice on breastfeeding and HIV**
>
> Exclusive breastfeeding should be protected, promoted and supported for 6 months. This applies to women who are known not to be infected with HIV and for women whose infection status is unknown. When replacement feeding is acceptable, feasible, affordable, sustainable and safe, avoidance of all breastfeeding by HIV-infected mothers is recommended; otherwise, exclusive breastfeeding is recommended during the first six months of life.

---

trend as smoking in the high-income countries: it started out as a sign of status, but has now become a habit mainly of unprivileged groups. The interesting question is whether this is bound to happen in all countries as societies modernise and transform.

HIV constitutes a new challenge to the promotion of breastfeeding as up to one third of children born to HIV infected mothers may acquire the infection during pregnancy, delivery or through breastmilk. If resources are available the transmission can be reduced to 1–2 % if the mother is on antiretroviral treatment during the pregnancy, if the delivery is carried out by caesarean section and if breastfeeding is avoided. However, the risk for HIV transmission is reduced by exclusive breastfeeding as reflected in the present international policy shown in Box 2.5 (WHO 2001).

In spite of acknowledging the risk of bottlefeeding in poor settings the application in practice of these guidelines poses considerable problems, especially in rural parts of African low-income countries. The reason is that 'choice of infant feeding' is virtually unknown because breastfeeding is the cultural norm and bottlefeeding is too costly. Advice from the health service is

---

[1] www.ibfan.org

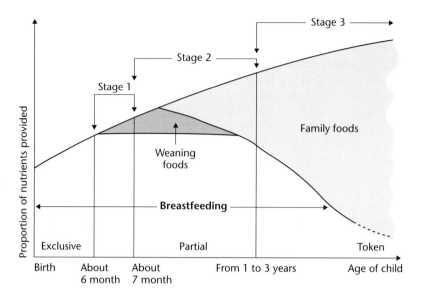

Figure 2.2 Complementary feeding.
Source: Savage King F, Burgess A. 1993.

often perceived as advice against breastfeeding and the UN Guidelines may in fact just become a vague promotion of feeding bottles. Furthermore, if a mother does not breastfeed questions about her HIV status will be asked with resulting severe stigmatisation. Many HIV-infected mothers may compromise by artificially feeding their babies at home and breastfeeding in public as a denial that they are HIV-infected. Thereby the advice to avoid breastfeeding may increase the risk of transmission of HIV through mixed feeding and increase the risk of diarrhoea through non-exclusive breastfeeding.

A vulnerable time in a child's life is when other foods are introduced into the child's diet. At about 6 months of age, the child's nutritional needs start to exceed the breastmilk production, which thus needs to be complemented with other food. This does not mean that the child should reduce the amount of breastmilk consumed per day. Typically, specially prepared 'educational foods' are given as token meals for the child to adapt to other foods. This process has

been referred to as weaning (Greiner 1996). At this time the maternal antibodies from birth are diminishing. The child is beginning to move on its own and, being exposed to more pathogens, is increasingly susceptible to infections. With time the specially prepared educational foods or complementary foods become a more important part of the diet and are progressively replaced by family foods (see figure 2.2).

The complementary foods need to be nutrient-dense, which means that they must provide a great mass of nutrients per gram. In addition the child needs frequent but small feeds. The stomach of a child is small and can only be filled to a certain volume. This volume does not correspond to its energy requirements if the child is only given three meals a day, like the rest of the family. A child under five years old needs at least five meals a day, plus extra snacks. The nutrient-density is particularly a problem in low and middle-income countries, where the diet consists mainly of bulky, energy-poor porridges and vegetables. The energy density can be improved by adding fat or sugar to the food, or by changing the consistency of the food by germination or fermentation.

UNICEF has pointed out that, in order to provide adequate nutrition for a child, a number of prerequisites must be met at different levels. At the basic level, the society needs sufficient human, organisational and economic resources and control of these resources along with adequate knowledge. This in turn could promote household food security, adequate maternal and childcare, sufficient health services and a healthy environment. These are the underlying determinants of an adequate dietary intake and good health, which will prevent the child from developing malnutrition or even save it from death.

2.3 Water

The supply of sufficient amounts of safe water is a fundamental health determinant for human populations. The reason is not only that water is essential for the life processes within the human body; water is also essential for daily personal and domestic hygiene. It is also a requirement for food preparation. Production in agriculture and industry requires large amounts of water. In emergency situations, such as in refugee camps, *a minimum supply of five litres of safe water is needed for each person per day* to stop excess mortality. Two to three litres of water are needed for drinking and cooking, and the remaining two litres for washing and cleaning. Within weeks, in the post-emergency phase, a daily ration of 20 litres per person per day has proven necessary to avoid the transmission of major water-borne diseases. In contrast to these minimum requirements, the average Swedish citizen uses 200–300 litres of drinking water per day for their personal use, which includes frequent use of flush toilets (Yassi 2001). It is interesting to note that a country like Sweden has such an unlimited supply of high quality drinking water that it is used

---

Box 2.6

Minimum daily survival requirements per person

5 litres of safe water & 0.5 kg cereal equivalents of food

---

for flushing toilets into the public sewage system.

Water is a prerequisite for health, but can also be a vehicle of disease. Communicable diseases associated with water can be divided into water-borne, water-washed and water-related vector diseases. Water may transmit virus, bacteria, parasites and worms. Contaminated water can cause water-borne diseases such as dysentery, cholera and other diarrhoeal diseases (WHO 1992).

Water-washed diseases result from water scarcity, which impairs personal hygiene. The inability to wash can result in the spread of lice and mites, and eye diseases like trachoma and bacterial skin infections.

Water-related vector diseases are caused by microbes that are transmitted by water dependent vectors (i.e. insects that transmit the disease). The most prominent of these diseases is malaria, which is transmitted by mosquitoes that need water for replication. Another prominent water-related vector disease is schistosomiasis. This disease is caused by a parasite that is excreted in human urine and reproduces in a snail that lives on the shores of freshwater lakes and rivers. The transmission of schistosomiasis can be reduced if the population refrain from urinating in the water. It can also be controlled if the number of snails is reduced and if infected humans are treated with available drugs.

Water may also be the vehicle of toxic substances that cause disease. Substances such as arsenic naturally occur in the soil in certain areas, and humans will be exposed when drinking water from wells containing natural arsenic. This has been the unfortunate side effect of drilling for microbiologi-

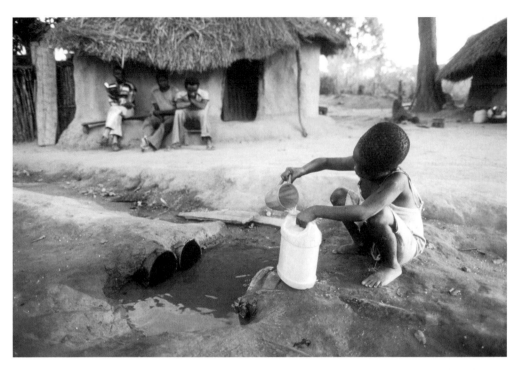

ZAMBIA. Water is taken from the broken water pipes.
© Trygve Bølstad/PHOENIX.

cally safe drinking water in Bangladesh and in a number of other Asian countries. Substances such as nitrates may enter the water from industrial waste, and agricultural activity may result in water being contaminated by toxic pesticides. Toxicological contamination is a severe local health problem in many areas. However, on a global scale, the communicable water-borne diseases give rise to a much higher burden of disease than the toxicological ones. It seems that toxicological contamination from naturally occurring substances occurs mainly in low-income countries and in deprived populations who cannot afford to make arrangements for a safe water supply. Toxicological contamination from agriculture and industry tends to increase gradually when the country develops economically and gains the economic resources to buy and produce such toxic substances, but not enough to control them. Populations in high-income

countries are, despite intensive industrialisation, very rarely exposed to any toxicological contamination in their drinking water. These countries have sufficient resources to avoid the introduction of toxic substances into their drinking water supply.

As a country develops socio-economically, the use of freshwater increases dramatically. This is due to the increased use of water in mechanised agriculture, industry and domestic consumption. The modern agricultural sector is by far the largest consumer of freshwater, followed by the industrial sector. The total freshwater reserves of the earth exceed the requirements for both the present and the foreseeable future. However, the geographical distribution of the human population and the availability of freshwater are extremely uneven. The Middle East and North Africa have the lowest availability of water, but paradoxically their economies have one of the highest dependencies on agriculture. With further population growth and economic development these regions will need to import real or virtual water in the future. Virtual water import means importing food products that require a lot of water for their production. In such areas there is an urgent need to improve water management. Efficiency in the use of water must be increased by targeted irrigation and industrial water conservation, as well as recycling water for domestic needs. The prevention of leakage in water systems in urban areas is another effective measure. The quality of the water supply needs to be maintained by the control of sewage and wastewater. Wastewater from industrial, agricultural and urban areas poses direct health risks. It may also indirectly impair health by polluting fishing waters.

The organisation of the water supply is as important for health as the volume of water available in a community. Many poor people in the world still draw their drinking water from rivers, streams and open, unprotected wells. The safety of a drinking water supply can be greatly improved by protecting the wells. This means building a rim and a cover so that rainwater does not transmit dust and dirt into the well. Animals also have to be stopped from using the same well as humans use. The way water is withdrawn from the well is also important. The introduction of a special well bucket that is never set down on the ground but only used to pour the water into other buckets, is an important improvement of water safety. A completely covered well with a hand pump pouring safe, clean water directly into the vessel of each household is the next step in improvement. Thereafter, the community may strive for a motorised pump and piping, so that each household can have a tap at the house, and ultimately a tap inside the house.

Such improvements in water supply also have indirect effects on health, besides keeping the microbes away. Fetching water is a very time and energy consuming task, carried out mainly by women. The provision of piped and tap water relieves women from a lot of hard work, giving them time to care for their children and themselves. The provision of an improved water supply is also linked to better facilities for washing clothes. There are several steps of gradual improvement on the path from washing in rivers to the use of modern electrical washing machines that reduce working time and effort, mainly for women, and increase the availability of clean clothes.

Though difficult to quantify, it seems that the main environmental health problem in the world is still unsafe, microbial contaminated water for drinking and household use, combined with a lack of adequate sanitation for the disposal of waste, faeces and urine.

Table 2.6 Percent of population using safe water and sanitation in different regions in 2000.

Region	% with improved drinking water		% with adequate sanitation	
	urban	rural	urban	rural
East Asia and Pacific	93	67	73	35
CEE/CIS and the Baltic states	95	82	97	81
Latin America and Caribbean	94	66	86	52
Middle East and North Africa	95	77	93	70
South Asia	94	80	67	22
Sub-Saharan Africa	83	44	73	43
High income countries	100	100	100	100

Source: State of the world's children 2004. UNICEF.

Water safety can be secured by relatively simple technologies, such as protective wells and hand pumps as mentioned above. In drier areas the drilling of deep-water wells and the installation of mechanised pumps and piping may be necessary to supply safe water.

In the last decades of the 20th century, an estimated 2 billion people in low and middle-income countries have gained access to safe water, and 400 million have gained access to basic sanitation. The 1980s was the International Drinking Water Supply and Sanitation Decade (UNDP 1998). During this decade many international organisations put great efforts into research and into building latrines and safe wells even in remote villages. The percentage of populations with access to safe water and adequate sanitation in different regions of the world is shown in table 2.6. In Sub-Saharan Africa about half of the population has access to safe water, while access to adequate sanitation is least frequent in South Asia, where these needs are met for only a third of the population. However, 1.3 billion people, corresponding to one-fifth of the world's population, still lack access to safe water, and 2.5 billion (40 % of the world's population) lack access to adequate sanitation. These will remain the main environmental problems in the world for many years to come.

2.4 Sanitation

Faeces constitutes a major route of transmission of communicable diseases in human populations. Urine transmits only a few, but nevertheless important parasitic diseases. The ways in which the excreta—the joint term for faeces and urine—are disposed of is therefore a most important health determinant. The disposal of excreta and other wastes is referred to as sanitation. In all societies there are in fact a number of culturally determined taboos linked to defecation practices and excreta disposal and each

---

Box 2.7

Requirements for quality sanitation

1 Protect against disease transmission.
2 Eliminate the bad smell of faeces and urine.
3 Stop insects from breeding on the excreta.
4 Provide the privacy needed for the comfort of the user.
5 Return the nitrogen and nutrients in excreta to the field where food is grown.
6 Use limited amounts of water and energy.

---

community has varying degrees of hygienic rules and practices for defecation and urination.

The practice of defecating or urinating in the bush or in the fields may not pose any significant health or environmental problem in scarcely populated areas or among nomadic populations living in an environment that is conducive to this practice. However, as the population density increases, all human societies have had to develop technical solutions and special practices for excreta disposal.

Unfortunately, even seemingly simple latrine construction remains relatively expensive for the poorer part of the population in low and middle-income countries. This explains why more than 40 % of the world's population still live without access to proper sanitation. The estimated percentage living without improved sanitation facilities is 20 % in Latin America and 40–50 % in Africa and Asia. Latrines can solve a number of problems (Box 2.7).

There is no best latrine or toilet solution for the whole world. The modern flush toilet is probably not the best option for providing most households in the world with improved sanitation facilities. The flush toilet offers the perfect solutions to issues 1 to 4, but fails completely on 5 and 6. There are a

78

number of different latrine constructions, adapted to various environments, income levels and cultures (Esrey 1998). Two examples are worth mentioning.

In rural Vietnam, the population density is high, and due to the irrigation of rice fields, the water level in the ground is high. Faced with these realities and very limited economic resources, Vietnam's public health professionals still managed to develop an appropriate latrine solution, known as the *Vietnamese double septic tank.* The latrine is built in brick and has two containers for faeces. It enables the urine to be separated through a half-pipe of bamboo or metal, to be collected in a vessel outside the latrine. When one septic tank has been filled with faeces, it is sealed for several months and left to ferment while the other tank is used. When the time has come to seal the second tank, the first one is opened. The now fermented faeces can be used as fertiliser in the fields. The urine is also used for targeted fertilisation, putting nitrogen back to the cultivated land. The success of this latrine in Vietnam is not only that it protects against infectious diseases but also that it helps maintain soil fertility and agricultural production. Whether a latrine is appropriate and accepted in a community depends jointly on technical, environmental, cultural and economic factors.

In Zimbabwe, the Blair Institute developed the *ventilated improved pit latrine,* which is appropriate for many settings in Africa, although still too expensive to afford for most rural families. It is a covered pit latrine that has the disadvantage that the excreta are not returned to agricultural production, but many other advantages. A cement floor covers the latrine pit. The floor has a central hole for defecation and a smaller hole at the side for ventilation. A pipe is placed in the smaller hole, like a chimney. The pipe leads the airflow from the latrine pit up above the roof of the latrine, thus removing the bad smell. The latrine house is built in a spiral, so that light never enters through the central hole. The wind blowing across the top of the latrine and the sun heating the pipe will make the air flow travel down through the central hole into the pit and hence up and out of the pipe. A net covering the top of the pipe stops flies from getting out, but the light shining down through the pipe into the latrine pit attracts the flies to fly up into the pipe. The flies reach the net, where they are trapped and die. This latrine is thus free of both smell and flies. The disadvantage is that this latrine is rather expensive.

With such smart solutions, as exemplified above, it is hoped that almost all households in the world will gain access to improved sanitation within one or two decades. This would break the transmission of many infectious diseases and provide a major contribution towards better world health.

2.5 Other environmental determinants

Unsafe water and sanitation remain the main environmental health determinants in the world. In the following section, we will describe additional environmental determinants of human health: housing, occupation, traffic, air, climate and natural disasters.

2.5.1 Housing

Housing is a basic health determinant, as it contributes to the physical, mental and social well being of individuals. The house also protects families and their assets from violence and theft. At least 600 million urban dwellers and more than 1 000 million rural inhabitants in Africa, Asia and Latin America live in shelters or under precarious housing conditions in neighbourhoods that pose severe threats to life and health (WHO 1998). In addition tens of millions of people are homeless. In high-income countries, the

---

Box 2.8

Summary of WHO's definition of a Healthy House

- structurally sound and free from accidental injury hazards,

- sufficient space for all normal household activities for all members of the family,

- adequate supply of potable and palatable water,

- sanitary means of collection, storage and disposal of all liquid and solid wastes,

- appropriate installed facilities for personal and household hygiene,

- weatherproof and watertight with proper protection from the elements,

- indoor environment which is healthful and comfortable,

- free from excessive noise from both interior and exterior sources of the structure,

- natural and artificial means of illumination that are adequate for all household activities,

- free from toxic and/or noxious odours, chemicals and other air contaminants or pollutants,

- adequate but not excessive solar radiation,

- adequate protection from insects and rodents,

- health, welfare, social, educational, cultural and protective community services.

---

problem of housing largely concerns considerations of light, insulation, ventilation and the psychosocial environment in the surroundings, since the basic needs of water, cooking, washing, food storage and waste disposal are solved. The World Health Organization has identified the requirements for healthy housing (Box 2.8).

Most housing in low-income countries and a considerable part in middle-income countries fall outside the basic standards of safety or protection against ill health. The combination of overcrowding with high levels of virus, bacteria and disease vectors in particular increase the risk of severe respiratory infection and measles, as well as many other diseases. Historical data from Sweden in the 19th century show that overcrowding was associated with a three times greater risk of measles mortality, after controlling for young age, low social class and being born out of wedlock (Burström 1996). Tuberculosis is another airborne disease that is spread easily in conditions of overcrowding in combination with poor ventilation and malnutrition—a combination affecting millions of people living in low and middle-income countries today. Disease vectors in the surrounding of human settlements can be restricted by locating houses away from mosquito breeding places, restricting the access of mosquitoes and flies with screens over windows and doors, preventing access to food, disposing of waste and repairing cracks in walls and floors. Actions from many sectors of society are needed to solve the problem of unhealthy living conditions. Both public and private services are needed to construct healthy living conditions in safe neighbourhoods.

Today about 48% of all people in the world live in urban areas. An estimated increase from 2.6 billion to 4 billion urban settlers is expected between 1995 and 2015. Urbanisation has both positive and negative effects on human health. In low- and middle-income countries, it appears as if the positive effects are the greatest. Even if poor segments of the population live in miserable conditions in the big cities, the majority of them would have been in a worse situation if they had remained in rural areas. In most countries, industrialisation and economic growth lead to urbanisation. Unfortunately

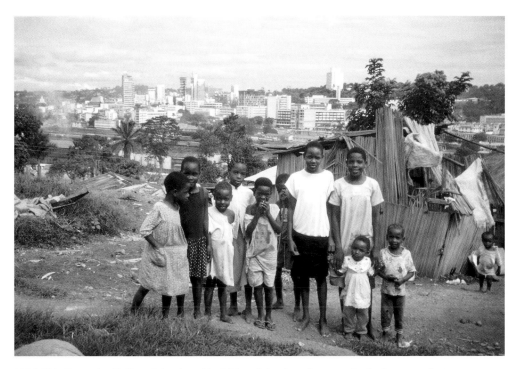

UGANDA, Kampala. Skyline of the city with children living in a slum area in the foreground.
© Sean Sprague/PHOENIX.

the development of water and sanitation systems and safe housing is not paralleled by the increasing number of people that move to the rapidly growing cities in low and middle income countries.

Today urbanisation in the world is occurring mainly in low and middle-income countries (Table 2.7). It should be noted that

Table 2.7 Urban population as % of total population by region in 1975 and 2002.

Regions	1975	2002
East Asia and Pacific	19	40
Europe and Central Asia	56	64
Latin America and Caribbean	61	76
Middle East and North Africa	45	57
South Asia	20	28
Sub-Saharan Africa	19	35
High income countries	72	78

Source: World Development Indicators 2002, The World Bank and State of the world's children 2004, UNICEF.

the continents with the best health status have the highest proportion living in urban areas, while in Africa and South Asia, having the worst health status, less than one-third of the population live in urban areas. Less than half of the world's population earn their living from agriculture, and the number of people who produce food is fewer than the number who only consume (Figure 2.3).

Poverty, population growth, war and natural disasters, and shortages of land are some of the main reasons why people move to urban settlements. Changes in social and cultural values are also contributory factors.

The people who move to urban areas need employment, housing, education, fuel, as well as social, sanitary and medical facilities. Few of the low and middle-income countries can keep up with the supply of these services. It is the poorest population that suffers most from living in growing shantytowns without basic services. In many parts of the

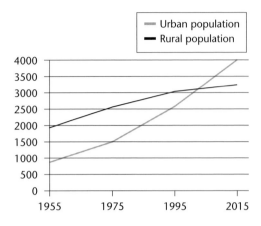

Figure 2.3 The world's urban and rural population in millions 1955–2015.

Source: World Health Report, 1999. WHO.

world, urban settlement is followed by severe social problems such as increased alcohol and drug use, increased crime rates and prostitution, fuelled by the lack of social control and the anonymity of large cities.

2.5.2 Occupation

The right to employment is part of the Universal Declaration of Human Rights, but far from all people are guaranteed this right. About 120 million people in the world are registered as unemployed, but this is a gross underestimate. Unemployment in urban areas is as high as 50 % or more in some low-income countries. The urban poor make their livelihood in the so-called informal sector, as street vendors or car attendants, as casual labour, in personal services such as shoe-shining, etc. The informal sector refers to economic activity beyond government regulation and taxation. Many or most of the underemployed in the informal sector suffer from poverty, inequality, loss of self-esteem and reduced psychosocial well-being, due to a lack of proper employment. The majority of the world's population work in the agricultural sector and the informal sector. In low-income countries, these types

of work offer little possibility to escape poverty. In fact, it has recently been recognised that the informal sector in cities in low- and middle-income countries is much larger than formerly realised. It has been suggested that the lack of the right to property among the entrepreneurs in the informal sector is the main obstacle to economic development in most low and middle-income countries (de Soto 2000).

In high-income countries, unemployment rates vary from less than 5 % in Japan and Luxembourg to more than 20 % in Spain. In low-income countries, unemployment rates may be as high as 45 %. It is obvious that these high unemployment rates do not imply that this half of the labour force is not involved in economic activities. The mechanisms and obstacles of the informal economic sector have emerged as a major research area in development studies in recent years. In all countries unemployment among urban youth breeds severe psychosocial problems, with delinquent behaviour, violence and social disintegration (WHO 1998).

Almost all occupations and income-generating activities are linked to health risks. Most risks are known to occupational medicine and can be prevented if the workplace is designed for safety. However, this is not often the case in low-income countries. Deficient occupational safety is also common in middle-income countries, but not in high-income countries. The use of pesticides in agricultural plantations is a drastic example. Their toxicity is well known, and in high-income countries their use is carefully regulated, and adequate protection is offered to all workers handling these toxins. In plantations in Latin America, Asia and Africa, however, acute toxicity and chronic effects of pesticides constitute a growing health problem. The same pattern can be seen in almost all occupations. While risks are controlled and accidents and exposures are kept to a minimum in high-income countries, exposure to occupational hazards are greater in middle-income, and even more so in low-income countries. In poor countries the threat posed by industrialisation is not limited to workers. Through the leaking of toxic substances to food, water, air and the environment at large, the rapid ongoing industrialisation in Asia in particular is bound to increase toxicological and other environmental problems in the near future (Yassi 2001). Environmental lead, arsenic, mercury and other heavy metals released from industrial activities enter the food chain and can cause serious toxic effects. They may also deplete body stores of iron, vitamin C and other essential nutrients, leading to decreased immune defences and other disabilities associated with malnutrition.

2.5.3 Air and Energy

Air pollution is estimated to kill about three million people each year through lung and heart diseases. A common misconception is that most of these deaths are due to outdoor air pollution in cities in rich industrialised countries. On the contrary, 90 % of deaths are estimated to occur in low and middle-income countries, and more than half of them are estimated to occur as a result of indoor air pollution, due to poor housing in rural areas (WHO 1998). Accordingly the burden of disease from air pollution mainly affects poor women and children in rural areas, and particularly girls involved in cooking food indoors. Poorer populations burn biomass such as dung, wood and coal for cooking and indoor heating in large areas of Sub-Saharan Africa and Asia. Open fires without appropriate stoves or chimneys to conserve heat and reduce air pollution are used by poor households rather because they cannot afford them than due to lack of knowledge.

Outdoor air pollution is also increasing in the world, and mostly in low and middle-income countries, because of rapid industrialisation and the spread of motorised vehicles without proper control mechanisms for emissions. More than 70 % of all deaths caused by outdoor air pollution occur in low and middle-income countries. Forest fires are another reason for air pollution. In 1997 a large forest fire in Indonesia caused the deaths of more than 1 000 people and respiratory problems among more than 20 million people in large areas of South East Asia.

Acid rain has been presented as another threat to human health and livelihood. Fossil fuel burning power stations with high chimneys, to avoid air pollution among the local population, spread sulphur and nitrogen oxides, which are converted to sulphuric and nitric acid, giving rise to acidic precipitation far away from the point of emission. However, the consequence of this acidification is unclear. The death of areas of forest experienced in Central Europe have been attributed to acid rains, but a combination of cold winters and the planting of inappropriate eco-types of pine trees in high-altitude forests may have caused the deaths. Acidification mobilises metals such as lead, mercury, cadmium copper and aluminium in the soil, and these may eventually enter freshwater and the food chain.

Fossil fuels such as oil, coal and natural gas are used as raw materials for 90 % of the world's commercial energy production. Oil remains the dominant source of energy supplying about 40 % of global energy needs. The high-income countries use over 70 % of the world's fossil-fuel consumption. Adverse health effects of fossil fuel include air pollution due to burning oil and coal, as described above, and most probably the greenhouse effect. If the coal is impure when burning, residual metals including lead, cadmium, mercury and arsenic may spread. Eastern Europe and China use coal to a large extent, and in combination with inadequate control of emissions this poses a serious environmental problem (WHO 1992).

Hydroelectric power stations cause adverse health effects through indirect effects on the environment and by displacing people to make room for building the large dams. The dams may provide water for drinking and irrigation, but in tropical regions dams may enhance the transmission of vector-borne parasitic diseases.

Nuclear power can cause severe health effects if accidents occur; otherwise this is, in environmental terms, a fairly safe energy supply, as regards human health. The detrimental health effects following the Chernobyl accident in 1986 were of different kinds. A total of 31 emergency workers died from acute radiation injuries, 300 others became severely ill from high levels of radiation, and some ultimately died from these effects. Increased rates of thyroid cancer in children were noted in southern Belarus in the following years. More than 100 000 people were permanently evacuated from the contaminated area in Ukraine. The resulting psychosocial distress probably caused more ill health than the direct effects of radiation. Several distant areas of Europe became contaminated with radioactivity. The long-term effects of these lower degrees of contamination in remote countries have not yet been clearly linked to any substantial adverse health effect. Low doses of radiation have been detected in the environment around nuclear power plants, but no clear correlation to increased disease frequency has been proven.

The final disposal of high-level radioactive waste may pose a problem for future generations if safe storage cannot be achieved. It is a delicate task to assess these obvious long-term risks in relation to the likely positive short-term benefit to health that a cheaper energy supply without carbon dioxide emission may offer in many countries.

Better-quality energy sources with fewer negative health effects and new technologies for increased production efficiency and energy consumption are continuously under trial. Even with new energy-saving techniques, alternative energy sources and lower the per capita energy consumption in the future, the projected global population growth will demand more energy than is currently produced in the world.

2.5.4 Climate

Is climate in itself a determinant of health? For certain diseases, such as the severest type of malaria, falciparum malaria, there is a strong link to tropical climate (See Chapter 1.3). Whereas a warm climate increases the transmission of certain vector-borne diseases, a cold climate may also have negative health effects. In poorer populations, cold climate leads to very crowded living conditions during winter, and this greatly increases the transmission of poverty-related diseases such as leprosy and tuberculosis, which do not require any insect vector. In fact a better term for the so-called tropical diseases is 'diseases of poverty', but the infectious diseases affecting poor people are partly determined by the climate they live in. Parasitic diseases are not exclusive to tropical countries but also affect populations in cold climates (Britton 2003).

Human activities affect climate in a long-term perspective. Destruction of the stratospheric ozone layer will increase exposure to ultraviolet radiation, which is a contributing factor to skin cancer and cataracts. Ozone is continuously being produced and destroyed in the stratosphere, but human consumption of certain types of gases causes a thinning of the ozone layer. The detrimental gases are chlorofluorocarbons (CFC's), used in refrigerators, aerosol propellants and fire extinguishers, and methyl bromide, a chemical used in pesticides. Emissions from high-flying aeroplanes add further gases. International efforts are being made to reduce or ban the use of these compounds. Preventative measures involving cautious exposure to the sun, through the use of protective clothing, sunscreen and sunglasses, are recommended.

Global warming is caused by the 'greenhouse effect', meaning the increased concentration of carbon dioxide (CO_2), methane and certain nitrogen-containing gases in the atmosphere. These gases create an energy trap around the earth, because they absorb the re-emitted energy from the earth's surface, but admit incoming heat from solar radiation like a greenhouse—hence the name. Because of the rising concentration of these gases, a global warming effect in the atmosphere has been confirmed, but the future magnitude and impact is still uncertain. Therefore the potential effects of global warming on health are poorly understood. It may act through effects on agricultural production, freshwater shortages and a rising sea level. Harvests may be reduced in some areas and increased in others, as the effects most probably will be very unequally distributed. Africa, South Asia and Latin America will have less rainfall and lower crop yields, while Europe and Canada will benefit from increased rainfall and better harvests. Deserts are expected to spread in Sub-Saharan Africa, South Asia and the Arab States.

The high-income countries account for most of the emissions of greenhouse gases produced by burning fossil fuels, but it seems as if the least developed regions of the world suffer the most from the environmental changes. International organisations have agreed on treaties to deal with this threat to environmental change by phasing out the use of chlorofluorocarbons, and many governments support research into and the introduction of alternative energy sources. It is annoying to have to conclude that the expected health effects of global warming range from close to none to very severe (Yassi 2001).

2.5.5 Natural disasters

Drought and floods occur repeatedly in many parts of the world, causing displacement and hunger due to damaged harvests. Ethiopia, Sudan and Bangladesh are just three of the countries that have been afflicted many times by droughts and floods leading to starvation and epidemics of diseases such as cholera. In Sudan in 1998 a combination of war and natural disasters caused widespread starvation. The extent of the impact of natural disasters on health is dependent on countries' levels of develop-

ment and the capacity and willingness of their social and political structures to cope with crises. Bangladesh suffers from being flooded during monsoon periods, some years (as in 2004) more severely than others. This densely populated low-income country repeatedly battles against floods. However, disaster preparedness has gradually improved during recent decades. Another positive development is the sharp drop in fertility rates that have slowed the population growth rate so that Bangladesh may relatively soon achieve a 'two child family' level and eventually a stable population. Without this there will always be very poor people that have to cultivate and live on land suffering from frequent flooding.

Tornadoes, typhoons, hurricanes, volcanic eruptions and earthquakes are familiar natural disasters, which are obviously not preventable. Prevention of the health effects of these natural disasters depends on the emergency preparedness for humanitarian assistance in the affected countries. In Central America in 1998, Hurricane Mitch killed over 10 000 people and destroyed extensive parts of the infrastructure, causing damage corresponding to decades of development. Natural disasters may contribute substantially to local mortality and human suffering, but their joint health effects remain surprisingly small on a global scale compared to how much time is allocated to natural disasters in TV news. The earth is a relatively safe place for humans, were it not for the health risks related to poverty.

2.6 Behaviour

The effect on health of the determinants described so far is modified by a person's individual behaviour. An example is provided by the way a person handles food and water before eating. Apart from hygienic practices, there are a few factors that strongly and directly influence health status. These are tobacco, alcohol, sex, and traffic; they are reviewed in the following sections. Another important behavioural determinant is the degree of physical activity, which is reviewed in chapter 6.

2.6.1 Tobacco

The health hazards of tobacco smoking are well established. About one billion people in the world today are regular tobacco-smokers. Each year three million people are estimated to die from lung cancer and cardiovascular diseases caused by tobacco smoking. Tobacco use was estimated to cause 4 % of the total burden of disease in the world in the year 2000 (WHO 2002), when measured as disability-adjusted life years lost (DALY's) (Chapter 3.6). In the high-income countries and former socialist countries of Europe, as many as 15 % of deaths are mainly due to tobacco use. But in many high-income countries, there has been a decrease in tobacco use during recent decades, which contributes to the decreased mortality from coronary heart disease in these countries. In the 1990s, smoking increased among young females, and smoking is becoming increasingly common in the lower socio-economic strata of high-income countries. In parallel with the habit of bottle-feeding babies, the habit of smoking has trickled down through the socio-economic strata, from the well paid, highly educated to becoming an indicator of psychosocial deprivation. In high-income countries smoking is also changing from being a male to being a female habit.

Unfortunately, a rapid increase of tobacco use has taken place in low and middle-income countries over the last 30 years. The tobacco-related mortality in the world is predicted to rise to 8 million yearly by the year 2020. This is largely the direct effect of the determined marketing policy of the tobacco industry, which is seeking new markets as those in Europe and North America are shrinking. Interventions are urgently needed to counteract this catastrophic effect on global health status. Public health programmes for the prevention of tobacco consumption should support and inform the individual, but simultaneously, public policies such as an age limit for buying cigarettes, taxation on cigarettes and laws to control the tobacco industry's marketing practices are helpful in limiting the use of tobacco. Following determined efforts by the former Director General, Gro Harlem Brundtland, WHO Member States concluded a groundbreaking public health agreement in 2003. This Framework Convention on Tobacco Control sets out new rules for curbing tobacco advertising and promotion, and illicit trade in tobacco products.

A sad and paradoxical fact is that many of the poorest low-income countries depend heavily on the export of tobacco for their economic viability. A reduction in the price of tobacco and lower export volumes will have an indirect adverse health effect in these countries.

2.6.2 Alcohol and illicit drugs

Alcohol has been consumed in human populations for millennia. It has negative health and social consequences via intoxication, dependence and long-term biochemical effects. Intoxication is a powerful mediator for acute outcomes, such as road traffic accidents or domestic violence. Alcohol dependence is a disorder in itself. It is estimated that 120 million persons worldwide suffer from alcohol dependency, which is strongly associated with higher rates of violence, accidents, cirrhosis of the liver, some types of cancer and mental disorders. Alcohol abuse caused 4 % of all DALYs lost in the world in 2000. In contrast to tobacco, alcohol consumed in moderation is believed to slightly reduce the risk of cardiovascular disease. The abuse of alcohol and narcotics is already a very severe and growing health problem around the world. The religious ban on alcohol in Islamic countries considerably reduces the adverse health effects from alcohol, but this is partly replaced by a frequent use of narcotic drugs in some of these countries. Iran is estimated to have a

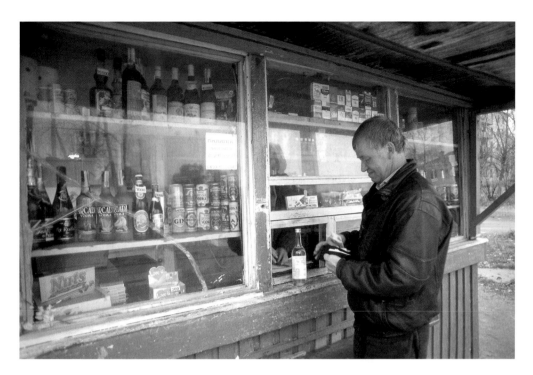

RUSSIA, Vazhini. Man buying liquor in the kiosk.
© Sean Sprague/PHOENIX.

relatively limited alcohol problem, but the country has several hundred thousand intravenous drug users. See further chapter 7.1.6.

Global alcohol consumption has increased in recent decades, with most of this increase occurring in low and middle-income countries, where alcohol is being marketed increasingly. Both average volume of alcohol consumption and patterns of drinking vary dramatically between different parts of the world.[1]

The estimated prevalence of illicit drug use varies considerably across WHO regions. The most hazardous use patterns are found among dependent users who typically inject drugs daily or nearly daily over periods of years. Injecting opioids is associated with increased overall mortality from HIV/AIDS, overdose, suicide and trauma. Other adverse

[1] www.ias.org.uk/theglobe

health and social effects that could not be quantified include other blood-borne diseases such as hepatitis B and C, and criminal activity associated with the drug habit. Globally, 0.2 per cent of deaths (86 000/year) are attributed to illicit drug use. Illicit drugs account for a high proportions of the disease burden in men among countries in the Americas, Eastern Mediterranean and European regions.

2.6.3 Sex

Unsafe sex accounted for 6 % of DALYs lost in the world in 2000 (WHO 2002). Before the appearance of the HIV virus, the prevention of sexually transmitted infections (STIs) was given low priority in most national health policies. The HIV epidemic has forced governments to act, and in some countries, where governments have been open about the problem, such as Brazil,

Thailand and Uganda, it appears as if actions by the public sector and the civil society have curbed the epidemic. In Africa unsafe sex is currently estimated to cause about 20 % of DALYs lost, mainly due to HIV/AIDS. This means that unsafe sex is now as important a cause of disease as is under-nutrition, the other major cause of preventable morbidity and mortality. In the most severely affected countries, such as Botswana, unsafe sex is the absolute dominant cause of human suffering from disease and premature death. See further chapters 5 and 9.

2.6.4 Traffic

Injuries from traffic follow a pattern similar to that of occupational hazards. Although the populations of high-income countries have more vehicles and travel more kilometres per person per year, their risk of being injured or dying as a result of traffic is smaller than in both middle- and low-income countries. In fact, the risk of dying as a result of traffic is highest in densely populated middle-income countries. It is in these countries that the economy is good enough to allow quite intense traffic, while resources are not sufficient to make this traffic safe (see further chapter 8). Although the risk per car or transport kilometre is greater in low-income countries, the relative impact of traffic on the general mortality and morbidity is less. Hence, traffic is a health determinant that in relative terms causes most suffering in middle-income countries. It also seems that making traffic safe is a lengthy process. The rebuilding of roads to make them safe and the establishment of the monitoring and regulation that is needed to ensure car safety and careful driving habits take decades. Hence, newly rich countries such as the United Arab Emirates and other Gulf States are today high-income countries with extremely high mortality and morbidity from traffic.

Similarly, Sweden had its highest number of deaths due to traffic 50 years ago in the first decade of a long period of strong economic growth. This is in spite of a much greater number of cars on the roads today. Five decades ago, Sweden already had good economic resources, but it took careful research, advocacy, legislation and mass communication to make the traffic environment as safe as it is today. Still, traffic is a major cause of death and disability among the young and middle-aged in Sweden and other high-income countries. The reduction of mortality due to road traffic accidents in high-income countries has not come about automatically. It is a combined effect of safer

---

Box 2.9

Successful actions for traffic safety in Sweden

In 1948 the National Society for Road Safety, a non-governmental organisation, commissioned Swedish authors to write short stories that promoted traffic safety. Stig Dagerman wrote, "To kill a child" (http://hem.passagen.se/iblis/dagerman.html). This short story has become one of the most read texts in the Swedish language. Few of the millions of readers realised that this powerful story about the unnecessary death of child in a traffic accident was commissioned in the cause of health education.

The reduction from more than 1 300 annual traffic deaths in Sweden 40 years ago to 535 deaths in 2002 came about in spite of a steep increase in the number of cars. This successful health promotion was achieved through a number of actions that ranged from cultural highlights to technological innovations and various legislations. It serves as a good example of how public health actions should be directed at many points and levels in the causational web of a specific disease or injury.

---

cars, better roads, more monitoring of traffic and strict legal regulation of the traffic environment. It also required a major shift in attitudes regarding safety and preventive measures in the general population. In fact traffic safety may also be regarded as a cultural issue e.g. how acceptable it is to drink and drive (Box 2.9).

2.7 Health services

Health service is not the most important prerequisite for good health. The other six determinants mentioned in this chapter are more fundamental to human health than health services. However, it is difficult to estimate the relative importance of health services for the health status of a specific population based on scientific evidence. One of the main reasons is that the access and utilisation of health care jointly vary with the other determinants in most parts of the world. There are in fact very few instances in which it is possible to isolate the effect of health services from the other health determinants in an intelligent way. A classical study by Thomas McKeown (1979) compared the decline in mortality from infectious diseases in Western Europe with the availability of antibiotics and anti-tuberculosis drugs. In a time series analysis, he argues that, since most of the decline in mortality occurred before the introduction of these drugs, general social factors played a more important role than drugs for the decline in mortality. However, it was not the same combination of factors as one century earlier in Europe, that caused the impressive decline in child mortality in middle and low-income countries over recent decades. The recent decrease in child mortality has occurred following modest improvement in socio-economic and nutritional determinants. It is therefore assumed that the improved child survival in the world in the last few decades is largely due to the improved access to vaccines and antibiotics, and to oral rehydration therapy for the treatment of acute diarrhoea. It has even been suggested that the unregulated and unofficial sale of antibiotics at village markets by medically untrained persons is largely responsible for the improved child survival in the poorest parts of the world. We are consequently unable to provide the reader with an estimate of the relative importance of medical services for the present global health situation. We strongly encourage further readings and studies of this issue (Merson 2001, Beaglehole 2003).

The term medical services mostly refers to curative services for sick patients, whereas health care includes preventive, curative, and rehabilitation services. The terms health service and health care are more or less synonymously used. Health system is a wider concept and includes health actions outside the health care sector. The types of health care provided in a country may be classified as public, private, traditional or informal. The first two are supposed to be evidence-based activities supported by scientific studies, often referred to as modern medicine. Traditional care is sometimes easily classified based on long standing cultural tradition but today this is often no longer the case. It includes completely new forms of alternative treatment and also merges with activities referred to as informal care. In many countries the conventional dichotomy between modern and traditional medicine is no longer a reality. The informal sale of drugs on local markets or in small clinics by untrained persons merges with traditional medicine in many low-income countries. Untrained persons that provide similar services as those selling drugs on local markets staff many small private clinics in low-income countries. Officially these clinics should provide evidence based medical care by qualified professionals. Careful health system analysis is needed to understand the health care in a country, especially in a low-income country where the situation today is far more complex than the old concepts of 'modern and traditional medicine' (see chapter 11).

2.7.1 Modern medicine

Access to health care is measured as the percentage of the population that can expect evidence-based treatment for common diseases and injuries, including treatment with essential drugs within one hour's walk or travel. In almost all high-income countries and in many middle-income countries, such as Poland, Cuba and Costa Rica, access to health care is nearly 100 %. In other middle-income countries, such as Thailand, it is estimated to be about 60 %, while in most low-income countries, less than half of the population is estimated to have access to health care. In many low and middle-income countries, the percentage with access to health care is not known or difficult to estimate. Even when a community has access to modern medical services, the utilisation of available services depends on price and quality of services, on people's faith in and perception of modern health care as such, in the way they have had to pay and how they have been treated in the past.

Modern medicine can now provide a wide range of treatments for most diseases but access to these treatments depends mainly on affordability. The most drastic example is the antiretroviral treatment that can prolong life for many years for those infected by HIV. The care and drugs needed are available for all infected in high-income countries, for many of the infected in middle income countries but only for about 1 % of those infected in low-income countries.

The ways health care is financed in each country is documented in National Health Accounts (WHO 2002). Per capita spending on health care in current USD is 100 times higher in the high-income countries than in the low-income countries in South Asia and Sub-Saharan Africa. The United States is now the country with the highest percentage of GDP spent on health care (13 %); a total of USD 4 500 per capita is spent annually on health care. In Sub-Saharan Africa the annual spending on health services varies between 4 to 30 USD per capita. Cuba and Russia spend about USD 100 per capita.

The disparity in access to and quality of the health care and the level of health care expenditure in different populations, vary greatly throughout the world (World Bank 2003).

The access to health care for an individual patient depends on three factors. The economic level of the country, the financing system for the health service in the country and the economic resources of the patient. Almost all countries have a mixture of public and private health care provision, as will be reviewed in chapter 11. Cuba and North Korea only have a public health system, as private practice is not allowed and the informal medical practices are relatively limited.

The organisation of the health care system in most countries is based on a chain of referral (table 2.8). Preventive work and basic care are performed by the primary health care as close to the family and community as possible. The most common diseases should be treated at primary level, and major preventive interventions such as immunisation are also performed at that level. The primary level should be served with training and supervision from higher levels of the health care system, and they should be able to refer patients suffering from more complicated disease conditions efficiently to either the secondary or tertiary level of care. The secondary level is the basic hospital service and the tertiary level deals with the advanced treatment of special conditions. Remember that outlined above is a model system, and that reality in most countries is different. The demand for secondary and tertiary care is often great, leading directly to an over-burdening of emergency rooms in the hospitals with patients that could have been treated at the primary level. Economic limitations lead to shortage of staff and lack of drugs at the primary level in low-income countries. This also leads to people directly seeking care at hospitals—or perhaps more often going directly to the local market to buy their drugs from informal drug sellers. The information flow back and forth along the chain of referral concerning

Table 2.8 Health care and staff according to economic level.

Level of Health care and population per facility	Activities	Low-income countries	Middle-income countries	High-income countries
Home care	Family actions like child care, breastfeeding, home care of disease, water and sanitation	Family and social network	Family and social network, some places home visits by health care staff	Family and home visit of health care staff when needed
Primary health care 2 000–5 000	Immunisation, maternal and child clinic, family planning, health education and treatment of common diseases	Nurses with few years training	Nurses with many years training	Specialised physicians and nurses
First referral level 100 000–200 000	District hospital for curative care and emergency services	1 or 2 physicians and limited resources	Team of specialised physicians and nurses	Team of many specialised physicians and nurses
Second referral level 0.5–1 million	Teaching hospital with sub-specialities for advanced treatment	Specialised physicians for those affording transport	Care for all but advanced care only for fee	Very advanced care for almost all in need

the patient's condition is deficient in many low-income countries; for most patients the referral chain is a fiction. In middle-income countries the access to referral depends on the economic resources of the patient's family. The public hospitals in low and middle-income countries can often offer most patients basic treatment for delivery and accident care, but most advanced examinations and treatments require extra payment from the patient.

Private health care can be provided for profit or by non-profit organisations such as churches or charities. The care offered may be in the form of private hospitals offering tertiary specialised care, smaller hospitals with basic care, or outpatient clinics, all depending on the demands and economic resources of the local community.

The access to cost-effective life-saving drugs to cure major infectious diseases such as malaria, acute respiratory infections and tuberculosis is exceedingly unequal in the world. An estimated one-third of the world's population lack access to essential life-saving medicines for diseases that can be cost-effectively cured following a short examination for diagnosis. Drugs for life-saving treatment of chronic conditions such as HIV, di-

abetes and hypertension are even less accessible in low-income countries. However, successful management of these life long diseases requires regular clinical and laboratory check-ups that are almost as costly as the drugs. Beside the problems of financing, the production and distribution of the drugs needed by poor patients, there are three major obstacles regarding the supply of essential drugs to those who need them.

The first obstacle occurs when the drug has been developed during the last 20 years and the producing company has a valid patent and sells the drug at a high price. The price should cover the cost of synthesis of the active molecule, the production of the tablet, the cost of the research for the drug in question and for other drug projects that failed, and finally the profit for the investors. The lack of access is determined by high prices, which simply excludes most of the population of the world. Patents encourage the pharmaceutical industries to invest in the development of new drugs, but it makes new drugs very expensive during their first 20 years of production, when their patents are valid. Many new drugs are useful against the major infectious diseases but cannot be used by those affected because the price is too high. A two level price system whereby the high income countries would pay for the research and middle and low-income countries would only pay for the synthesis of the substance and making of the tablet would solve the situation. There are presently intense discussions in the World Trade Organisation (WTO) to reach a solution to this most unethical situation (see chapter 12).

A second obstacle may occur with drugs that were developed more than 20 years ago for which no patent exists. Most drugs used in middle and low-income countries are of this type, the reason being that the prices are markedly lower because consumers do not have to pay for the research. The main cost is the synthesis of the active substance which is today mainly carried out in middle-income countries, while the final production of the tablets may be carried out in low-income countries, which greatly reduces the price. However, drugs that are only needed for diseases affecting poor communities, such as the parasitic disease sleeping sickness, may still be too expensive to produce with the available funds. Such drugs may even go out of production because the market is not large enough to generate profit. This was the case for eflornithine, a drug for the treatment of sleeping sickness, until the drug was recently found to be effective in the 'treatment' of female facial hair. This market is enormous in the rich countries and production of eflornithine was resumed.

The third obstacle is that the drugs do not exist due to a lack of research. For malaria and tuberculosis, we still use drugs developed 50 years ago. Increasing resistance makes these drugs increasingly ineffective. Research and development of drugs for malaria and tuberculosis is virtually non-existent. During the last 25 years, only 13 out of 1,233 newly developed drugs were for diseases affecting mainly the poorer populations of the world (Pecoul 1999). This lack of research investment in drugs for the diseases of the poor constitutes a clear 'market failure' that is partly being addressed by the formation of the Global Fund to Fight AIDS, tuberculosis and malaria (see chapter 12.3). Of course, access to drugs cannot in itself solve the problem of ill health in poorer countries, but it is one important factor for the reduction of morbidity and mortality.

The main sources of financing in health care are shown in table 2.9. The World Bank changed its policy during the 1990s to also include financing the social sector. In most countries in Africa and South Asia, public health care has traditionally been free for the consumer. Revised financial systems are now on trial in most middle and low-income countries, including user fees for both health care services and drugs. Studies show that in most communities there is a great willingness to pay for good health care within their economic potential. User fees have the advantage of discouraging unnecessary consumption of health care, which is the motive for their use in the public health care system in high-income countries. The serious disadvantage of user fees in low- and middle-income countries is that the poor-

Table 2.9 Main sources for financing of health care*.

Public health care financing	Private health care financing
Taxation	User fees
Custom duties and other revenues of the national and local government	Revolving drug funds
Compulsory social insurance	Private insurance

* Health expenditure per capita = the sum of private and public health expenditure as a ratio of total population in current USD. Public health care expenditure includes government spending, borrowings and donations from international organisations and health insurance funds. Private health care expenditure includes household spending, private insurance, charitable donations, and direct service payments by private corporations.

Table 2.10 Public, private and total health expenditure in current USD in 2000.

Region	Public as % of GDP	Private as % of GDP	per capita in current USD
East Asia and Pacific	2	3	44
Europe and Central Asia	4	2	108
Latin America and Caribbean	3	4	262
Middle East and North Africa	3	2	170
South Asia	1	4	21
Sub-Saharan Africa	2	3	29
High income countries	6	4	2,735

Source: World Development Report 2004, The World Bank.

est, most sick and most vulnerable populations may become excluded from receiving assistance, even when fees are minimal. Systems that exempt the poorest populations from user fees represent an attempt to decrease inequalities. A sustainable solution to the financing problem of a public health care system can only be found within the contexts of sound economic growth and public policies that include a willingness to finance health care.

As shown in table 2.10, there is an almost even balance between private and public health expenditure in Latin America and the Caribbean, in the Middle East and North Africa. In East Asia and the Pacific, Sub-Saharan Africa and South Asia, private health expenditure is higher, while in Central Asia and in the high-income countries, public spending dominates. This will be further discussed in chapter 12.

2.7.2 Traditional and complementary medicine

The majority of the people in Africa and other low-income countries use traditional and complementary forms of medicine. These are also popular in middle and high-income countries, in the latter, especially among highly educated women. However, the utilisation of traditional and complementary forms of health care varies greatly between countries. In France, for example, an estimated 75 % of the population has used traditional or complementary medicine at least once (WHO 2002).

The concept of traditional medicine merges with that of alternative or complementary medicine. These are more or less well-defined systems of curative and preventive care that are propagated beside the scientific medicine that is developed and taught in medical schools. Medical practitioners of different types have existed in all societies. In the ancient Chinese civilisa-

---

Box 2.10

WHO definition of traditional medicine

"Diverse health practices, approaches, knowledge and beliefs incorporating plant, animal, and/or mineral based medicines, spiritual therapies, manual techniques and exercises applied singularly or in combination to maintain well-being, as well as to treat, diagnose and prevent illness."

Source: WHO traditional medicine strategy 2002

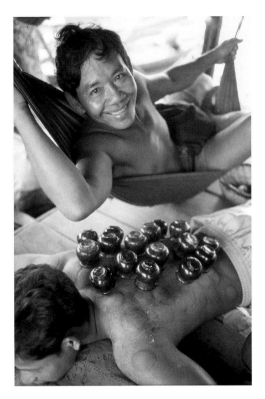

CAMBODIA, Siem-Reap. Man is being treated with cupping glasses.

© Jean-Léo Dugast / PHOENIX.

tion, a variety of written traditional systems of medicine exist, some as much as 5 000 years old. In India, the Ayurvedic system is used by large parts of the population, either for conditions where evidence-based treatment is not available or because such treatment is not affordable or acceptable to the family or community. Both these systems from the ancient Asian civilisations represented the best evidence-based knowledge up to a point in time when they gradually became stagnant schools to which no further advances were added.

Homeopathy is a separate system of complementary medicine that originated in Germany only a century ago and has spread to many other countries. It prescribes a wide variety of extremely dilute solutions to treat a variety of illnesses. Today, practitioners of homeopathy successfully compete with traditional Ayurvedic practitioners in India. It is interesting to see that, in the era of globalisation, alternative systems of medicine are very successful in crossing wide geographical and cultural gaps. It even seems as if an exotic factor makes other countries' traditional systems of medicine especially popular where they are not part of the local tradition, as is the case with homeopathy in India and Chinese traditional medicine in Europe.

Traditional Chinese medicine, like acupuncture, is today widely practised and accepted in Europe, and herbalists of all kinds practise widely across the globe using both traditional herbal drugs and exotic imports from remote countries. In the discussion about the effects of traditional herbal drugs, the malaria drug quinine is an interesting example. Those who think that traditional drugs are not effective should note that quinine remains the best drug against one of the main diseases of the world. However, the active substance has been purified over many years, tested and integrated into scientific medicine. Those who think that herbal drugs are safer than synthetic should note that quinine is responsible for many severe side effects and deaths. This is why few if any use it in the herbal form, in which there may be considerable variations in concentration of the active substance. A drug that can interfere in a disease process in the body can also cause side effects, whereas drugs without any type of side effect rarely have beneficial effects on the pathological processes of a disease.

In many countries, traditional and modern types of medicine and also surgical procedures are utilised for different kinds of disease conditions, or they may be used simultaneously for the same condition. They can also be harmful, as when homeopathy is used to treat children with life-threatening pneumonia, instead of life-saving antibiotics. Herbal drugs can be lethal, due to hepatotoxicity. The traditional practice of uvulectomy involves cutting the tip of the soft palate of an infant in the belief that this

94

will reduce the incidence of diarrhoea. This is a very strongly established practice in Eritrea, and has no known benefits but implies considerable risk for the child and expense for a poor family. Female genital mutilation is a very harmful practice that like many other traditional practices has more than health motivations in the local culture. However, in general, alternative and traditional practices are biologically neutral but can still be quite costly for poor families; for example, the practice to tie a thread with an amulet around the arm or foot of a child in India or Africa in order to protect against diseases. Although they are biologically neutral, such actions may have great psychological advantages for the worried mother. In many African nations, pure herbalists may offer their services at very modest costs or free of charge, whereas diviners may charge high prices for their services, sometimes even more expensive than biomedical treatments. Traditional treatments will therefore contribute to poverty in many households. It should be remembered that poor families spend almost all of their small economic resources on food, education and health care.

During recent decades attempts have been made in low-income countries, especially in Africa, to promote co-operation between the traditional practitioners and the modern health care system. One example involved measures to educate traditional birth attendants to use clean practices and tools. Other challenges, according to the newly adopted WHO traditional medicine strategy, are to produce national policies and a regulatory framework, guaranteeing safety, efficacy and quality as well as access and rational use of traditional medicine.

In conclusion, access to cost-effective evidence based health care is an important determinant for health. The access depends on the economic level of the country and of the family. It is also dependant on whether the country has a fair policy for financing health service. That means the healthy help to pay for the treatment of the sick and the rich help to pay for the treatment of the poor. Access to health service also depends on cultural, gender and social factors as well as if the mix of public, private, traditional and informal health service is rational or not. The access to drug treatment is heavily influence by global trade policy. Globalisation may be beneficial for the poor if WTO will make it possible for poor countries to access patent drugs for treatment of life-threatening conditions (Smith 2003).

References and suggested further reading

Aleman J, Liljestrand J, Pena R, Wall S, Persson LA. Which babies die during the first week? A case control study in a Nicaraguan hospital. Gynecol Obstet Invest. 1997;43:112–5.

Allen T, Thomas A (eds.). Poverty and development into the 21st century. Oxford University Press; 2000.

Antonsson-Ogle B, Gustavsson O, Hambreus L, Holmgren G, Tylleskar T. Nutrition, agriculture and health when resources are scarce. 2nd revised edition. Uppsala: Uppsala University; 2000.

Basch P. Textbook of International Health. Second edition. Oxford University Press; 1999.

Beaglehole R. (ed) Global Public Health: A new era. Oxford University Press; 2003.

Britton S. Linneus, Armauer Hansen, and Nordic research on some neglected diseases. In: Akuffo H, Linder E, Ljungström I and Wahlgren M (eds). Parasites of the colder climates. Taylor & Francis; 2003.

Burstrom B. In: Risk factors for measles mortality. Ph D thesis. Stockholm: Karolinska Institutet; 1996.

Caldwell P. Child survival: Physical vulnerability and resilience in adversity in the European past and contemporary Third World. Soc. Sci. and Med. 1996;43:609–619.

Caldwell P, Santow G. Selected Readings in the Cultural, Social and Behavioural Determinants of Health. Health Transition Series; 1989. (http://htc.anu.edu.au/html/htsl.htm)

De Soto H. The Mystery of Capital: Why Capitalism Triumphs in the West and Fails Everywhere Else. Times Books; 2000.

Chaloner EJ, Mannion SJ. Antipersonnel mines: the global epidemic Ann R Coll Surg Engl 1996;78:1–4.

Cleland JG, van Ginneken JK. Maternal education and child survival in developing countries: the search for pathways to influence. Soc. Sci. and Med. 1988;27: 1357–1368.

Cohen S, Syme SL. Social support and health. London: Academic press; 1985.

Cohan JE. How many people can the world support? Norton; 1995.

Evans T, Whitehead M, Diderichsen F, Bhuiya A, Wirth M (eds). Challenging Inequities in Health – From Ethics to Action. Oxford University Press; 2001.

Esrey S, Gough J, Rapaport D, Sawyer R, Simpson-Hebert M, Vargas J, Winblad U. Ecological Sanitation. Swedish International Development Co-operation Agency (Sida); 1998.

Greiner T. The concept of weaning: definitions and their implications. Hum Lact. 1996;12:123–8.

Helman CG. Culture, Health and Illness. 3rd edition. Butterworth Heinemann, Oxford; 1996.

Human Rights Watch. Global Report on Child Soldiers, 2001.

ISI (International statistical institute) World fertility survey: major findings and implications. 1984.

Last JM. Public health and human ecology. Prentice-Hall International Editions, Appleton & Lange, USA; 1987.

Lomborg B. The sceptical environmentalist. Measuring the real state of the world. Cambridge University Press; 2001.

Marmot M, Wilkinsson RG. Social Determinants of Health. Oxford University Press; 1999.

McKeown T. The Role of Medicine, (2nd edition). Oxford University Press for the Nuffield Provincial Hospitals; 1979.

McMichael T. Human Frontiers, environments and disease. Cambridge University Press; 2001.

Merson MH, Black RE, Mills A. International Public Health. Aspen; 2001.

Park K. Textbook of Preventive and Social Medicine. 15th edition. M/s Banarsidas Bhanot Publishers: Jabalpur, India; 1997.

Pecoul B, Chirac P, Trouiller P, Pinel J. Access to Essential Drugs in Poor Countries. A lost battle? JAMA 1999;281:361–67.

Ramalingaswami V, Jonsson U, Rohde J. The Asian Enigma. Progress of Nations, UNICEF; 1996

Sachs JD. Report of the Commission on Macroeconomics and Health. Macroeconomics and Health: Investing in Health for Economic Development. Geneva: World Health Organisation; 2001.

Savage King F, Burgess A. Nutrition in development countries. 2nd edition. Oxford: Oxford University Press; 1993.

Sen A. Development as Freedom. Oxford University Press; 1999.

Sen G, Georg A, Ostlin P. Engendering International Health: The Challenge of Equity. MIT Press; 2002.

Smith RD, Beaglehole R, Woodward D, Drager N. Global Public Goods for Health. Health economics and public health perspectives. Oxford University Press; 2003.

Todaro MP. Economic Development. 6th edition. Longman; 1997.

UNESCO 2002, Education for all – monitoring report; 2002.

UNDP, Annual Report, 1998.

UNICEF, State of the World's Children, 2003, 2004.

Wamala SP, Lynch J. Eds. Gender and Social Inequalities in Health – A Public Health Issue. Lund, Sweden: Studentlitteratur; 2002.

Whaley RF. A textbook of World Health. A practical guide to global health care. Parthenon Publishing Group; New York: 1995.

World Bank, World Development Indicators. 2001 and 2002.

World Bank, World Development Report 2003, Sustainable development in a dynamic world. Oxford University Press; 2002.

World Bank, World Development Report 2004, Making Services Work for Poor People. Oxford University Press; 2003.

WHO, Our planet, our earth: report of the Commission on Health and Environment. Geneva; 1992.

WHO, Female Genital Mutilation: Report of a WHO Technical Working Group: Geneva: 17–19 July 1995. Geneva: World Health Organisation; 1996.

WHO, World Health Report (WHR). 1998–2004.

WHO, Climate Change and Human Health: Impact and adaptation. WHO/SDE/OEH/001. May 2000.

WHO, New data on the prevention of mother-to-child transmission of HIV and their policy implications: conclusions and recommendations. WHO Technical Consultation on behalf of the UNFPA/UNICEF/WHO/UNAIDS Inter-Agency Task Team on Mother-to-Child Transmission of HIV. Geneva: World Health Organisation, 2001. Report No. WHO/RHR/01.28.

WHO, Traditional Medicine Strategy 2002–2005. WHO/EDMrTRM/2002.1

Yassi A, Kjellstrom T, de Kok T, Guidotti TL. Basic Environmental Health. Oxford University Press; 2001.

Öyen E, Miller SM, Samad SA. Poverty, a global review. Scandinavian University Press; 1996.

3   Health indicators

> *For me a good life is to be healthy.*
>
> An old man, Ethiopia

The basic health indicators, such as child mortality and life expectance, are as crucial for understanding the health situation in a country as are the pulse rate and body temperature for the diagnosis of an individual patient. A health indicator is a variable that provides a single numeric measurement of an aspect of health within a population for a special period of time, normally a year. Many of the United Nation organisations such as WHO, UNICEF, UNDP, UN Statistical Division, UN Population Division and the World Bank annually publish health indicators for all countries of the world.

Health indicators are of two types. The first type is summary measures of survival/mortality, such as child mortality and life expectancy. The second type is measures of the burden of specific diseases or risk factors. The analyses of global variations in disease occurrence have been greatly influenced by the pioneering work of Christopher Murray and Allan Lopez. They started the global burden of disease study at The Harvard School of Public Health. Between 1996 and 2003 they published five major books (Murray 1996, 1998, 2003) with the first coherent estimates of the occurrence and impact of all major diseases in all countries of the world. When Murray was head of health statistics at the World Health Organization (WHO) he further developed new measures for health system performance. These measures induced an intensive debate (Murray 2002). The critique focused on the quality of the data used and was partly correct, as the new concepts were used before sufficient data had been made available. However, Murray and Lopez have left a lasting intellectual imprint in the field of global public health.

They turned global public health into an area of innovative and debated research from having been dominated by doubtful diplomatic compromises about numbers to be used in mass-media-oriented advocacy. But how well do the internationally published numbers from different countries reflect the health reality in each country? It is often asked if we can trust the numbers. This is the wrong question. The provided number for child mortality in a given country is not right or wrong, it is more or less correct. Therefore the question that always should be asked is: "What is the degree of uncertainty of each number for a certain indicator, country and year?" Murray and Lopez also started to provide such a systematic assessment of uncertainty intervals for some of the health indicators (WHO 2002).

The quality of the data for a certain indicator from a certain country depends both on the method used for its collection and on how well this method was applied that year in the country. The authority and the methods used to collect and compile national health and demographic statistics differ between countries, as does the quality of the primary data collection. The Ministry of Health or the National Statistical Bureau supplies the international organisations with national statistics on demographic and health indicators. It is very important to note that countries can use different ways to obtain data for the same health indicator and international organisations use different methods to edit and compile the information into numerical values for each year.

Civil registration, i.e. routine registration of all births, deaths and migrations, are clearly incomplete for more than 80% of the world's population, including China, India and large parts of Africa (Murray 1997). The absence of routine civil registration of births and deaths in a given country does not mean that nothing is known about health and mortality in that country. Child mortality can be used as an example. The data is obviously compiled from routine vital registrations of all births and deaths where that exist, but in the majority of countries child mortality is estimated through the use of other data collection methods.

National census of the whole population enables estimation of child mortality by the use of indirect demographical methods. A national census is only performed about every tenth year. The reason is the high costs of tracing and registering everyone in a country. The information about children that have died is often not obtained in the rapid interviews of a census.

Hospital and health facility registers provide data on deaths of children. However, health facility registers are of very varied quality. Their reliability depends both on the motivation and time available for the local health worker to fill in the forms, as well as on the proportion of the population in the area that are effectively covered by the service provided. In many countries most of the child deaths occur at home and are neither registered in hospitals nor reported to the authorities; the ceremonies around death are entirely a responsibility of the family. In countries like Sweden the authorities carry out almost all actions around a death and therefore have almost perfect statistics on the deaths and their causes.

Sentinel systems provide good estimates of the child mortality in some major countries such as China and India. The data on population changes and health are obtained through regular careful registration in a representative selection of small areas in the country. The complete civil registration in the small areas enables an extrapolation to the whole country as the small areas have been selected as representative of the country.

Demographic surveillance sites constitute a methodology that is similar to the sentinel system. The difference is that the area in which detailed information on demography, health and deaths is collected does not represent the country as a whole. Such sites are still useful for following the time trends and especially for doing community based research on different health interventions. INDEPTH is the name of a growing international organisation for the improvement of the quality of such surveillance sites, especially in Africa. More than a million people across Africa live in areas with complete registration of births and deaths and the quality on health indicators in Africa are steadily improving. INDEPTH is led by African scholars and is co-ordinated from Ghana.[1]

A national household sample survey is the most cost-effective method to estimate the national child mortality. Information is obtained from careful interviews of women in a group of households in a representative number of local communities. The women are interviewed regarding births and deaths of children during past years and a number of additional issues concerning the health of the family and their utilisation of health services. Such surveys are done at three to four year intervals in most low-income countries. Most receive technical and financial support from USAID and a company in the US that has developed impressive skills in conducting such surveys. These surveys are known as Demographic and Health Surveys (DHS). The actual surveys are undertaken by national agencies in each country but all data is provided free to the world.[2]

The data quality is not the only problem when using data from periodic household surveys to assess the general health status of low and middle-income countries. Another problem is that health and demographic indicators such as child mortality may vary considerably from one year to the next or from season to season. In low-income coun-

---

[1]   www.indepth-network.net
[2]   www.measuredhs.com

tries the harvests largely depend on sufficient rainfall. During a drought year the child mortality will increase considerably and following a year with good rains the child mortality decreases. The seasonal variations of mortality also mainly depend on weather. Malaria is just one of the diseases that increase in incidence during the rainy season, thus affecting the seasonal variation of child mortality. Natural or man-made disasters can quickly affect the health and demographic situation in a country.

Internationally published time series, with child mortality from low-income countries, show data for each year. However, these numbers are averages for the last three to five years. The data given for a specific year is often just an interpolation between estimations for different time periods. Unfortunately the way these interpolations have been made and the values used for the interpolations are not regularly provided. The data internationally published also lags a few years behind because of the retrospective character of the data collection and compilation. The health status also varies geographically within a country, between urban and rural areas and between different regions, depending on variations in socioeconomic status and access to health care. The conclusion is that when health indicators are used to assess the development of countries precautions must be taken because the method of collection used in most low

and middle-income countries results in varying degree of uncertainty. For many countries the uncertainty is relatively small and the available data are therefore most useful. For a few countries, especially very poor and war-torn countries, the uncertainty is very wide and the data is only available for a few indicators. For some health indicators, such as maternal mortality rate, the numbers for most countries have an uncertainty of up to plus/minus 50% (Hill 2001).

In the year 2000 WHO began to publish the uncertainty interval for some health indicators. Most country health indicators are unfortunately still published without any information about the uncertainty and usually without stating the method of data collection used in each country. It is therefore difficult to judge the level of uncertainty of the data and when making comparisons it is not fruitful to look at exact figures but rather in what range the indicators lie for each country. Whether the life expectancy is 45 or 65 years is interesting, but not whether it is exactly 64 or 66 years. One could say that most of the available data on major health indicators is useful for almost all countries in spite of varying degree of uncertainty. Cautious conclusions can be made about the general trend of the state of health in the countries of the world, but we should refrain from making detailed comparisons and ranking between countries that have almost the same value for an indicator.

Table 3.1 World Health progress over the last 40 years.

World Indicators	1960	2002
Infant mortality rate	126	56
Under 5 Mortality Rate	197	82
Life Expectancy	48	63
Total Fertility Rate	5.0	2.8
Maternal mortality ratio	...	400
Crude death rate	17	9
Crude birth rate	36	22
Population Growth Rate	2.0 (1965–1980)	1.5 (1990–2002)

Source: State of the Worlds Children; UNICEF 1997 and 2004.

This chapter explains the most useful health and demographic indicators that are needed for judgement of the health profile of a country. Most of the selected indicators are shown in Table 3.1. To these have recently been added disability-adjusted life years (DALYs), which measure the combined effect of mortality and disability of specific diseases. We also explain the measures of disease occurrence as well as anthropometrical indicators used to assess nutritional status. These numeric indicators constitute the basis for any understanding of the national health and demographic development of any country. By studying table 3.1, you will see the extraordinary positive gain the world has made in improved health status over the last 40 years!

3.1 Infant mortality rate

The annual number of children less than one year of age who die per 1 000 live births.

There has been an impressive decrease in infant mortality rates worldwide over the last half century. The infant mortality rate in the world in 2002 was estimated at 56 per 1 000 live births, less than half of the estimated rate of 126 per 1 000 live births in 1960. The reported infant mortality rates for countries today vary between 3 and 165 per 1 000 live-born babies. In 2002, the average infant mortality rate was 106 per 1 000 live births for Sub-Saharan Africa, 70 for South Asia, 46 for the Middle East and North Africa, 33 for East Asia and the Pacific, 27 in Latin America and the Caribbean, 33 in the former socialist countries of Europe and only 5 per 1 000 live births in the high-income countries (UNICEF 2004).

Each year an estimated 7.5 million children die during their first year of life in the world. Infant mortality can be divided into neonatal and post neonatal mortality (figure 3.1). The neonatal period stretches from birth to the 28th day of life. Survival is in this period highly dependent on the care of the mother during pregnancy, delivery and the postpartum period. After the 28th day, the main factors that determine survival are safe environment, good feeding practices and the quality of care. As the infant mortality rate in a country decreases, a greater and greater proportion of the infant mortality occurs in the neonatal period. The most common global causes of infant deaths in the neonatal period are pre-term delivery, birth asphyxia, infections and congenital malformations. These neonatal conditions cause most of the infant deaths in high-income countries. In the richest countries preterm babies down to 23 weeks of gestation today survive with high technology care—of course at very high costs.

The causes of post-neonatal mortality are mainly dependent on socio-economic, environmental, nutritional and care issues. As a country develops, living standards and nutritional status in the population improve and the infant mortality rate decreases. With enough political will to adhere to an appropriate evidence-based health policy, all middle-income countries could reduce the infant mortality rate to 50 per 1 000 live births. The policy should include literacy campaigns, primary education, safe water and sanitation, immunisation programmes, basic primary health care, health education, including promotion of breastfeeding and good weaning practices.

About 4 million stillbirths (deaths of the foetus before birth) occur worldwide every year. Of these, half are caused by complications during labour and delivery. These deaths are not included in the infant mortality rate, but they are included in the perinatal mortality. *Perinatal mortality* is defined as the total number of deaths of the foetus from a gestational age of 22 weeks to the seventh day of life of the newborn (figure 3.1). Perinatal disorders include preterm delivery, asphyxia, congenital anomalies, obstetric trauma and severe bacterial infection, including sepsis and meningitis. Chapter 9

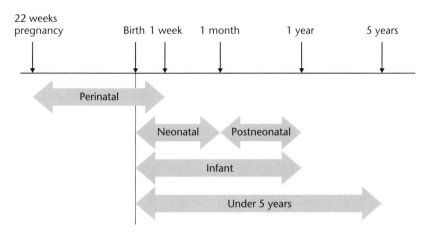

Figure 3.1 Definitions of childhood mortality.

discusses the causes of perinatal morbidity and mortality further. To care for newborn children after birth, a few basic factors are more vital than others: warmth, cleanliness, early and exclusive breastfeeding, eye care, and immunisation. It is also important to establish the early recognition and prompt treatment of infections (WHO 1998). With these few simple measures and with basic obstetric care, the majority of the perinatal and neonatal mortality in the world could be prevented.

The infant mortality rate is not only the most used health indicator but it is also widely used as a general indicator of the socio-economic development of a country. The reason being that rapidly growing infants are in the most vulnerable stage of life and their survival depends on a range of socio-economic factors (see chapter 2).

3.2 Under-five mortality rate

> *The annual number of children dying between birth and exactly five years of age, expressed per 1 000 live births.*

The world under-five mortality rate, like the infant mortality rate, is improving (Figure 3.2). It is currently estimated at 82 per 1 000 live births, a decline from 197 in 1960. In 1960, about 21 million children throughout the world died each year before their fifth birthday. In 2001, it is estimated that 10.4 million children died before their fifth birthday. It is estimated that national under-five mortality rates varied from 20 to 375 per 1 000 live births in 1960, and in 2002 it varied from 3 to 284 between the countries of the world (UNICEF 1998 and 2004).

Sub-Saharan Africa had the highest mean under-five mortality rate, amounting to 174 per 1 000 live births in 2002, followed by South Asia 97, the Middle East and North Africa 58, East Asia and the Pacific 43, Latin America and the Caribbean 34, and the formerly socialist countries of Europe 41. The high-income countries have a mean under-five mortality rate as low as 7 per 1 000 live births. There are great disparities between countries on the same continent. In 2021 the under-five mortality rate was 11 in Costa Rica and 41 in Nicaragua, 19 in Sri Lanka and 93 in neighbouring India, 67 in Namibia and 260 in Angola. Within countries, the under-five mortality rate differs between social groups in almost every society of the world.

As mentioned before, 10.4 million children die before reaching their fifth birth-

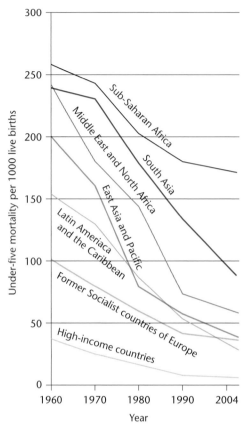

Figure 3.2 Trends in under-five mortality by region 1960–2002.

Source: State of the World's Children. UNICEF. 2006.

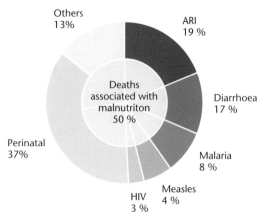

Figure 3.3 Major causes of death among children under five, worldwide, 2003.

Source: Bryce, 2005.

age are mainly accidents and late effects of congenital disorders.

Under-five mortality rate is more and more frequently used as an aggregate measure of overall socio-economic development of a country or a population group. The reason is that under-five mortality, even more than infant mortality, depends on socio-economic factors such as female education, access to preventive and curative health services, quality of water supply and sanitation, food security and diet. When living conditions improve, the incidence of death between one and four years decreases faster

day. The main direct causes are acute respiratory infection, diarrhoea, malaria, measles, malnutrition and perinatal disorders (Figure 3.3, Table 3.2). Malnutrition is also an important underlying cause of almost all other conditions causing child mortality. Of the global under-five mortality rate, about 70% is constituted by the infant mortality rate, which is to say that the majority of all deaths in children less than 5 years old occur during the first year. When child survival improves, the infant mortality rate gradually increases to constitute a greater part of the under-five mortality rate. In high-income countries the remaining causes of deaths in the period 1–4 years of

Table 3.2 The most common disease conditions causing Under-Five-Mortality* in 2001.

Acute respiratory infection	2.0 million
Diarrhoea	1.4 million
Measles	0.5 million
Malaria	0.9 million
Perinatal disorders	2.4 million
HIV	0.3 million
Other	2.9 million)
TOTAL:	10.4 million

* Annual number of children dying between birth and exactly 5 years of age expressed per 1 000 live births.

Source: Unicef, State of World's children 2004.

than the infant mortality rate. In Sweden, for example, the number of deaths between 1 and 4 years has been reduced almost to zero, while there are still 3 per 1 000 live births who die in the first year mostly due to pre-term delivery or malformation.

3.3 Life expectancy at birth

The number of years a newborn baby would live if subjected to the present mortality risks prevailing for each age group in the population.

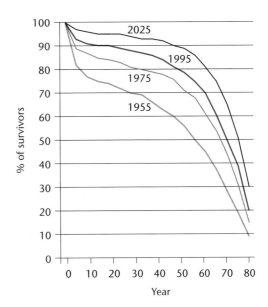

Figure 3.4 Survival curves for the world 1955–2025.

Source: World Health Report, WHO. 1999.

The worldwide life expectancy at birth is estimated to be 63 years. It was estimated to be 48 years in 1960 and is calculated to rise to 73 years by the year 2025. Regional differences in life expectancy at birth are great. Sub-Saharan Africa has the lowest life expectancy, 46 years. The high-income countries had an average of 78 years in 2002. Japan has the longest life expectancy, at an average of 81 years, partly explained by the healthy Japanese diet. Zambia and Sierra Leone are today countries with the lowest life expectancy at birth, around 35 years. The main reasons are poverty, together with AIDS and consequences of war, respectively.

As for child and infant mortality rates, life expectancy is an indicator of socio-economic development, and indeed they are

linked to each other. The survival curves in figure 3.4 show that much of the remarkable improvement in life expectancy is caused by the improved child survival in the world.

The definition of life expectancy at birth mentioned above is a complex calculation. Another, more simple way of explaining life expectancy at birth is: "the average number of years that would be lived by those born today if the current risk of dying at each age were to persist throughout their whole life".

Table 3.3 Life Expectancy by region in 1970 and 2002.

Region	Life expectancy in 1970	Life expectancy in 2002
Sub-Saharan Africa	44	46
Middle East and North Africa	51	67
South Asia	48	63
East Africa and Pacific	58	69
Latin America and the Caribbean	60	70
CEE/CIS and Baltic States	66	69
High income countries	72	78

Source: State of the World's Children, UNICEF 2004.

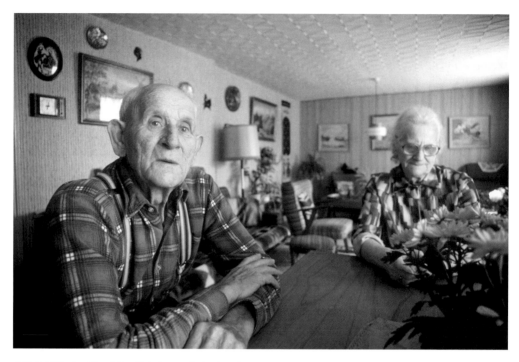

DENMARK, the island Fur. Elderly couple in their home.
© Jørn Stjerneklar/PHOENIX.

Life expectancy can also be calculated at other ages than at birth. Life expectancy at age 15 can be used to understand adult mortality. Life expectancy at 65 measures the changing conditions among the elderly in a country. Life expectancy is sensitive to social change, since the death rates in all age groups are included. Often, but not always, life expectancy co-varies with child survival rates.

Male and female life expectancy figures differ globally. In most countries in the world, women live longer than men (see also chapter 2 on gender). Russia has seen a drastic decrease in the life expectancy at birth for males over the last fifteen years. This has been due mainly to an increased use of alcohol and tobacco, and reflects the changing life conditions in Russia that results in increased rates of cardiovascular disease, suicide and accidents involving alcohol.

The size of the elderly population is increasing all over the world. With socio-economic and medical advancements, people not only live a longer life, but a healthier life as well. In the high-income countries, 13 % of the population, representing 135 million people, are over the age of 65 years, and 35 million are over the age of 80 (UNDP 1998). This success challenges the capacity of the health and social service system to provide good care for the elderly. However, with an increased life expectancy in most parts of the world, not only the rich nations of the world are experiencing an ageing of their population. In 2025, it is estimated that more than 800 million people in the world will be older than 65 years, and of these 65 % will be living in low and middle-income countries (WHO 1998).

3.4   Disease occurrence

> *Prevalence: The proportion of a popula-*
> *tion affected by a disease at a given point*
> *in time*
>
> *Incidence: Number of new cases of a dis-*
> *ease in a population during a specified*
> *time period*

So far this chapter has described the most useful summary health indicators. Before we go on to the demographic indicators, we will describe the most basic measures of occurrences of specific diseases; prevalence and incidence. *Prevalence* is the proportion of a certain disease in a given population, usually at a specific date or another given point in time. One example is the prevalence of tuberculosis in a village which is the number of cases of tuberculosis in the village at a certain point in time divided by the total number of persons in that village at the same point in time.

Incidence is the number of new cases of a disease occurring during a set time interval in a certain population. The incidence of tuberculosis in a village is the number of new cases of tuberculosis in the village during one year divided by the total number of persons in the village in the middle of that year. These two basic measures are related to each other and to the duration of the disease. A disease with very short duration can have high incidence and yet low prevalence. In contrast a disease with life long duration may have high prevalence but a low incidence. The relationship between incidence, duration and prevalence is as follows:

Incidence × duration = prevalence

By way of example, diarrhoeal episodes may have a high incidence in Uganda, i.e. many people fall ill during a year. However, most will have recovered in about one week, and the prevalence of diarrhoea will never be high. In contrast, the incidence of HIV is relatively low in Uganda, but the prevalence of HIV is high since HIV is a lifelong infection.

In high-income countries the prevalence of HIV is now increasing because the anti-ret-roviral treatment is so effective that few of those infected die of AIDS. As treatment increases the duration of the disease it will result in higher prevalence even in the absence of increase in incidence.

3.5   Maternal mortality ratio

> *Number of deaths of women from preg-*
> *nancy-related causes per 100 000 live*
> *births*

Around 500 000 women die of pregnancy-related causes throughout the world each year. These deaths occur almost exclusively in the low- and middle-income countries, as modern gynaecological and obstetric services have brought mortality to almost zero in high-income countries. The *Maternal mortality ratio* expresses the number of maternal deaths per 100 000 live births. This ratio (MMR) measures the risk of death among pregnant and recently delivered women. The strength of this measure is that it expresses the quality of pregnancy care and delivery care, 'safe motherhood'. MMR is not sensitive to fluctuations in fertility. Though very important for health policy this is an indicator that is presently measured with considerable uncertainty in most countries. The worldwide maternal mortality ratio is estimated to be 397 with a lower and upper uncertainty interval of 234 and 635, respectively, deaths per 100 000 live births.

Another measure used is the *maternal mortality rate*, which expresses the number of maternal deaths per year per 100 000 women aged 15–49. This expression, which is rarely used, reflects both the risk of death among pregnant and recently delivered women and the proportion of all women to become pregnant in a given year. It can consequently be reduced either by making pregnancies safer (like the maternal mortality ratio) or by lowering fertility. It measures the contribution of maternal mortality to the overall mortality among women of reproductive age.

Observe the difference between rate and ratio. Ratio is the value obtained by dividing one quantity by another: a general term of which is proportion. Rate is the value obtained by division when time is an element of the denominator. In this context ratio tells the proportion of 100 000 pregnant women that will die and the rate is how many pregnant women that will die during a year per 100 000 women in the reproductive age group.

Maternal mortality is difficult to estimate, especially in the countries with the highest mortality. Firstly, it is a comparatively rare event, since it typically occurs in only 0.5–1.5 % of deliveries even in low-income countries. Secondly, deaths related to sexuality and reproduction tend to be stigmatising events (e.g., clandestine abortions). Therefore, reporting is often incomplete, and under-registration a common problem. Thirdly, the denominator when maternal mortality is estimated would ideally be 'number of pregnant women', but this is impossible to calculate with any certainty. The convention is therefore to define a 'proxy denominator', which implies that the maternal mortality ratio is the quotient (ratio) between 'number of maternal deaths' in the numerator and 100 000 live-born babies in the denominator. The desire to assess changes in maternal mortality is hampered by the above-mentioned uncertainties. It has recently been estimated by Hill (2001) that the uncertainty of maternal mortality ratios for most low and middle-income countries are so wide that this indicator is useless for monitoring improvements in maternal health in periods less than a decade.

Instead of using an *outcome indicator*, such as maternal mortality ratio, to evaluate health programmes, a number of *process indicators* have been defined. The process indicators reflect access to and quality of care of pregnant women. Although the process in-dicator does not reflect the outcome of the care they are still preferred for monitoring because much better data is available for the process indicators. The most used process indicators are the assistance of a skilled attendant at delivery, trends in coverage of antenatal or delivery care, percentage of all deliveries in which caesarean section is carried out, and the percentage of women dying from a predefined disease affecting a pregnant woman. In a given setting, hospital or health unit, process indicators are more reliable as an expression of improvement of maternity care. Still, there is a need to make careful studies at the community level of the maternal mortality ratio. They should be carried out at long intervals, since they are costly and yet yield results with wide uncertainties. In most low and middle-income countries it is only meaningful to measure maternal mortality at five to ten year intervals.

Lifetime risk of maternal death measures the risk of maternal death over a woman's entire reproductive life span and is related to the total number of pregnancies. As a consequence of high infant and child mortality, the total fertility rate tends to be high for two principal reasons. Firstly, there is a psychological replacement effect aiming at substituting the loss of a child with a new pregnancy. Secondly, there is an endocrine effect: when a breastfed infant/child dies, the sucking stimulus on the nipple stops, with an ensuing reduction in circulating prolactin. Such a reduction implies return of ovulation, enhanced fertility and a probable new pregnancy. The final result is that the lifetime number of pregnancies tends to increase in societies with high infant and child mortality. The lifetime risk of maternal death is then increased, and the number of pregnancies per lifetime should multiply the individual risk associated with each pregnancy. In the least developed countries, the lifetime risk may be as high as one in ten, whereas in Northern Europe it is in the order of one in 10 000.

The global variation of national maternal mortality ratio (MMR) is even greater than that of infant and under-five mortality. The 2002 maternal mortality ratio was estimated at 2 000 /100 000 live births in Sierra Leone, meaning that one woman died per 50 births. The regional differences are great, from Sub-Saharan Africa 940/100 000 live births and 560 in South Asia, to 110 in East Asia and Pacific and 13 in high-income countries (UNICEF 2004).

Maternal mortality ratios have decreased enormously in Western European countries in the last 200 years. In Sweden, the decline started around 1750, with the ratio falling from 1 000 to 500 per 100 000 live births by 1850, and now being less than 5 per 100 000 live births. The major determinants for this decline were better obstetric practices, improved hygiene and nutrition, and declining fertility rates. Pregnancy-related mortality constitutes an important part of adult female mortality in low-income countries, but not the major part. In a typical Sub-Saharan population of 100 000 persons, around 4 000 children will be born each year. Around 500 of these children will die, as compared to around 40 women that will die of a pregnancy-related cause. The causes of maternal mortality are further elaborated in chapter 9.

3.6 Disability-adjusted life years (DALY)

> *A comprehensive indicator including both losses of healthy years due to disability and premature death*

Disability-adjusted life years (DALY) is an indicator that measures the disease burden in a population, taking into account not only premature mortality but also disability caused by disease or injury. Murray and Lopez (1994) developed the measure for their study on the Global Burden of Diseases. The DALY measure is used to present the health impact of all diseases and injuries

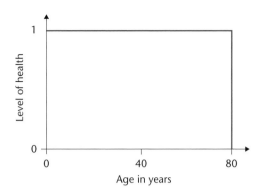

Figure 3.5 *Presentation of a life in full health until sudden death at the age of 80 years.*

Source: Stefan Peterson, Karolinska Institutet, Stockholm.

in a standardised and comparable way. This increased the validity of comparisons of the burden of different diseases between world regions and countries over time. In fact, the World Bank and the World Health Organization were the first to use the DALY measures to compare the burden of disease in different regions of the world and thereby the value of different health interventions (World Bank 1993). It became possible to estimate and compare the cost of avoiding the loss of a DALY for each intervention.

The method uses 107 diagnoses, covering all conceivable causes of death and 95 % of all possible causes of disability. As a basis for the DALY measure, a 'gold standard', or most desirable life, is defined as living in a completely healthy state until death at age around 80 years. Perfect health is 1 and death is 0 on the DALY diagram shown in figure 3.5.

As we all know, life is not usually like that. For each premature death, the number of years lost is counted up to 82.5 years for females and 80 years for males, which is the highest national life expectancy at birth in the world, i.e. Japan. For example, if a man dies in a car accident at 20 years of age (80–20 years); 60 years are lost due to this premature death. Such a measure of premature deaths in number of years lost is known as "years of life lost" (YLL).

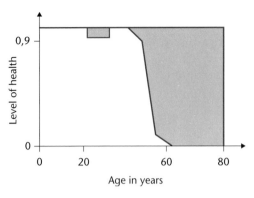

Figure 3.6 *Illustration of a person who gets a knee injury at the age of 20, recovers and later gets disabled from cancer and dies at the age of 60.*

Source: Stefan Peterson; Karolinska Institutet, Stockholm.

Injury and disease cause not only deaths but also varying time periods with morbidity and disability. The time period in years that is lived with a disability due to each disease is also added to the DALY measure. The disability is measured in length in years and in severity. Severity weights have been appointed for each disabling condition on a scale from one to zero. Schizophrenia was given a weighted severity loss of 0.8, whereas the common cold only causes a loss of 0.007. The disability severity weight for each disease reflects the average degree of disability a person suffers with each condition. Panels of healthy experts with knowledge about disease conditions have determined the weights. The severity weight is then multiplied by the average time a person is suffering from the disability from each disease.

Let us look at an example from a person's life, in figure 3.6. This man gets a knee injury at the age of 20 with a weighted severity of 0.1. During the years he suffers from the knee injury his health is only 0.9 of the maximum of 1.0. After a few years of knee disability he is successfully operated on and recovers completely. At the age of 45 he gets cancer, which disables him more and more until he finally dies at the age of 60 years. The

hatched area in figure 3.6 represents his life years lost due to disability and early death.

Another component of the DALY measure is that years lost due to premature death or disability are given different values at different ages. These differences in values are introduced in DALY calculations by what is called 'age weights'. The age weight used in the DALY calculations is obtained from a scale where the value of a year lost rises steeply from zero at birth to a maximum at 25 years of age, and then decreases progressively in older ages (Figure 3.7). This means that if a newborn girl dies, 32.5 DALYs are lost, if she dies at age 30 years, 29 DALYs are lost, and at age 60 years, 12 DALYs are lost. For males, the above figures will be slightly lower, because their shorter life expectancy is taken into consideration. Finally, the years lost in the future are discounted, so that years lost now are worth more than years lost in the future. This is a standard procedure in economics and in the DALY calculations a discount rate of 3 % per year is used.

The innovative Global Burden of Disease study calculated the total sum of the combined loss of all premature deaths that occurred in the world in 1990 and the loss of healthy life from disability in future years from specific diseases arising in that year (Murray 1994). The study used all possible data sources of recorded causes of death and

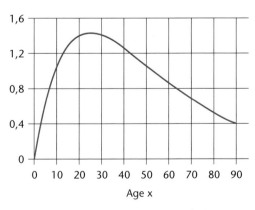

Figure 3.7 *Age weights in the DALY calculations.*

Source: World Bank; World Development Report, 1993.

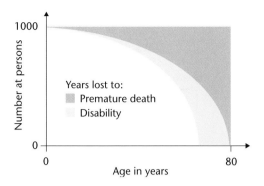

Figure 3.8 Illustrations of DALYs lost due to premature death and disability by a large population.

Source: Stefan Peterson; Karolinska Institutet, Stockholm.

prevalence and incidence of disease, as well as expert judgement when data were not available. By adding all the DALY's lost for a certain disease in a defined population, the DALY curve looks like the example in figure 3.8.

The DALY measure has been criticised because of the four built-in social preferences. These are (1) different weights for sexes, (2) different age weights, (3) discounting future years lost and (4) severity weighting of disabilities. Many argue that life years for men and women should be given the same weight. However, as has been described above the difference is small and only gives a slightly greater value for diseases that affects females. Some people argue that all years lost should be given the same value independently of the age at which the years are lost. Others argue that discounting years is wrong, because they value years now and in the future equally. In a complex measure like DALY, the built-in social preferences may conceal issues of inequity. However, sensitivity analysis has shown that the results of the Global Burden of Disease study are not greatly affected by these social preferences. Another problem is that the Global Burden of Disease study calculates DALY on data, which on some continents are of poor quality. Especially for the disability calculations, the data is of varied quality in different regions and for different disease conditions.

But bearing all these inherent weaknesses in mind, DALY is still an interesting measure, because it is the first comprehensive attempt made to summarise the world's burden of injury, disease and premature death. It has initiated a debate and new research to find even better complex indicators for global comparisons (Murray 2002). The DALY measure is useful to describe the disease burden across the world and to make projections for the future. At present, many countries are exploring the possibility of using DALYs as a measure of trends in disease burden and as a tool for cost-effectiveness studies and priority setting. The main results from the Global Burden of Disease study are presented in chapter 4.

Since Murray and Lopez moved to work at the WHO in 1999, WHO has started to include the DALY measure in their annual report. This allows for refinement of the results from the initial study because of new health data. From the year 2000, they also included a DALE, disability-adjusted life expectancy, which was renamed as the more cheery HALE, health-adjusted life expectancy, in 2002. This measure is based on life expectancy at birth, but includes an adjustment for the time spent in poor health. It is the equivalent of the number of years a newborn can expect to live in full health, based on current statistics of mortality and morbidity. In Japan, for instance, the HALE is 72 years, while in Afghanistan only 35 years. Many find this a measure that is instinctively easier to understand compared to DALY.

3.7 Total fertility rate

The number of children that would be born per woman if she were to live to the end of her childbearing years and bear children at each age in accordance with the prevailing age-specific fertility rates

The fertility rate measures how many children an average woman would give birth to if all through her own reproductive age pe-

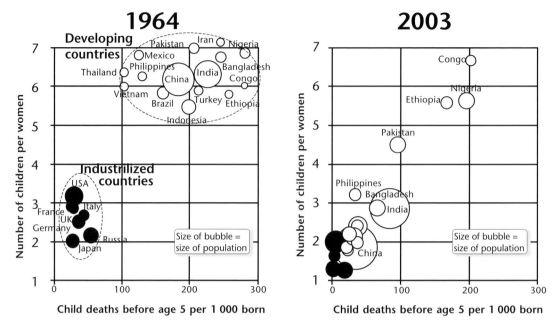

Figure 3.9 Changes in fertility rate and child in 22 countries with > 50 million people.
(See in moving graphics with all countries at www.gapminder.org)

riod she was to give birth each year at the rate of women in her country for a particular year.

If the total fertility rate is 2.1, the population is replacing itself, meaning that one man and one woman replace themselves with the same number of individuals in the course of their reproductive career. If all women on earth had a total fertility rate of 2.1, there would be no population growth. Unlike the crude birth rate, the total fertility rate is not affected by the age structure of the population. This makes total fertility rate more relevant for comparison of fertility across countries and times, whereas crude birth rate is needed for calculation of population growth rate.

The total fertility rate in the world has decreased dramatically from 5.0 in 1955 to 4.2 in 1975 and 2.8 in 2002. It is estimated to decrease further to 2.3 in 2025 (WHO 98, UNICEF 2004). Today, Sub-Saharan Africa is at the top of the list, with 5.5 children per

woman, as against 3.5 in the Middle East and North Africa, 3.4 in South Asia, 2.6 in Latin America and the Caribbean, 2.0 in East Asia and the Pacific, 1.7 in the former socialist countries of Europe and 1.7 in high-income countries. In all of these regions the fertility rates continue to decrease.

It is remarkable to see that all over the world the decreasing trend in under-five mortality rates occurs along with a decreasing trend in total fertility rates. This trend is created not in a straight causation chain but as a web of factors that affect both child survival and fertility. However, most scientists agree that a decline in child mortality precedes a decline in fertility, because mothers must be confident that their children will survive before they will go for two child families (Figure 3.9).

3.8 Crude birth rate

> *Number of births per 1 000 population during one year.*

The total number of births in the world in 2002 was about 130 million. The crude birth rate in the world is 22 births per 1 000 people per year, a decrease from 33 in 1970. The crude birth rate varies between the countries of the world from 8 children born per 1 000 population to 53 per 1 000 population. The sub-Saharan region has the highest figure, 41 births per 1 000 population. Middle East and North Africa has 27 per 1 000 population, South Asia 26, Latin America and the Caribbean 22, East Asia and the Pacific 17, the former socialist countries of Europe 13 and the high-income countries 12 (Table 3.4).

Crude birth rates have declined in all regions of the world over the last 30 years. In Sub-Saharan Africa, that decline has been the slowest, only from 48 to 41, while in East Asia and the Pacific region, the decline was from 35 to 17 in the same time interval. In 2002, many of the former Socialist countries of Eastern Europe and central Asia, Sweden, Switzerland, Austria, Greece, Italy and Germany had a crude death rate higher than crude birth rate, causing a negative population growth if immigration is insufficient to compensate. All other countries had higher birth than death rates.

Crude birth rate is dependent on the age structure of the population. A population with a large proportion in the childbearing age naturally has a higher crude birth rate than a population with predominance of either children or people beyond fertile age. So the high crude birth rate in Africa arises from the combination of high fertility and a young age structure.

3.9 Crude death rate

> *Number of deaths per 1 000 population during one year.*

On a global scale, crude death rate varies from 2 to around 20 per 1 000 population. The total number of deaths in the world in 2002 was about 57 million (WHO 2004). Sub-Saharan Africa has the highest crude death rate in the world, with 18 deaths per 1 000 population per year, but this still represents a decline from 21 in 1970. Crude death rates in the Middle East and North Africa regions were 17 in 1970 and 6 in 2002. During the same time period, crude death rate declined from 18 to 9 in South Asia, from 11 to 7 in East Asia and the Pacific, from 10 to 6 in Latin America and the Caribbean, and from 10 to 9 in the high-income countries, but increased from 9 to 11 in the former socialist countries of Europe (UNICEF 2003).

In refugee camps, the crude death rate is a useful indicator of the adequacy of emergency interventions. It is easy to calculate,

Table 3.4 Crude birth rate, crude death rate by region in 2002.

Region	Crude birth rate	Crude death rate
Sub-Saharan Africa	41	18
Middle East and North Africa	27	6
South Asia	26	9
East Asia and Pacific	17	7
Latin America and the Caribbean	22	6
CEE/CIS and Baltic States	13	11
High Income countries	12	9

Source: State of the World's Children, UNICEF, 2004.

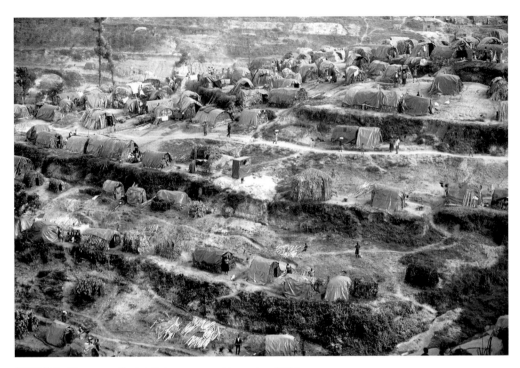

RWANDA, Gikongoro district. Refugee camp. November 1994.
© Trygve Bølstad/PHOENIX.

the total number of deaths during one year divided by the total population times 1 000, to get number of deaths per 1 000 population. Crude death rate is also sensitive to changing conditions in the life of the refugees, for example if a cholera epidemic has started. Since the health situation may change very rapidly in a refugee camp, death rates are mostly measured as the number of deaths per 10 000 populations *per day*. A decrease in crude death rate is always good in a high-mortality population.

Cause-specific death rates may also be useful for planning interventions. If, for example, there is an increase in death rate from diarrhoeal disease, one has to find out whether the deaths are caused by cholera, shigellosis or ordinary diarrhoea, and then plan to isolate and treat the patients correctly and try to discover and eliminate the source of contamination.

The highest crude death rate ever measured and published in modern times was

found in 1994 following the genocide in Rwanda among the population in the refugee camps of Goma in the present Democratic Republic of Congo. The reason was a cholera epidemic on top of the other sufferings of the refugees. The crude death rate was as high as 43 per 10 000 population per day (Paquet 1994). The regular death rate in Rwanda of 20 per 1 000 population per year corresponds to 200 deaths per 10 000 population per 365 days, about 0.5 deaths per 10 000 population per day. This means that the death rates had increased 80-fold among the refugees.

The risk of death varies with age. The highest age-specific death rates in life are seen in the first week of life, and especially the first 24 hours, and then above the age of 65 years, increasing progressively in older age (Figure 3.4). Because of this the crude death rate is very dependent on the age composition of the population. This is why crude death rate is a useless health indicator

Table 3.5 Crude death rate and Crude birth rate in United Arab Emirate and Sweden in 2002.

	Crude death rate	Crude birth rate	Life expectancy
United Arab Emirate	2	17	75
Sweden	11	10	80

Source: State of the World's Children, UNICEF 2004.

for international comparisons, as illustrated by the example of Sweden and the United Arab Emirates, in Table 3.5.

The United Arab Emirates have a crude death rate of 2 per 1 000 population, a decrease from 12 per 1 000 in 1970. Sweden has had an increase in crude death rate from 10 to 11 per 1 000 population since 1970. Does this mean that the risk of dying is lower in the United Arab Emirates than in Sweden? If the two population pyramids in the two countries are compared, one can see that the United Arab Emirates have a more broad-based population pyramid, meaning that the population is younger than in Sweden. In the United Arab Emirates the health has improved immensely because of a good economy and because the country has put efforts into developing the education system and the health services. With social and medical advancements, the health has improved but the risk of dying is not lower in any age group in UAE than it is in Sweden. The reason for the low crude death rate is only a different population composition with very few old people. In Sweden, where a large proportion of the population is over 65 years of age, the crude death rate is higher; because of a large proportion of the population belong to age groups where the risk of death is higher (Figure 3.10).

In conclusion, as a country experiences a positive socio-economic development, with increasing life expectancy and falling fertility rates, crude death rate will gradually fall from 30 per 1 000 to less than 5 death per

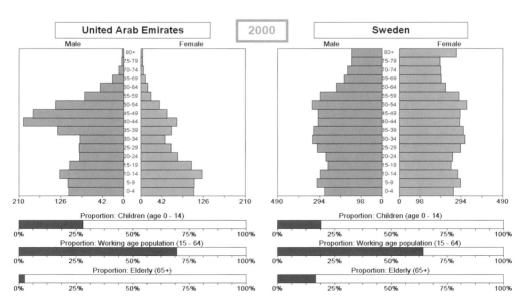

Figure 3.10 The population pyramides of Sweden and United Arab Emirate 2000.
Source: UN statistics 1996.

1 000 population. When the population pyramid changes to a less broad based distribution, the crude death rate will increase to around 10 per 1 000 population, despite continued improved life expectancy. Therefore, the crude death rate is useless as a health indicator for international comparisons.

3.10 Population growth rate

Growth of the population size in one year expressed in percent.

The annual population growth rate in percent between 1990 and 2002 varied globally from –1.4 % in Estonia to +4.2 % in Afghanistan. In shorter time periods, the variation in growth rate can be even greater. The world population growth rate was estimated at 1.5 % between 1990–2002, a decline from 1.8 % for the period 1970–1990. The regional differences in annual population growth rate are large (Figure 3.11).

The annual population growth rate in a country depends on three factors: death rates, birth rates and migration. Underlying these factors is a complex web of cultural, environmental and socio-economic factors like child survival, access to family planning, literacy rate, the status of women in society, etc. The speed of growth is better appreciated by calculating the doubling time at present growth rate. The doubling time of a population can be rapidly estimated from the equation

$$\frac{69}{\text{Annual population growth rate in \%}}$$

For example, Zimbabwe had an annual growth rate of 3.0 % between 1980 and 1996. 69/3 = 23, meaning that the population in Zimbabwe is doubling from 11 million to 22 million in about 23 years, if nothing happens to birth rate, death rate or migration. The doubling time concept is

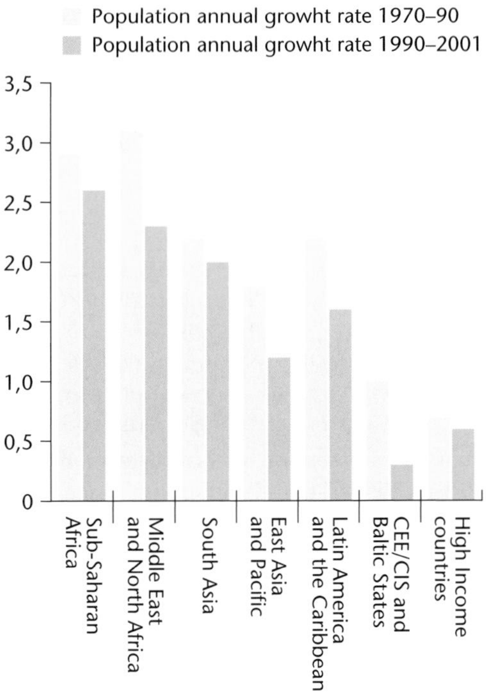

Population annual growht rate 1970–90
Population annual growht rate 1990–2001

Figure 3.11 Population annual growth rate by region between 1970–1990 and 1990–2000.

Source: State of the World's Children. UNICEF, 2003.

therefore useful to understand the force in population growth but it does not constitute an exact prognosis (see chapter 10).

One way of depicting foreseeable population growth is to plot the population pyramids of a country or region. When the pyramid has a large base, there is a high fertility. In contrast, high-income countries have a small base, and since survival is larger at all ages, the pyramid only slowly diminishes with higher ages.

3.11 Anthropometrical indicators

The most used method for the assessment of under or over nutrition in a population is to measure the size of the body of a representative sample of individuals from a specific age and gender group (Gibson 1990). The measurement of body size is called anthropometry. The word means 'to measure man', from Greek *anthropos = man* and *metrein = to measure*. In its simplest form it includes the measurement of the body weight and the body height. In adults over 18 years of age, the aim is to assess if the subject is thin, ordinary or overweight by comparing the weight with the height of the subject. This is done by combining these two measurements in the indicator called 'Body Mass Index' (BMI), which is a measurement of the shape of the body. The proportion of the population with a BMI below and above the normal range becomes the indicator of under and over nutrition.

Anthropometry in children is more demanding than in adults, because two aspects must be evaluated. First, just as with the adults the proportion of children with a body shape that is thin, ordinary or overweight. Second, the proportion of children that have normal and abnormal growth performance, respectively. Growth is specific to children. The difficulty with measurement of growth is that the child must be compared with a group of 'healthy' children of the same age and sex. A thin child is said to be *wasted* and the phenomenon is generally called *wasting*. If a child has impaired growth, she/he is said to be *stunted* and the phenomenon is known as *stunting*. The joint effect of stunting and wasting is that the child weighs less than normal for its sex and age and this is referred to as *underweight*.

Whenever anthropometric surveys of children are done, it should be made clear whether the objective is to assess shape or growth or perhaps both of these characteristics. With the basic measurements of a child, weight, height, age and sex, three major anthropometric indices can be calculated using for example free software called *Epi Info 2002*.[1]

3.11.1 Body mass index (BMI)

> *Proportion of overweight adults:*
> *% with BMI (kg/height in m^2) > 25*
>
> *Proportion of underweight adults:*
> *% with BMI (kg/height in m^2) < 18.5*

BMI is the most used anthropometric indicator of nutritional status in adults. It is calculated as the weight in kilograms divided by the height in metres squared. The BMI value reflects the balance between dietary energy intake and physical activity during the last few months or several years. Diseases that affect digestion and metabolism as well as infectious diseases that put extra energy demand on the body also influence BMI. Therefore BMI cannot distinguish between a person that is thin due to lack of food, due to AIDS or due to both.

Adults with a BMI between 18.5 and 25 tend to have fewer diseases and to live longer than persons with a lower or higher BMI. A person who is unhealthily thin is said to be *wasted,* and the phenomenon is generally known as *wasting*. In contrast, a

[1] www.cdc.gov

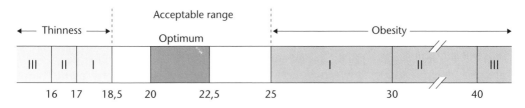

Figure 3.12 A schematic diagram outlining the optimum range of BMI and the cut-offs for warning grades of thinness and obesity.

Source: TALC, Teaching – aids at Low Cost.

person who is unhealthily fat is said to be overweight or obese. A BMI >25 indicates overweight, but this is not necessarily equivalent to obesity, as athletes with great muscle mass will also have a high BMI. Overweight is usually classified as grade 1: 25–30; grade II: 30–40; or grade III: >40. If BMI is below 18.5, the risk of death increases. It has also been suggested to classify adult wasting into three grades: grade I: 17–18.5; grade II: 16–17; and grade III: <16, the last bearing the highest death risk. If the number of individuals with low BMI in a population is increasing, it is likely that there is a food shortage.

One shortcut to assessing the shape of the body is to measure the mid-upper arm circumference (MUAC), assuming that a thin arm accompanies a thin body. This is quicker, but may still be good enough in emergency settings. It is useful for pregnant women, as the thickness of the arm is not affected by the pregnancy. It should be noted that BMI does not tell if a person or a population is tall or short. The attained height of adults is the best summary measure of life conditions during childhood and adolescence, as it is not further affected by what happens in adult life.

3.11.2 Weight-for-height (WFH), wasting in children

The proportion of wasting in children is the % of children in a specific age group with weight-for-height below –2 standard deviations of a reference group.

By relating the weight to the height of a child, an index called weight-for-height is derived. This index is often abbreviated as WFH. It is similar to body mass index and answers the question: "How thin is the child?" or "How wasted is the child?" Wasting is a condition in which a child has a low weight for its height and has lost muscle mass and fat stores. It is a sign of current and recent malnutrition or of 'over-diseasing',

meaning that the child has been frequently sick in the last weeks and months. In order to know whether a child has an acceptable weight-for-height, the index of a child must be compared with a population of 'ordinary' and 'healthy' children of the same age and sex as described below in section 3.11.3.

Mid-upper arm circumference (MUAC) is commonly used as a proxy for 'body shape', substituting for BMI in adults and weight-for-height in children. MUAC usually remains almost unchanged from the age of 1 to 5 years. The normal circumference at this age is around 16.5 cm. Below the cut-off point of 13.5 cm, the child is moderately wasted. A child with a MUAC below 12.5 cm is classified as being severely wasted.

3.11.3 Height-for-age (HFA), stunting in children

The proportion of stunting in children is the % of children in a specific age group with height-for-age below –2 standard deviations of a reference group.

If the height is related to age, the index is called height-for-age (HFA). This index assesses the child's growth performance and answers the question: "How short is the child for his age?" or "How stunted is the child?" If the child's HFA is low, he/she is classified as 'stunted'. Stunting is a condition in which the child is short for his/her age. This condition seems to reflect overall socio-economic conditions and has no immediate connection with the diet, because too many other factors also influence growth performance. It is often erroneously said to be a sign of hunger and lack of food, but stunting is mostly not caused and cannot be treated by better diet alone.

In order to know whether a child has an acceptable height-for-age, the height of the child must be compared with a population of 'healthy' children of the same age and sex. But how should one select 'ordinary, healthy children'? For a long time, it was

118

thought that each ethnic group needed its own reference or standard. However, it has been found that children from different ethnic and genetic groups grow at the same rate if they are living in 'well-to-do' circumstances. In contrast, wide differences are found within countries between the well-to-do children and the poorest children in the same ethnic and genetic group. In India the mean height in 7 year-old boys differ by more than 10cm between the upper and lower income groups. In Sweden, this socio-economic gap in height between poor and rich closed some decades ago, when children from families with low income reached the same growth performance as children in the upper income groups.

The nutrition unit at WHO co-ordinates a multi-centre study on how children grow in well-to-do groups around the globe. WHO recommend the use of an American reference database until the new data will become available as a worldwide reference. The recommended database was collected and compiled by the National Centre for Health Statistics in the United States. It is referred to as the WHO/NCHS database and is used as a reference in anthropometric studies of children around the world. When comparing a child's weight-for-height with the weight-for-height of the children of the same age and sex in the reference population, there are three mathematical ways to express any deviation: (1) Standard deviation (SD) scores are also called z-scores, (2) percent of median and (3) centiles.

Standard deviation scores (SD scores), are the best to use but a little complicated to explain. A 'normal value' is defined as a value of any of the three child anthropometric indices falling within –2 and +2 standard deviations from the median. Any value outside –2 and +2 standard deviations is considered abnormal.

The percent of median is simpler to understand. For example, a child has a height of 87cm and the median for his age is 100cm. By considering the median to be 100%, it is possible to calculate what per-

centage of median the child's height is: 87/ 100 = 87%. So the child is 87% of median in WFH. The lower cut-off used for height (HFA) is 90% and the child is thus stunted according to this definition. The cut-off used for weight (WFH and WFA) is 80%.

A third method sometimes used is the calculation of percentiles of the reference population. The cut-off for the percentile of any of the indices is usually below the 3rd centile.

A child who is below –2 SD score in WFH is wasted, and if the child is below –3 SD score or has symmetrical oedema (i.e. swelling) of the feet and legs he/she is severely wasted and in immediate danger. Such a child should be admitted to hospital where he/she can be observed, treated and fed day and night. A child that has a very low height-for-age but a normal weight-for- height has a chronic problem that must be alleviated but the child is not in urgent need for care.

3.11.4 Weight-for-age (WFA), underweight in children

> *The proportion of underweight in children is the % of children in a specific age group with weight-for-age below –2 standard deviations of a reference group.*

A third common index is derived by combining weight and age to weight-for-age, WFA. This index summarises in a way the two previous indices, the body shape and the growth performance. This index answers the question: "How underweight is the child for his/her age?" This index is easily perceived as the most straightforward as it is what is frequently done in clinical examination of sick children. However, this index is not very useful as an indicator of the health and nutritional status of a child population because it is a messy mix of wasting that is mainly linked to nutrition and stunting that is only partly linked to nutrition. In spite of this the weight for age index is unfortunately frequently used as an indicator of 'malnutrition'. This is probably because malnutrition indexes are mainly used to advocate for action rather than to analyse which action is needed. In populations where stunting rates are high, such as in India, the weight for age indicator will identify a lot of children as malnourished. A project to improve the diet in such an area is highly unlikely to influence the stunting rate and might easily be said to have failed when it is found that the stunting rate remains almost the same. In contrast an increased rate of underweight young children that have suffered the effects of a war can be almost exclusively due to increased wasting due to prevalent diarrhoea and lack of food during the previous weeks. It is usually better to separate the assessment of body stores of energy and growth performance by the two other indices: weight-for-height (WFH) for wasting and height-for-age (HFA) for stunting.

The World Health Organization has established a Global Database on Child Growth where all major surveys on child anthropometry are gathered.[1]

The percentage of wasted children (weight-for-height below –2 SD of WHO/NCHS reference value) in low-income countries ranges from 25 % in Afghanistan and 16 % in India

[1] www.who.int/nutgrowthdb

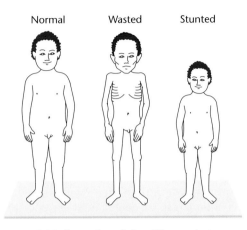

Figure 3.13 *llustration of the difference between a normal child, a wasted child and a stunted child of the same age. A child could also be simultaneously stunted and wasted. The priority for nutrition intervention is on wasted children.*

down to 1–2 % in South America. On a global basis, 10 % of children in low-income countries are wasted, which means the situation is poor. Different kinds of disasters may raise the figures dramatically in affected areas. This is a disturbing picture of under-nutrition among children under five in underprivileged populations. These children should be an important target group for any kind of nutrition intervention undertaken in these countries.

Table 3.6 *Classification of under nutrition.*

	Moderate undernutrition	**Severe undernutrition**
Symmetrical oedema	No	Yes (oedematous undernutrition)[*]
Weight-for-height		
Z-score	Between –2 and –3 Z-score	Below –3 Z-score
% of median	Between 70 to 79 %	Below 70 %
	(moderate wasting)	(severe wasting)[**]
Height-for-age		
Z-score	Between –2 and –3 Z-score	Below –3 Z-score
% of median	Between 85 to 89 %	Below 85 %
	(moderate stunting)	(severe stunting)

* This includes kwashiorkor and marasmic kwashiorkor in older classifications. However, to avoid confusion with the clinical syndrome of kwashiorkor, which includes other features, the term "oedematous malnutrition" is preferred.
** This corresponds to marasmus (without oedema) in older classifications. However, to avoid confusion, the term "severe wasting" is preferred.

Table 3.7 Global estimates for the prevalence* of wasted, stunted and underweight children in different regions 1995–2004.

Region	% wasted	% stunted	% underweight
Sub-Saharan Africa	9	38	29
Middle East and North Africa	6	21	14
South Asia	14	44	46
East Asia and Pacific	–	19	15
Latin America and the Caribbean	2	16	7
CEE/CIS and Baltic States	3	14	5
High Income countries	–	–	–

* % below –2 SD of WHO/NCHS reference value.

Source: State of the World's children, UNICEF 2006.

Stunting (height-for-age below –2 SD of WHO/NCHS reference value) is widespread among children in low-income countries. It ranges from 52 % in Afghanistan and 46 % in India to 16 % in South America. The global average prevalence of stunting among children in low-income countries is 32 %. Increasing evidence shows that stunting is associated with poor developmental attainment in young children and poor school achievement or intelligence levels in older children. The underlying causes of this growth retardation are poverty and lack of education.

3.11.5 Low birth weight

> *The proportion of newborns with low birth weight is the % of children born with a weight less than 2,500 grams.*

Low birth weight is defined as a weight less than 2,500 grams at birth, regardless of whether the child is born pre-term (i.e. before the end of the pregnancy) or not. The birth weight is strongly correlated to the chances of survival of a newborn baby. Low birth weight may be caused by low food intake and hard work by the mother during the pregnancy. It may also be caused by diseases such as malaria that have affected the mother during pregnancy or because she has suffered from physical violence. Other reasons are smoking and placental insufficiency. At the population level, low birth weight is mainly a reflection of the health, social, nutritional, and cultural status of the pregnant women. Poverty and low social status cause malnutrition in women. A woman may be working hard in the fields and have too many children, too close together, without access to fertility regulation methods. Recurrent episodes of malaria deplete her stores of iron, and her general nutritional status may be poor even before a new pregnancy. The prevalence of low birth weight varies between regions, from 30 % in South Asia, 15 % in Africa, 8 to 10 in middle-income countries and 7 % in the high-income countries. (UNICEF 2004). The strong association between poverty and low birth weight is confirmed by the fact that 95 % of all low-birth-weight babies (20 out of 21 million per year) are born in low-income countries. The fact that the proportion of low birth weight and underweight in children in South Asia is so much higher than in Africa, where infant mortality is higher, has not been well explained.

References and suggested further reading

Antonsson-Ogle B, Gustavsson O, Hambreus L, Holmgren G, Tylleskar T. Nutrition, agriculture and health when resources are scarce. 2nd revised edition. Uppsala: Uppsala University; 2000.

Bryce J et al, Can the world afford to save the lives of 6 million children each year? Lancet, Vol 365, 2005; pp. 2193–2200.

Gibson RS. Principles of Nutritional Assessment. Oxford University Press; 1990.

Hill K, AbouZahr C, Wardlaw T. Estimates of maternal mortality for 1995. Bulletin of the World Health Organization 2001;79: 182–98.

Jamison DT, Breman JG, Measham AR, Alleyne G, Claeson M, Evans DB, Jha P, Mills A, Musgrove P. Disease Control Priorities in Developing Countires. Oxford University Press, 2006.

Last JM. A Dictionary of Epidemiology. Oxford University Press; 1983.

Lopez A, Mathers CD, Ezzati M, Jamison DT, Murray CJL (eds) Global Burden of Disease and Risk Factors, Oxford University Press, 2006.

Murray CJL Quantifying the burden of disease: the technical basis for disability-adjusted life years. Bulletin of the World Health Organization 1994;72:429–445.

Murray CJL, Lopez AD, Jamison DT. The Global Burden of Disease 1990: summary results, sensitivity analysis and future directions. Bulletin of the World Health Organization 1994;72:495–509.

Murray CJL, Lopez AD. The Global Burden of Disease: A comprehensive assessment of mortality and disability from diseases, injuries, and risk factors in 1990 and projected to 2020. (Global Burden of Disease and Injury, No 1) Harvard School of Public Health, World Health Organization, World Bank 1996.

Murray CJL, Lopez AD. Global Health Statistics: A Compendium of Incidence, Prevalence and Mortality Estimates for over 200 Conditions. (Global Burden of Disease and Injury, No 2) Harvard School of Public Health, World Health Organisation, World Bank 1996.

Murray CJL, Lopez AD. Health Dimensions of Sex and Reproduction: The Global Burden of Sexually Transmitted Diseases, HIV, Maternal Conditions, Perinatal Disorders, and Congenital Anomalies. (Global Burden of Disease and Injury, No 3) Harvard School of Public Health, World Health Organisation, World Bank 1998.

Murray CJL, Salomon JA, Mathers CD, Lopez AD (eds). Summary measures of population health. WHO 2002.

Murray CJL, Lopez AD. The Global Epidemiology of Infectious Diseases (Global Burden of Disease and Injury, No 4) Harvard School of Public Health, World Health Organisation, World Bank 2003.

Murray CJL, Lopez AD. The Global Epidemiology of Non-communicable Diseases: The Epidemiology and Burdens of Cancers, Cardiovascular Diseases, Diabetes Mellitus, Respiratory Disorders, and Other Major Conditions (Global Burden of Disease and Injury, No 5) Harvard School of Public Health, World Health Organisation, World Bank 2003.

Paquet C, van Soest M. Mortality and malnutrition among Rwandan refugees in Zaire. Lancet 1994:823.

State of the World's Children. UNICEF 1997–2004.

World Bank, World Development Report 1993. Investing in Health. 1993.

WHO, World Health Report, 1998–2004 (www.who.int/whr.en).

4 Health transition

Health transition is a concept that describes the change in disease patterns that occur during socio-economic development (Omran 1971). Health transition is composed by two interlinked components: *demographic transition* and *disease transition*. The disease transition is sometimes called the epidemiological transition.

The health transition is caused by the changes in life conditions and environment that occur during development. These changes decrease the occurrence of some diseases and increase the occurrence of others, but the occurrence of diseases also change as a result of the new composition of the population. During socio-economic development the proportion of children and adolescents will fall and the proportion of old people will increase as a result of the demographic transition. The health transition starts from a disease pattern dominated by malnutrition and infectious diseases in a society with high fertility where half the population is less than 15 years of age. It proceeds gradually to a society with low fertility, where a quarter of the population is more than 65 years of age and where non-communicable diseases prevail.

The driving forces behind the health transition are socio-economic changes, welfare policies, public health actions, and cultural and behavioural changes that jointly lead to a new age distribution and a new pattern of disease in the population (Figure 4.1). Increased use of health technology may also be added but it should be noted that the access to vaccines and antibiotics occur at different stages of socio-economic development in different countries. The analysis of the different driving forces has favoured the socio-economic factors as the most important for the early health transition in West Europe (McKeown 1983). However the spectacular improvement of health in the world during the last 50 years is to a large part, perhaps up to 50 %, attributed to new health technologies.

The socio-economic development of a country may reverse during war, political conflicts and long-standing economic declines. Recent analysis has noted that achieved health improvements are surprisingly resistant to economic backlashes and deteriorations of access to medical technology. This made Murray and Chen (1993) suggest that the joint effect of socio-economic improvements, behavioural changes that favour hygiene and use and provision of health service even in difficult periods are due to accumulated "health assets" in the society. These assets are the professional and personal knowledge, skills and traditions in society that promote health and favour the needs of the vulnerable in times of scarcity. This view parallels the interpretation of multidimensional development presented in chapter 1.9.3. An example of this is when Cuba suffered a severe and prolonged economic decline during the 1990s. The background was the sudden loss of favourable trade conditions with The Soviet Union when the latter nation dissolved. The resulting economic crises resulted in some negative health effects but the child mortality and life expectancy continued to improve in Cuba throughout the decade. Another example is Sweden during the same decade when economic recession resulted in increased unemployment and budget cuts in the public health service system. In spite of

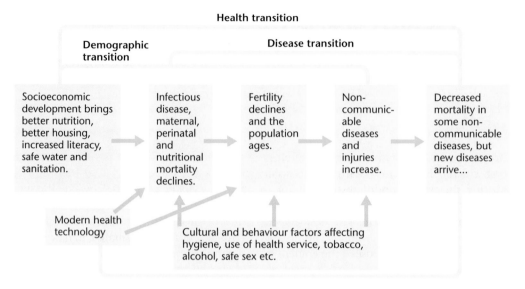

Figure 4.1 The health transition, showing the relationship between the demographic and the disease transition.

Source: Adapted from Mosely et al., 1997.

these economic difficulties the child mortality fell during the entire decade and life expectancy increased for both men and women. A third example is Sri Lanka that had suffered a prolonged civil war during the last two decades and in the same time period the formerly low child mortality has continued to fall in the country.

The health transition occurs at different times and speeds, depending on the pattern and rate of social and economic development in the country. Even within a given country, the transition often occurs at different time periods in different population groups. High-income countries, which today are post-industrial societies, are still undergoing a health transition due to changes within the group of non-communicable diseases. The earlier dominance of cardiovascular diseases and cancer is being replaced by an increasing burden of Alzheimer's disease and osteoporosis. This is both due to a decrease in the age specific incidence of the first two types of diseases and to a continued increase of the proportion of very old in the population.

The countries of the world are at very many different stages of health transition. To understand the different stages of health transition it no longer makes sense to classify countries into the two groups; industrialized and developing (see chapter 1.10). This chapter explains the reciprocal effects between general development, disease occurrence and demographic changes. We focus first on the disease transition and then the demographic transition even though they are closely interlinked. We will thereafter review the disease pattern in the world of today and point to future projections as well as discuss the future implications for the health sector in countries at different stages of socio-economic development.

4.1 Disease transition

Little is known about disease patterns in pre-agricultural societies. It is assumed that when human societies passed from living on hunting and gathering to practising agriculture as the main means of subsistence, the mortality decreased and the fertility increased. However, agriculture had its periodic failures and it made people live close together in daily contact with domestic animals. Infections and periodic hunger dominated the disease pattern. The denser population settlements in agricultural societies led to severe hygienic problems, especially when urban settlements emerged. Trade and travel over long distances formed the basis for countrywide, continental and later pandemic (the whole world) diseases. One of these epidemic diseases was plague, and wide spread epidemics are known as pestilence.

Based on the main causes of mortality in each historical period the disease transition is arbitrarily divided into four stages (Omran 1977; Olshansky 1986).

1 pestilence and famine
2 receding pandemics
3 non-communicable diseases
4 delayed degenerative diseases

Broadly speaking, these four historical stages are in the modern world represented by the dominant disease patterns in (1) collapsed countries, (2) low, (3) middle and (4) high-income countries, respectively. However, this is a didactic simplification. Many countries today have population groups that represent two, three or even all four of these stages at the same time.

4.1.1 Stage of pestilence and famine (today's collapsed countries)

At this stage in development, mortality is high and mainly determined by infectious diseases, malnutrition and pregnancy & birth related disorders. Some of the infections, such as the Plague and smallpox were spread in epidemics. Fertility rates are high, and pregnancy-related mortality is also significant. Population growth is slow or non-existent because the high fertility is counterbalanced by high mortality. During this period, life expectancy at birth fluctuates between 20 and 40 years of age.

This stage persisted in Europe until around the second half of the 18th century. Large parts of the populations in some of the least developed countries suffering from complex emergencies are still in this stage. These are "collapsed" countries (or parts of countries) such as Sierra Leone, Somalia and Afghanistan, and they may still be regarded as being in this stage of the health transition.

4.1.2 Stage of receding pandemics (today's low-income countries)

In this stage of health transition, mortality declines but fertility remains high, with a resulting exponential population growth. The life expectancy at birth is between 30 and 50 years of age. Larger epidemics become less frequent, but infectious diseases, maternal disorders and malnutrition are still the main causes of mortality.

Most of the low and middle-income countries entered this stage in the end of the 1940s. Many of the low-income countries are still at this stage today, especially those in Sub-Saharan Africa. Following the severe impact of the HIV/AIDS epidemic some countries in Africa may be considered to have reversed to the pestilence stage of health transition. Europe and North America entered the stage of receding pandemics towards the end of the 18th century and emerged from it about 100–200 years later.

It is during this stage that the major demographic changes known as the demographic transition occur. Above all, women and children benefit from the decline in mortality and fertility, since they previously suffered the greatest burden of infectious diseases and maternal complications, in combination with malnutrition.

4.1.3 Stage of non-communicable diseases (today's middle-income countries)

This stage is entered through socio-economic development, improved living conditions and targeted health interventions. With declining mortality due to infectious diseases, life expectancy at birth increases to 70 years of age and beyond. With an ageing population, the disease panorama changes from a high prevalence of infectious diseases to a greater degree of chronic and non-communicable diseases. When people survive communicable diseases, they may live long enough to contract the non-communicable diseases. As a result, the ageing population dies mainly from heart attacks and strokes, resulting from arteriosclerosis, and from other non-communicable diseases, such as diabetes, cancer and obstructive pulmonary disease. In this stage, injuries become a great public health problem.

Most middle-income countries in the world have entered this stage of the health transition now. In some middle-income countries a growing part of the population are already in the fourth stage. At the same time the more affluent parts of the population in today's low-income countries have entered into the stage dominated by non-communicable diseases.

4.1.4 Stage of delayed degenerative diseases (today's high-income countries)

This stage designates a new pattern of chronic diseases. This pattern gradually emerges when the mortality due to ischaemic heart disease and certain common types of cancer start to decrease. When tobacco smoking decreases and the dietary fat intake is reduced people will die from Alzheimer's disease instead of a heart attack and instead of suffering from chronic obstructive pulmonary disease they will live 10 years longer and then suffer from osteoporosis. Mortality from injuries also tends to decrease due to preventive measures, better trauma care and improved rehabilitation. This results in a greater relative importance of chronic diseases such as Alzheimer's disease and osteoporosis, and other conditions, which are common in old age.

The increased burden of delayed degenerative diseases is partly a result of successful public health actions resulting in an awareness of the importance of physical activity and the risks of smoking. Also, the curative aspect of medical science has become more successful in keeping people with chronic diseases alive longer, at least when the society can afford these treatments. Many high-income societies have also experienced an increased occurrence of allergy, eating disorders and several emerging psychosocial disorders of unclear aetiology, such as "electromagnetic allergy", "sick house syndrome" and "chronic fatigue syndrome". These new emerging disorders in the "post-industrial society" have tentatively been summarised as confidence insufficiency disorders as they are believed to mainly have psychosocial causes.

Many high-income countries have low fertility, often far less than 2 children per women. This result in an increased proportion of very old in the population and together with the disease transition the stage of delayed degenerative diseases puts a heavy economic burden of care for the elderly on the post-industrial societies. Only high-income countries with substantial immigration such as the United States maintain a high fertility rate in the post-industrial period and thereby the economic burden of care for the elderly is relatively less in the USA than in Western Europe.

4.2 Demographic transition

The transition of a society from equally high birth and death rates with a stable size of the population to equally low birth and death rates, and once more a stable size of the population, almost always involves a stage of rapid population growth. The reason is that birth rates tend to fall later than death rates. This sequence, stable population, falling death rates, population growth, falling birth rates, and once more stable population, is known as the demographic transition. It occurs at different rates and in different time periods in the countries of the world. It is

Table 4.1 Simplistic overview of the present stage of the demographic transition in different types of countries.

Type of country	Number born	Number dead	Surviving	Size of the next Generation
Collapsed countries	6	4	2	Equal
Low income countries	6	2	4	+200%
Middle income countries*	4	1	3	+150%
High income countries	2	0	2	Equal

* Some former communist countries have a low birth rate and therefore a decreasing size of next generation.

differently related to the socio-economic development in different countries. Table 4.1 shows an overview of the average number of children that are born and that die from every women at each economic level in development; collapsed countries, low, middle and high-income countries, respectively.

Three different patterns of demographic transition have been described as (1) classical, (2) accelerated and (3) delayed, respectively (Omran 1971). The classical transition in Western Europe occurred over a period of almost 200 years. In contrast the accelerated transition in Japan lasted less than one century and several middle-income countries now appear to be making an even faster demographic transition.

The transition in low-income countries, especially in Sub-Saharan Africa, is designated as delayed. This means both that the onset of the decline in mortality occurs at a late stage in history and that the decline in fertility is further delayed in relation to a relatively rapid decline in mortality, assumed to be due to the provision of new technologies through the health service. This has resulted in very fast population growth in many African countries of the last 20 years. However, the HIV epidemic is changing this in several, but not all Sub-Saharan African countries. To the three earlier categories of demographic transitions must now be added a new category resulting from the severe impact of the AIDS epidemic in populations where HIV have infected 25–50% of the adult population. This new model, which may be called reversed demographic

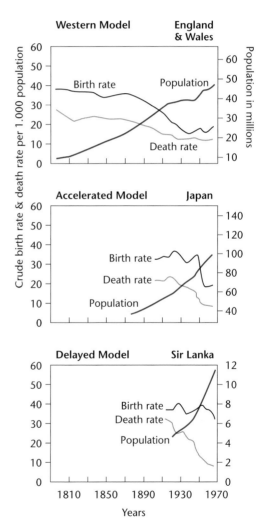

Figure 4.2 Demographic transition in three different patterns, 1810–1970.

Source: Omran AR. The epidemiological transition. Midland Memorial Fund, 1971.

transition, i.e. a reverse to death rates almost as high as the birth rates and thereby a decrease and almost stop of the population growth (Figure 4.2).

4.2.1 Classical transition—socio-economically driven

The *classical (or "Western")* type of transition took place in Europe over a period of 200 years. It mainly depended on socio-economic changes in the society. The crude death rate gradually decreased from about 30 per 1 000 population to 10 or less per 1 000 population, and the crude birth rate decreased from about 35 to less than 20 per 1 000 population. This decline in mortality started at the time when Edward Jenner made the smallpox vaccine available, but more than a century before medical science provided antibiotics.

Up to the 18th century in Europe, crowded living conditions with small, poorly ventilated apartments increased the likelihood of spread of diseases such as typhus, tuberculosis and measles. Sweden and Finland have maintained a thorough registration of vital events since the mid 18th century. From this data, a decrease in mortality is seen as early as the 1750s. Improved nutritional status and living standards, with better sanitation and access to clean water due to economic growth and social policy, were responsible for much of the decrease in the panorama of infectious diseases in Europe and North America. The elucidation of the transmission of cholera by John Snow in 1855, the discovery of the tuberculosis bacterium by Robert Koch in 1882 and the development of vaccine against rabies by Louis Pasteur in 1885 exemplifies the rapid increase in understanding of the infectious diseases. Diagnosis and treatment gained a solid scientific basis, and the preventive measures were implemented. These preventive measures, together with a gradually decreasing family size and improved economy yielded better housing that promoted a decline in the incidence of tuberculosis and other airborne diseases. Literacy, as described in chapter 2, is one of the important determinants of the decline in mortality. The age at marriage, trends in breastfeeding practices and ultimately the changing roles of women are social and cultural changes that took place over long time periods, but they are important parts of the social changes affecting the disease transition (Murray 1993).

In Europe and North America, mortality began to decline during the age of receding pandemics at the end of the 18th century, and the decline in fertility followed some 50–75 years later. But fertility initially increased to some extent, because of better health and survival, and therefore young people survived and had a longer fertile age interval. A small family norm gradually emerged and it improved child survival, education and the emancipation of women. This reduced the population growth in Europe, in combination with the emigration to other continents. Almost 25 % of the population of Europe left for North America, Latin America, South Africa, Australia and New Zealand in the 19th and the early 20th centuries.

Industrialisation and the mechanisation of agriculture brought economic growth, but also adverse health effects, due to pesticides and occupational hazards. Urbanisation disrupted much of the social context, was associated to high unemployment rates, increased risk of accidents, and resulted in what has been termed 'social pathology'. Examples of social pathology are alcoholism, increased drug use and antisocial behaviour, with violence and rising crime rates. Behavioural change following urbanisation has also increased the prevalence of risk factors such as unsafe sex, smoking, and eventually a diet with a high content of sugar and saturated fats. These behavioural changes have increased the risks of developing some of the non-communicable diseases, such as the neuropsychiatric and cardiovascular diseases.

4.2.2 The accelerated model—medicine- and technology-driven

The accelerated type of transition occurred in Japan, Eastern Europe and the former Soviet Union. It started later than the classical model, on the basis of the late start of social changes. However, the accelerated model was also catalysed by the worldwide improvements in medical science and technology, not the least in the introduction of contraceptive methods and safe induced abortion, which rapidly lowered birth rates. Mortality decline commenced at the beginning of the 20th century in Japan, well before some of the major inventions of excellent medical technology such as immunisation, antibiotics and oral rehydration solution, but the introduction of these innovations caused the mortality curve to decline more steeply. What took the high-income countries more than 100 years to achieve has taken many of the 'accelerated' countries less than 50 years.

Smallpox vaccination made a significant contribution to the decline in mortality since Jenner invented it in 1796. In Europe, the last epidemic of smallpox was in 1870–72, and thereafter, with the introduction of vaccination, disease surveillance and the isolation of infected cases, the disease disappeared. In Sri Lanka, mortality in the postwar period declined rapidly, largely due to a malaria control programme using the new chemical technologies, DDT against the mosquito and chloroquine as a drug against the malaria parasite. With other medical innovations, such as the manufacture of insulin, not only mortality rates but also survival rates of chronic diseases have improved. Demographic change can be very fast when people find that their children survive and when acceptable family planning methods are available. Modern family planning methods, in use since the 1960s, represent an important advancement in medical technology, which has affected both the demographic trend in those areas with access to the technology and the role of women when planned pregnancies became a reality.

4.2.3 The delayed model—population growth and medical advances

The *delayed* model refers to the transition that is taking place in low and some middle-income countries. This is characterised by a decline in mortality over the last 50 years, probably largely driven by medical advances and public health programmes, but where social change and fertility decline lag behind, due to poverty. The decline in fertility occurs but has not been rapid, and there is very little possibility of emigration. Therefore the population growth remains high. The transcontinental emigration in historic Europe is urbanisation in contemporary Sub-Saharan Africa. In the *classical* and *accelerated* models, the population growth was seldom higher than 0.7–1 %, but in the *delayed* model, in some low-income countries, it is still as high as 2.5–3.5 %.

Demographic transition is further described in Chapter 10. It describes the change in mortality and fertility that a country experiences when undergoing socio-economic development. In summary, the transition is from high fertility and high mortality in less industrialised societies, to low fertility and low mortality in highly industrialised societies. If the decline in mortality exceeds the decline in fertility, for example due to access to medical interventions, population growth will increase rapidly. Many of the countries undergoing the *delayed* type of transition were at this stage of rapid population growth when they were stricken by the HIV/AIDS epidemic.

4.2.4 The reversed model—HIV induced

Many but not all low-income countries have been severely affected by HIV/AIDS, especially in Eastern and Southern Africa, including the middle-income countries South Africa and Botswana. The HIV epidemic has in these countries slowed down the population growth due to a considerable increase in mortality from AIDS. In 1960 the life expectancy at birth in Botswana is estimated to have been 47 years. Due to successful

Table 4.2 Birth, death and growth rate of the population in Botswana.

Rate per 1 000 population	1960	1987	2002
Crude Birth Rate	52	40	31
Crude Death Rate	19	8	20
Growth Rate in %	3.2	3.2	1.1

Source: State of the World's Children, UNICEF, 2004.

socio-economic development and development of preventive and curative health services life expectancy increased to 61 years by 1987. All of this improvement and more has now been lost due to HIV/AIDS. Today the life expectancy in Botswana is estimated to be around 40 years. Botswana is probably the country that has been most severely affected by HIV in the whole world. Presently 39 % (sic!) of pregnant women are found to be HIV infected. The corresponding demographic rates for Botswana are shown in Table 4.2. The table shows that the birth rate continues to decrease in spite of the increased number of AIDS deaths. This gener-

ates a new pattern in most countries severely affected by HIV. They have a very slow population growth due to the combined effects of high mortality and a simultaneously slight fertility decline that results in birth rates that are only slightly higher than the death rates, and hence there is a very slow population growth. (See also Chapter 5.2).

4.3 Global Burden of Disease

As a consequence of the different speed of the health transition, the contemporary disease patterns vary considerably between the regions of the world. The Global Burden of Disease study by Murray and Lopez (1997) was the first extensive study of the worldwide occurrence of all major diseases and of their impact on disability and mortality in the human population. The study was done in collaboration between the Harvard School of Public Health, the World Bank and the World Health Organization. Murray

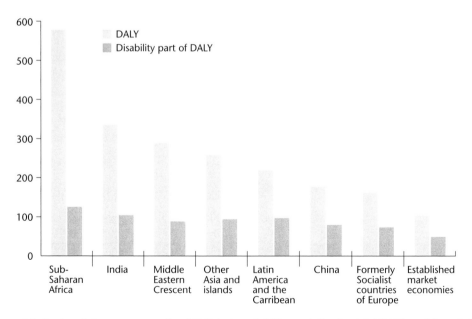

Figure 4.3 Burden of disease measured as DALYs lost per 1 000 population for total DALYs and for only the disability part of the DALY indicator by region in 1990.

Source: World Development Report; World Bank 1993.

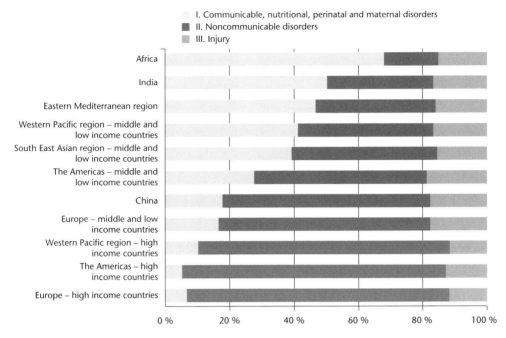

I. Communicable, nutritional, perinatal and maternal disorders
II. Noncommunicable disorders
III. Injury

Figure 4.4 The burden of disease by broad cause group as percentage of total for the region in 1998. Relative importance of group I, II and III disorders.

Source: World Health Report; WHO 1999.

and Lopez developed the DALY measure to be able to compare the disease burden in different regions of the world (defined in chapter 3.6). Figure 4.3 describes the total burden of DALYs lost in 1990 in the eight world regions. This graph shows that already in 1990 the health transition had decreased the total disease burden in many regions of the world. The region of Sub-Saharan Africa had the largest burden of disease per population, followed by India. The other regions had a decreasing disease burden in parallel to their socio-economic development. Figure 4.3 also shows that the mortality part of the DALY measure declines more rapidly in the beginning of the transition.

The Global Burden of Disease study classified diseases into a first group, including *communicable diseases, maternal, perinatal and nutritional disorders,* a second group, including *non-communicable diseases,* and finally a third group, including *injury.* In all high-income countries, as well as in China

and the low- and middle-income countries of Central and Eastern Europe, the non-communicable diseases dominate as the causes of mortality and DALYs lost. These countries have advanced furthest in the disease transition and switched from a high prevalence in the communicable disease group to a disease pattern where non-communicable diseases prevail (Figure 4.4). In India, Sub-Saharan Africa and the Eastern Mediterranean region, in contrast, communicable, perinatal, maternal and nutritional disorders dominate. In the low and middle-income countries of the Western Pacific and Southeast Asian regions, the burdens of communicable and non-communicable diseases are nearly equal. The proportion of injury as a cause of mortality and DALYs lost varies the least between regions. Between 7–10% of the deaths in the world are caused by injury, and between 11–14% of the DALYs lost are due to injury.

In conclusion, there is a great variation in disease patterns according to region, and because of different socio-economic developments and differential application of public health measures, the countries of the world show a great variation in their paths through the health transition. Many of the low and middle-income countries will not have the privilege of dealing with one major disease group at a time, but have to fight the communicable and non-communicable disease groups simultaneously. This, of course, has a profound influence on the health sector.

4.4 Future projections

The Global Burden of Disease study (Murray 1997) calculated the total number of deaths and DALYs lost in 1990 and produced lists of rank order for the diseases and disorders causing most deaths and DALYs lost. Murray and Lopez also calculated the projected change in the rank order of the most common causes of death from the year 1990 to the year 2020 (table 4.3 modified to include the DALY data from the update for 2002). Ischaemic heart disease and cerebrovascular disease are projected to continue as the two main causes of deaths in the world. The communicable diseases (diarrhoeal disease, respiratory infection, measles and malaria) and the perinatal disorders are projected to decrease considerably.

HIV was projected to rise from 30th place in 1990 to 9th place in 2020, but HIV has already, in 2002, reached number four as most important cause of death (Table 4.3). With an estimated 3 million deaths and 5 million newly infected by HIV in 2003 it is most probable that even before 2020 HIV will turn out to be the worst disease in the world. Tuberculosis will probably remain the same or increase as a consequence of the increasing prevalence following the HIV epidemic. The injury group is also projected to rise in the list of causes of death.

Table 4.3 Ranking for the most important causes of death in 2002 and expected change in ranking to 2020.

Disorder	% of deaths in 2002	Estimated Ranking in 2020
1. Ischemic heart disease	13%	1
2. Cerebrovascular disease	10%	2
3. Lower respiratory infections	7%	4
4. HIV/AIDS	5%	9
5. Chronic obstructive pulmonary disease	5%	3
6. Perinatal disorders	4%	16
7. Diarrhoeal diseases	3%	11
8. Tuberculosis	3%	7
9. Malaria	2%	29
10. Lung cancer	2%	5
11. Road traffic accidents	2%	6
12. Diabetes mellitus	2%	19
13. Hypertensive heart disease	2%	–
14. Self-inflicted injuries	2%	10
15. Stomach cancer	2%	8

Source: Murray 1997 & World Health Report, WHO, 2004, and
www3.who.int/whosis/menu.cfm?path=whosis,burden&language=english

Table 4.4 The diseases estimated to cause most loss of healthy life years (DALYs) in the world in 2002.

Diseases or disease groups	% of total DALYs lost	Millions of healthy life years lost (DALY)	Millions of deaths
1. Perinatal disorders	6%	97	2.5
2. Lower respiratory infection	6%	91	3.9
3. HIV/AIDS	6%	84	2.8
4. Unipolar major depression	4%	67	0.0
5. Diarrhoeal diseases	4%	62	1.8
6. Ischemic heart disease	4%	59	7.2
7. Cerebro-vascular diseases	3%	49	5.5
8. Malaria	3%	46	1.3
9. Road-traffic accident	3%	39	1.2
10. Tuberculosis	3%	36	1.6
11. Maternal disorders	2%	34	0.5
12. Chronic obstructive pulmonary diseases	2%	28	2.7
13. Congenital anomalies	2%	27	0.5
14. Measles	1%	21	0.6
15. Violence	1%	21	0.5
16. Self inflicted injuries	1%	21	0.9
17. Alcohol use disorders	1%	20	0.1
18. Protein energy malnutrition	1%	17	0.3
19. Falls	1%	16	0.4
20. Diabetes mellitus	1%	16	1.0
21. Schizophrenia	1%	16	0.0
22. Osteoarthritis	1%	15	0.0
23. Asthma	1%	15	0.2
24. Cirrhosis of the liver	1%	14	0.8
25. Bipolar disorders	1%	14	0.0
26. Pertussis	1%	13	0.3
27. Anaemias	1%	12	0.1
28. Sexually transmitted diseases except HIV	1%	11	0.2
29. Trachea/Bronchus/ lung cancer	1%	11	1.2
30. Drowning	1%	11	0.4
31. Alzheimer and other dementia	1%	10	0.4
Major disease groups			
Communicable, maternal, perinatal & nutritional	41%	610	18.3
Non-communicable	47%	697	33.5
Injuries	12%	182	5.2
Total in the world	100%	1490	57.0

Source: World Health Report, WHO 2004 and
www3.who.int/whosis/menu.cfm?path=whosis,burden&language=english

If we look instead at the DALYs projected lost to different disease groups, an interesting pattern arises. In its World Health Report 2004, the World Health Organisation published a list of DALYs lost in 2002 (ranked in table 4.4). On the basis of health data from 1990, Murray and Lopez also projected the relative significance of each disease group for the year 2020. Ischaemic heart disease is projected to advance to first place for most DALYs lost in the high-income countries, as well as middle and low-income countries. Unipolar major depression will take second place. In 2020, 14 % of DALYs lost are projected to be caused by neuropsychiatric disorders in low and middle-income countries, and 22 % in high-income countries. Of the DALYs lost, 13 % are expected to be due to all types of injury in high-income countries, and 21 % in low and middle-income countries, by the year 2020. Only 4 % of the DALYs lost will be due to communicable, perinatal, maternal or nutritional disorders in high-income countries and 22 % in low and middle-income countries.

Some have criticised the Global Burden of Disease study precisely because it projects so clearly the rise in the burden of non-communicable diseases and injury in the world. Many believe that the study may lead to an excessive focus on non-communicable disorders and injuries, and that the group of communicable, perinatal, maternal and nutritional disorders that mainly affect the poorest may be forgotten in the planning and management of health-care services. As we will show in the next four chapters of this book, many of the most common diseases in all three disease-groups can be prevented, and many can be treated and potentially cured. The future will tell to what extent Murray and Lopez have been right in their projections. Even if the world will be able to alleviate poverty and reduce the burden of the communicable diseases, the now low-income countries will still face a steep increase in non-communicable diseases (Laxminarayan, 2006).

4.5 Impact of the health transition on health services

The change in disease pattern that is triggered by the health transition has a fundamental impact on the demands on the health care sector. In many low and middle-income countries, this change is occurring rapidly, and the already strained human and financial resources of the health sector are insufficient to keep up with the demands for health care. Cost-effective choices and priority setting of the past must be revised when the non-communicable disease burden rises (Mosley 1997).

The total burden of disease measured by DALY will decrease per 1 000 population as shown in figure 4.3. However, it should be noticed that the burden from disability as a percent of total burden increases as a country undergoes socio-economic development.

Non-communicable diseases and disabilities caused by injury increase the complexity of the demand for healthcare services. The diversity of services needs to increase, and the staffs need new qualifications and probably more diverse levels of specialisation. Childhood diseases will continue, demanding their share of primary health care as before in low and middle-income countries. However, the rehabilitation of victims of injury, counselling of AIDS patients and good surveillance of diabetes patients are all complex and demanding health interventions that also need consideration in the future. When it comes to demand on curative services HIV infection is similar to diabetes. The new anti-retroviral drugs must be taken for life and require careful check-ups with laboratory testing. In this sense the HIV epidemic just increases the demand for chronic treatment in the same way as most non-communicable diseases do.

The paradox is that a greater demand for health services can be predicted at the later stages of the health transition. This is triggered by increased health care needs for chronic non-communicable diseases, which are not as easily preventable or curable as communicable diseases. It is also triggered by the increased awareness of a better educated population, in which people know the causes and possible treatments for different diseases, and can thus demand their rights to health care. As the mass media become more pervasive, health notices will reach a greater population. Urbanisation will decrease the physical distance from health care facilities and further increase the demand for health care.

For the reasons listed above, all the changes throughout the health transition will result in increased costs for health care. The higher costs will be mostly in the demand for secondary and tertiary level care. Hospitals in many of the low-income countries are already filled with patients with non-communicable diseases.

The solution for the rising cost of health care as a consequence of the health transition may actually lie partially outside the health care sector. As has been discussed in chapter 2, the causes of mortality, morbidity and disability can be found and prevented at different levels, from the structure of the society via the individual behaviour to biological mechanisms. The debate in public health on the best level of action for preventing disease and promoting health will continue forever. For example, to prevent lungcancer and other tobacco-related diseases individuals may benefit from health education on the adverse effects of smoking. At the societal level, restrictive laws on tobacco marketing and taxation may be efficient. The low and middle-income countries can probably not afford to abstain from using all possible measures to lower the impact of tobacco smoking on the burden of non-communicable diseases. But tobacco use prevention is just one example of how public policy must tap in to modify the effects of the health transition. Public policy must accept an increase in government health expenditures, and other sectors involved in promoting health and preventing disease must meet the increased costs and demands on the health care services following the health transition.

References and suggested further reading:

Caldwell JC. Health Transition: The cultural, social and behavioural determinants of health in the Third World. Soc. Sci. Med. 1993;36:25–135.

Chen L, Kleinman A, Ware N. Health and social change in International Perspective. Harvard University Press; 1994.

Cleland J. Population Growth in the 21st Century: Cause for Crisis or Celebration? Journal of Tropical Medicine and International Health 1996;1:15–26.

Laxminaraya R. et al, Advancement of global healh: Key messages from the Disease Control Priorities Project. Lancet Vol. 367, 2006; pp. 1193–1208.

McKeown T. Looking at diseases from the light of human development. BMJ 1983; 283:594–596.

Mosley, Bobadilla, Jamison. Disease Control Priorities in Developing Countries: An Overview and The Health Transition: Implications for Health Policy in Developing Countries. Oxford Textbook of Public Health; 1997.

Murray CJL, Chen LC. In search of a contemporary theory for understanding mortality change. Social Science and Medicine 1993;36:143–155.

Murray CJL, Lopez A. Mortality by cause for eight regions of the world: Global Burden of Disease Study. Lancet 1997;349:1269–76.

Murray CJL, Lopez A. Regional patterns of disability-free life expectancy and disability-adjusted life expectancy: Global Burden of Disease Study. Lancet 1997; 349:1347–52.

Murray CJL, Lopez A. Global mortality, disability, and the contribution of risk factors: Global Burden of Disease Study. Lancet 1997;349:1436–42.

Murray CJL, Lopez A. Alternative projections of mortality and disability by cause 1990–2020: Global Burden of Disease Study. Lancet 1997;349:1498–1504.

Omran AR. The Epidemiologic Transition: A Theory of the Epidemiology of Population Change. Milbank Memorial Fund Quarterly 1971;49:509–38.

Omran AR. The Epidemiologic Transition in the US: The Health Factor in Population Change. Population Bulletin 1977;32:3–42. (Population Reference Bureau, Inc., Washington, D.C. 1977).

Olshansky SJ. and Ault AB. The fourth stage of epidemiologic transition: The age of delayed degenerative diseases. Milbank Quarterly 1986;41:155–178.

Rogers RG. Hackenberg R. Extending Epidemiologic Transition Theory: A New Stage. Social Biology 1987;(3–4):234–43.

World Bank. World Development Report 1993.

WHO, World Health Report, 1998–2004 (www.who.int/whr.en).

5 Communicable diseases (30%)*

> *Take the death of this small boy this morning, for example. The boy died of measles. We all know he could have been cured at the hospital. But the parents had no money and so the boy died a slow and painful death not of measles but of poverty.*
>
> A man, Ghana 1995

Most of the global burden of human communicable diseases is caused by a relatively small number of microorganisms. These few are microorganisms of all different types. Some are viruses, some are bacteria, others fungi, protozoa or worms. These major infectious diseases of different types cause a wide variety of signs and symptoms, but with the exception of HIV/AIDS they all have one thing in common: the fact that scientific advances have made it relatively easy and cheap to reduce mortality by preventive and curative actions.

This reduction of mortality from communicable diseases has already taken place in high-income countries. It is currently taking place in most middle-income countries. The reduction in mortality has been achieved both through improved life conditions and better nutritional status of the population, as well as through vaccination, correct diagnosis and effective treatment with anti-microbial drugs at an early stage of the illness. The remaining high morbidity and mortality from infectious diseases in low-income countries is closely related to poverty and malnutrition. However, as a result of successful implementation of immunisation the burden of the vaccine-preventable diseases, such as measles and polio, has also been decreased in low-income countries. Even in war-torn southern Sudan it has been possible to eradicate polio. Unfortunately, the decreased occurrence of the vaccine-preventable diseases in low-income countries is replaced by increased occurrence of malaria

and HIV. Communicable diseases therefore continue to be the main part of the disease burden in the poorest countries (WHO 2004).

Some of the major infectious diseases, such as lower respiratory tract infection and diarrhoea, remain common all over the world, but due to general access to effective treatment at the primary health care level these two diseases cause limited suffering and almost no deaths in high-income countries. Other major infectious diseases, such as tuberculosis, measles and many of the sexually transmitted diseases, are today also rare in high-income countries. This is due to improved living conditions, as well as effective control, treatment and vaccination that have jointly reduced their transmission. The major parasitic diseases, of which malaria is the most prominent, occur almost exclusively in low-income countries. These parasitic diseases are often referred to as 'tropical' diseases. One of the reasons for this label is that the transmission of some of the most important parasites requires the passage through an insect, known as a vector, which only survives in tropical climates. This is the case for sleeping sickness, or trypanosomiasis, which is transmitted by a tropical insect known as the tsetse fly.

A large part of the severe poverty among humans today is found in tropical regions. In these countries poverty is partly due to the occurrence of the parasitic diseases and the occurrence of these diseases is also caused by poverty. This vicious circle of pov-

---

* % in parentheses is the share of the global burden of disease estimates by WHO in 2002.

erty and parasitic diseases has been broken in several tropical countries. Parasitic diseases have been successfully eliminated by economic and social development in combination with special disease control programmes in tropical countries such as Singapore, Malaysia, Mauritius, Sri Lanka and Cuba. Some types of malaria parasites were a century ago a public health problem in sub-Arctic countries such as Sweden, when housing conditions did not protect the population from frequent bites of the Anopheles mosquito. During summer the malaria-transmitting mosquito is still common in Sweden, but the malaria parasite was eradicated one century ago through drainage of mosquito breeding sites, improved housing and access to treatment. Socio-economic advances can counteract the burden of parasitic diseases. But the poverty related parasitic diseases constitute an extra cost for development in low-income countries.

The World Health Organization has a special research programme for 'tropical diseases'.[1] The reason being that the absence of these parasitic diseases in high-income countries makes the research oriented pharmaceutical companies reluctant to invest in research about human parasitic diseases. The term 'tropical diseases' thus refers to parasitic diseases that, for reasons of both biological and socio-economic circumstances, occur exclusively in tropical countries. However, these 'tropical diseases' do not constitute the main burden of disease in these countries. They do not even constitute the main burden of communicable diseases in tropical low-income countries. In these countries the burden of each of the four main communicable disease groups (lower respiratory tract infections, diarrhoea, HIV and tuberculosis) is bigger or in the same range as that of malaria. However, these four main communicable diseases also occur in middle- and high-income countries. Therefore the high-income countries allocate considerable amounts of money for research

into these diseases. It should be noted that several nutritional diseases, such as under-nutrition and deficiencies of vitamin A and iodine, have a similar global distribution as the tropical diseases, i.e. today they mainly occur in tropical low-income countries.

When considering the classification of diseases, it should also be noted that the line dividing communicable and non-communicable diseases is becoming less clear-cut. The reason being that several diseases, which used to be classified as non-communicable, have been found to be caused by microorganisms. It has been shown that cancer and cirrhosis of the liver are induced mainly by chronic infection with hepatitis virus type B or C. Cancer of the cervix of the uterus, one of the most prevalent types of cancer in women, is induced by the human papilloma virus. Chronic infection with Helicobacter pylori bacteria has been found to cause peptic ulcer and some related disorders of the stomach.

In this chapter we review the communicable diseases that cause most suffering, i.e. most DALYs lost in the world. For each type of disease we review its occurrence, causation, clinical features, requirement for diagnosis, and possible treatment and prevention. The small world maps show how many millions of DALYs are lost due to each disease. A similar review is performed in the following four chapters, concerning nutritional disorders, non-communicable diseases, injuries and reproductive health, respectively. The percentage in parentheses in each subtitle shows the proportion of the global burden of disease in DALY caused by each condition.

5.1 Acute lower respiratory tract infection (6 %)

Acute lower respiratory tract infections may be regarded as the second worst disease in the world in DALYs lost, preceded only by perinatal disorders (see chapter 9). Acute

[1]   www.who.int/tdr

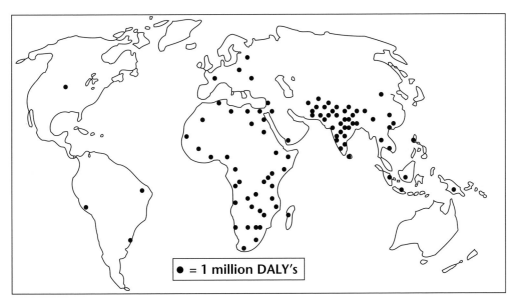

Map 5:1 Lower respiratory tract infections cause 90 million disability adjusted life years (DALY) lost per year.
Source: WHO, 2002.

lower respiratory tract infection was estimated to cause 6 % of the total loss of healthy years of life in the world (see Table 4.4) (WHO 2004). More than half of this loss of healthy years of life occurred in India and Sub-Saharan Africa, in spite of acute lower respiratory tract infection being common in all countries of the world. Most infections of the lower airways and lungs are also called 'pneumonia'. In 2002, pneumonia ranked as number one cause of death in children under the age of five years in the world. This is in spite of life-saving treatment with penicillin and other antibiotics having been available for more than 50 years. Pneumonia still causes the death of two million children each year due to lack of access of a treatment discovered half a century ago! Of these 5 000 child deaths per day, almost all occur in low and middle-income countries. The main reason why lower respiratory tract infection remains one of the worst killers in the world, is that lifesaving antibiotic drugs are not available to those in greatest need of these medicines. Pneumonia is a deadly disease in poor children because they suffer

from impairment of the immune system due to concomitant malnutrition (see chapter 6).

Children all over the world are estimated to suffer from about five episodes of acute respiratory tract infection per year. These episodes of cough, fever and runny noses put an enormous strain on their families and on the health services in all countries. The acute respiratory tract infections are divided into three groups. Upper respiratory tract infections include the common cold, ear and throat infections, tonsillitis and sinusitis. These diseases are very common, but rarely lethal. Many of the mid-respiratory tract infections, which are restricted to the trachea and larynx, may be life threatening, but do not occur as frequently as the upper and lower infections. The acute lower respiratory tract infections, which in strict medical terminology may be divided into pneumonia, bronchiolitis and alveolitis, are both common and serious.

Microorganisms that are spread by air or by direct contact commonly colonise the upper respiratory tract. The disease often starts as a viral infection of the mucosa of the nose and throat and then proceeds to become a lower respiratory infection, leading to a secondary bacterial pneumonia. About half of all patients with bacterial pneumonia show evidence of a previous viral infection. The types of bacteria that cause pneumonia are surprisingly similar throughout the world and their occurrence is independent of climate. The main bacteria are Streptococcus pneumoniae, Haemophilus influenzae and Staphylococcus aureus. The viruses that cause most acute respiratory tract infections are also quite similar throughout the world. The most common are the measles virus, respiratory syncytial virus, influenza virus, parainfluenza virus and adenovirus. While viral infections of the respiratory tract are frequent throughout the world, the incidence of pneumonia is higher in children in low- and middle-income countries than in children in high-income countries.

Acute lower respiratory tract infection no longer needs to constitute a serious threat to life, since we have the necessary antibiotics. However, it is vital that a correct diagnosis is made, that adequate treatment is prescribed, that the drug prescribed is available to the sick person and that the drug is correctly taken. It is thus the weakness in the health service system that mainly explains why two million children still die each year from this disease.

The first difficulty in reducing the incidence of child death due to lower respiratory tract infection is thus to enable caregivers and primary health care workers to diagnose the life-threatening lower respiratory tract infections among the vast number of children presenting with cough, fever or breathing difficulty. A major advance in the management of acute lower respiratory infection was the demonstration that the diagnosis of pneumonia in a child is possible without a medical doctor or x-ray, but by observing the breathing rate and counting the number of breaths per minute. It has been convincingly shown in controlled studies that primary health care staff can learn to diagnose pneumonia with high accuracy without using a stethoscope, x-ray or any fancy laboratory tests, the medical examiner only needs to count the number of breaths per minute. Between 1 and 5 years of age a breathing rate above 40 per minute is considered a sign of pneumonia and the child should be given antibiotics. The observation of subcostal and intercostal chest indrawings and five other 'danger signs' help to determine the severity of the pneumonia. If subcostal or intercostal chest indrawing is observed, the pneumonia is considered to be severe. The infection is classified as very severe if the child shows any of the five danger signs: unconsciousness; convulsions; lethargy; inability to drink or breastfeed; or vomiting everything eaten (Box 5.1).

Good case management of lower respiratory tract infection is being promoted throughout the world by a WHO programme called 'Integrated Management of Childhood Illnesses'[1]. Good case management consists of prompt identification of children who need antibiotic treatment through proper diagnosis and severity classification of children with pneumonia, and correct administration of the antibiotics. The recommended management also includes treatment to reduce fever and measures to secure adequate breastfeeding, as well as adequate intake of fluid and food during the illness (Lambrechts 1999).

WHO's guidelines for treatment are thus based on the severity of the pneumonia. If the child only shows signs of increased breathing frequency without chest recession or danger signs, the child can be treated at home. WHO recommends the use of cotrimoxazole, an antibiotic with few side effects that is effective against most bacteria causing pneumonia. An equally important reason is that this drug has become very cheap since the expiry of the patent. If it is purchased in large quantities by the National Health Service and distributed rationally to

[1]   http://www.who.int/child-adolescent-health

Box 5.1

Integrated management of childhood illnesses

Integrated management of childhood illnesses (IMCI) is a world-wide WHO programme. The main objective is to lower the mortality due to the five major childhood diseases.

- lower respiratory infection
- diarrhoeal disease
- malaria
- measles
- malnutrition.

Formerly WHO had separate programmes for lower respiratory infection, diarrhoeal diseases and malaria. However, the main problems for peripheral health staff in low and middle-income countries in diagnosing these diseases have been that many of the sick children only present with general symptoms like fever and weakness. These symptoms may be compatible with all these major diseases. Sometimes sick children may have two or all three of these diseases at the same time. It is thus very relevant of WHO to combine these programmes into one for integrated management of the main childhood illnesses. This has lead to more rational guidelines for the peripheral health worker in low and middle-income countries and hopefully to more relevant courses and instruction material for the primary health care staff in those countries.

The main activities of the IMCI programme are to assist Ministries of Health to formulate national guidelines and to arrange short courses for health staff on how to implement the national guidelines in their daily work with sick children. The home page of WHO's department of child and adolescent health contains extensive information about IMCI (www.who.int/child-adolescent-health).

The model chapter for textbooks and the information package for IMCI are especially recommended for reading.

---

peripheral units of the health service system, the necessary one week treatment for one child costs less than 0.5 USD. However, if purchased in a non-rational way, it can be several times more costly for the health service, or for the paying family in countries where patients have to cover the costs of drugs. The challenge to reduce child deaths from pneumonia is thus very much the challenge of improving the access to and correct use of antibiotics. It is a tragic paradox that the current over-use of antibiotics promotes the development of resistance to these life-saving drugs. Unfortunately, resistance to cotrimoxazole is now rather common among pneumococci, one of the most important bacteria that kills children by causing pneumonia.

Children with severe or very severe pneumonia should, whenever possible, be referred urgently to a hospital for treatment.

As many as 25 % of patients under two years of age with malnutrition develop a pneumococcal sepsis, i.e. the bacteria spread from the lungs to the blood. This condition has a high mortality. WHO recommends that these children should be treated with the form of ordinary penicillin that can be injected intramuscularly, known as procaine penicillin, or with some form of broad-spectrum penicillin, such as ampicillin or amoxycillin. Chloramphenicol is an alternative, cheaper type of broad-spectrum antibiotic for very severe pneumonia with good absorption when taken orally. It is today rarely used in high-income countries, because it can cause a rare but serious dysfunction of the bone marrow.

Based on WHO recommendations each Ministry of Health decides which antibiotics should be recommended for treatment of acute lower respiratory infections in its own

ASSESS AND CLASSIFY THE SICK CHILD
AGE 2 MONTHS UP TO 5 YEARS

ASSESS   CLASSIFY   IDENTIFY
                                             TREATMENT

ASK THE MOTHER WHAT THE CHILD'S PROBLEMS ARE

- Determine if this is an initial or follow-up visit for this problem.
  - If follow-up visit, use the follow-up instructions on *TREAT THE CHILD* chart.
  - If initial visit, assess the child as follows:

CHECK FOR GENERAL DANGER SIGNS

ASK:
- Is the child able to drink or breastfeed?
- Does the child vomit everything?
- Has the child had convulsions?

LOOK:
- See if the child is lethargic or unconscious.

A child with any general danger sign needs URGENT attention; complete the assessment and

THEN ASK ABOUT MAIN SYMPTOMS:
Does the child have cough or difficult breathing?

IF YES, ASK:
- For how long?

LOOK, LISTEN, FEEL:
- Count the breaths in one minute.
- Look for chest indrawing.
- Look and listen for stridor.

CHILD
MUST BE
CALM

Classify
COUGH or
DIFFICULT
BREATHING

If the child is:	Fast breathing is:
2 months up to 12 months	**50 breaths per minute or more**
12 months up to 5 years	**40 breaths per minute or more**

USE ALL BOXES THAT MATCH THE
CHILD'S SYMPTOMS AND PROBLEMS
TO CLASSIFY THE ILLNESS.

SIGNS	CLASSIFY AS	TREATMENT (Urgent pre-referral treatments are in bold print.)
• Any general danger sign or • Chest indrawing or • Stridor in calm child.	**SEVERE PNEUMONIA OR VERY SEVERE DISEASE**	➢ *Give first dose of an appropriate antibiotic.* ➢ *Refer URGENTLY to hospital.*
• Fast breathing.	**PNEUMONIA**	➢ *Give an appropriate antibiotic for 5 days.* ➢ Soothe the throat and relieve the cough with a safe remedy. ➢ Advise mother when to return immediately. ➢ Follow-up in 2 days.
No signs of pneumonia or very severe disease.	**NO PNEUMONIA: COUGH OR COLD**	➢ If coughing more than 30 days, refer for assessment. ➢ Soothe the throat and relieve the cough with a safe remedy. ➢ Advise mother when to return immediately. ➢ Follow-up in 5 days if not improving.

Figure 5.1 Integrated management of childhood illnesses. Assessment, classification and treatment of pneumonia.

Source: IMCI programme at WHO.

country. In addition to general information about efficacy and side effects, these national antibiotic policies are based on information about the pattern of bacterial resistance, treatment tradition, and availability and prices of different drugs as well as on the funds available to buy the drugs. This is a difficult choice for low-income countries. Should a cheaper antibiotic with a slightly greater incidence of side effects be recommended because it is the only drug that the country and the families can afford? In other words, should a few deaths from side effects be accepted in order to save many more lives from life-threatening lower respiratory tract infections? With good reason, many Ministries of Health find that the answer is "Yes." It should be realised that technical decision-making on drug policy in countries with very limited resources actually requires more skill and consideration than in countries that can afford the more simplistic approach that "only the best is good enough for us".

The number of deaths due to lower respiratory tract infections can also be reduced through improved housing, better nutrition, and partly through vaccination. Indoor air pollution and crowding in small houses are well-known risk factors for pneumonia in children. This air pollution comes from cooking food and heating the house without having the benefit of a chimney, probably for economic reasons. In fact this air pollution from poverty seems to kill more persons each year than the more talked about air pollution from industry and traffic in major cities. This explains why economic development and increased equity in countries and in the world will indirectly reduce the incidence of severe pneumonia in children.

Health education can contribute by promoting breastfeeding and good nutrition. Malnutrition during foetal life, as reflected by a low birth weight, is a risk factor for severe pneumonia. A low intake of vitamin A has been identified as another major nutritional reason for high mortality from pneumonia in low and middle-income countries. Regular distribution of vitamin A to children in low-income countries has been shown to considerably decrease mortality in acute lower respiratory tract infections (chapter 6.4.2).

Immunisation with existing vaccines against measles, diphtheria and pertussis prevents a proportion of deaths due to lower respiratory tract infections. A new vaccine against Haemophilus influenzae type B bacteria has shown a 100 % protection rate against lower respiratory tract infection due to this type of bacteria. This is of great significance, as this type of bacteria is the second most common cause of acute respiratory disease in the world. It is sad that the high price of this new vaccine, USD 2.70 per dose, with three doses needed for full protection, still restricts its use to the richer part of the world. If the financial issues could be solved, this vaccine could be included in ongoing immunisation programmes in low and middle-income countries, thus saving many thousands of children around the world from dying of pneumonia. The same is the case for a new and expensive vaccine against the very common Streptococcus pneumonia.

The efforts needed to reduce the burden of acute lower respiratory tract infections thus span from politics, economics, nutrition and health education to health service organisation, immunology and microbiology.

5.2 HIV infection and AIDS (6 %)

By the year 2002 HIV/AIDS was the disease that caused the third greatest number of healthy life years (DALYs) lost in the world (table 4.4). This new disease of the human immune system was named 'Acquired Immuno Deficiency Syndrome' (AIDS), when first described in United States in August 1981. The causal human immunodeficiency

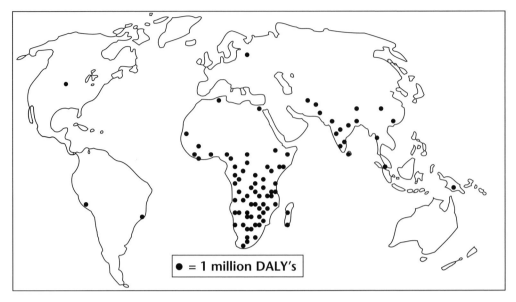

Map 5:2 HIV/AIDS cause 88 million disability adjusted life years (DALY) lost per year.
Source: WHO, 2002.

virus type 1 (HIV-1) was identified in 1983 and in 1985 it became possible to test whether a person was infected. This was first done by the identification of antibodies to the virus in the blood. A second type of the virus, HIV-2, was identified in 1986 and by then the main ways of transmission were elucidated. There is evidence that HIV transmission had already started in 1958 (Zhu 1998), and clinical cases of AIDS have in retrospect been identified in the 1970s (Bygbjerg 1983). It is assumed that the virus as all other major human epidemics passed from animals to humans. This may have occurred as early as 1940, but how it occurred is not confirmed. In spite of the rapid research achievements following the rapid spread in the beginning of the 1980s, AIDS has today become one of the main diseases of the world. At the end of 2003 an estimated 38 million people were infected with HIV, corresponding to about 1 % of the adult population of the world. More than two-thirds of those infected were living in Africa south of the Sahara. In 2005 it was estimated that 3.2 million became infected with HIV and that 2.4 million died of AIDS, of whom half a

million were children. About 12 million African children are today orphans because of the AIDS epidemic.[1] Worst of all, while the HIV epidemic seems to have been curbed in most high-income countries and in many middle-income countries, the situation continues to deteriorate in many low-income countries as shown in Table 5.1.

The highest identified HIV prevalence is found in some parts of African countries. Around 60 % of the adult population (15–49 years old) are infected in the most affected areas. In the demographic situation of most countries in Sub-Saharan Africa the population growth will stop at an adult HIV prevalence of about 50 %. This is now happening in parts of some countries, such as Botswana. In parts of Zimbabwe, it has been found that 58 % of women between 19 and 40 years are HIV-positive. This constitutes a hitherto unprecedented effect of disease in contemporary world history. In South Africa around 50 000 newly infected individuals are registered every month, and in Swaziland about 25 % of the adults of fertile age

[1] www.unaids.org

Table 5.1 Estimated occurrence of HIV and deaths in AIDS in 2005.

Region	People living with HIV in millions	Newly infected by HIV in 2002 in millions	% HIV prevalence rate in 15–49 year olds in the end of 2003	Number of deaths in AIDS during 2003 in millions
Sub-Saharan Africa	25.8	3.2	7.2	2.40
North Africa & Middle East	0.5	0.07	0.2	0.06
South and South-East Asia	7.4	1	0.7	0.48
East Asia	0.8	0.1	0.1	0.04
Latin America	1.8	0.2	0.6	0.06
Caribbean	0.3	0.03	2.4	0.025
Eastern Europe & Central Asia	1.6	0.3	0.9	0.06
Western Europe	0.7	0.02	0.3	0.01
North America	1.2	0.04	0.7	0.02
Oceania	0.07	0.00	0.5	0.00
TOTAL	*40.3*	*4.9*	*1.1*	*3.10*

Source: UNAIDS www.unaids.org, AIDS Epidemic Update, 2005.

are now estimated to be HIV-positive. To date the greatest impact of the pandemic of HIV/AIDS has been in Central, Eastern and Southern Africa. The burden of HIV/AIDS in some West African countries is only one tenth of that in the most affected countries in southern Africa. The good news is that careful studies show a falling HIV incidence in some formerly heavily affected areas (Kwesigabo 2000).

In Asia and the Pacific region the progression of the epidemic has been rapid since the late 1980s (table 5.1). In India alone there are 5 million infected persons, probably the highest number in any one nation, and in China, about half a million people are infected. HIV is now spreading in the world's two biggest countries. In China the transmission is largely through commercial sex and intravenous drug use, but with a significant contribution from the transfusion of blood derived from unregulated professional blood donors. In the Americas there are more than two million infected persons but the number of newly infected is no longer increasing, neither in North America nor in Latin America. Heterosexual transmission remains the most important means

of infection, followed by homosexual transmission and intravenous drug use. The latest estimates from UNAIDS are shown in table 5.1 (UNAIDS 2005), but readers are advised to look for updates.[1]

The scenario is also alarming in Eastern Europe and Central Asia. This is considered to be the area with the most rapidly growing HIV epidemic. The rapid growth is thought to be due to both the high prevalence of other sexually transmitted infections and concomitant high rates of infection through widespread intravenous drug use. In high-income countries, the epidemic has also reached ominous proportions; more than 75 000 people acquired HIV infection in 2002, bringing the total number of infected people in high-income countries to 1.6 million.

At present, vertical (mother-to-infant) transmission accounts for approximately one-fifth of all cases of AIDS seen in Sub-Sahara Africa, and it is anticipated that a similar scenario will prevail in Asia. The outcome for the infected newborn is poor without modern advanced treatment. In Africa

[1] www.unaids.org

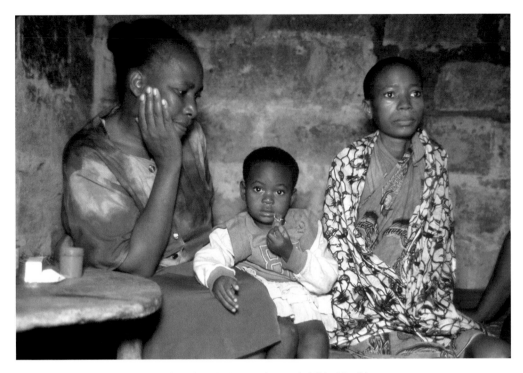

TANZANIA, Dar-Es-Salaam. Social worker visiting mother and child with aids.
© Sean Sprague/PHOENIX.

up to 40 % of infected newborns die in the first year of life, and up to 75 % die before the age of 5 years. Only a few will survive into adolescence. A study in 39 countries in Sub-Saharan Africa indicates that about 8 % of the deaths in children below 5 years of age are directly caused by HIV/AIDS. However, the proportion of child deaths directly caused by HIV varies from 1 % to 42 % between the African countries. The relative impact of HIV is greatest in Botswana and other countries in Southern Africa that have a better economy and that have successfully reduced child death from other causes.

The incidence of tuberculosis is increasing throughout the world, and the main factor responsible for this is immunosuppression due to HIV infection. About 7 million individuals are simultaneously infected with HIV and Mycobacterium tuberculosis. Throughout the world HIV-infected subjects run a 30–50 % lifetime risk of acquiring tuberculosis, while HIV-negative individuals have a lifetime risk of 10 %. At present most of the patients diagnosed with pulmonary tuberculosis in Central, Eastern and Southern Africa are HIV-positive.

HIV infection and its spread are no longer seen through the medical lens alone, but also through the social and economic lenses. It is becoming a disease of the marginalised and impoverished of the world. The vulnerable groups are commercial sex workers, intravenous drug users, women living in oppressive relationships, where sexual contact is not negotiable, and the poorest, which are deprived of access to health education. HIV/AIDS remains a severe social stigma in many societies. This influences how and if people avoid transmission and seek help from health services. A significant effort remains to be done to fight prejudice. A political commitment and will to stop the epidemic is crucial. In spite of the general increase in HIV infection in low-income countries, several studies show a positive effect of prevention, especially when both political actions and economic resources are present. A clear reduction of transmission has been shown in many community-based projects run by NGO's. Examples are programmes to supply condoms to commercial sex workers in Thailand, Tanzania and the United States, which have decreased the expected spread of the infection. For prevention to be effective, it is necessary to influence sexual behaviour and reinforce the individual's opportunity to make healthy decisions. It is necessary that the health and social services provide education, care and social support to the most vulnerable groups if the epidemic is to be stopped. As it is probable that pre-existing sexually transmitted illnesses (STIs) increase the risk of acquiring HIV infection, an important aspect of the prevention strategy is to reduce the occurrence of STIs.

Vaccine research efforts are being conducted, but no vaccine has yet been shown to be clinically effective. The present judgement among specialists is that for the foreseeable future no vaccine will be available to stop the HIV epidemic. However, effective antiretroviral drugs are now available but only as a life long complicated and costly treatment. When available this treatment has dramatically reduced mortality from HIV infection in high-income countries and large efforts are being made to make these drugs available for the more than 38 million that are infected. The drugs have also been successfully made available in some middle-income countries where HIV prevalence is around 1 % and a relatively well functioning health system exists, e.g. Brazil. The high cost of the drugs, the laboratory tests and medical consultations needed still make it impossible to treat the majority of the HIV infected in the low-income countries with prevalence above 20 % in adults. It should be noted that Brazil has a 10 times better economy than Zambia whereas Zambia has 20 times higher HIV prevalence. It is thus a much higher challenge to provide antiretroviral treatment in Zambia compared to Brazil. Highly affected middle-income countries like Botswana and South Africa are presently trying to make the anti-retroviral drugs available but the impact of these attempts has not yet been studied.

The tragic widespread incidence of HIV in Southern and Eastern Africa especially has lead to a heated debate on what to do about it. It seems as if too many arguments in this debate lack an evidence base. This is the case with claims that AIDS may not be due to HIV as well as suggestions that all those infected should get access to anti-retroviral treatment. Evaluation of the impact of different actions against the spread of HIV as well as cost effectiveness analyses is important for the decisions on global, national and local policy for HIV control. Policy also depends on many factors other than evidence and cost, but the ten to hundred fold differences in cost per life saved (Creese 2002) between different HIV interventions makes it important to always include some cost assessments when choosing interventions (Table 5.2).

The widely different costs per healthy year of life saved with the different interventions (Table 5.2) are due to the differences in HIV prevalence and the health system coverage as well as all the other differences between the affected societies. Standard solutions against the epidemic should be doubted. Adoption to local context appears to be crucial for successful curbing of the epidemic. Facing the real sexual behaviours behind the epidemic in each country, as well as the clandestine use of intravenous drugs is the main challenge to tailor the right preventive interventions. All interested in the control of the global HIV epidemic must have basic knowledge about both the biological and clinical aspect of the disease as well as of the socio-economic, political and cultural contexts in which the epidemic occurs. Section 5.2.1 provides the basic facts about the human immune system and the HIV virus infection.

Table 5.2 Estimated cost effectiveness of different interventions against HIV/AIDS in Africa.

Intervention	Reduce the main HIV transmission	Cost in US dollar per healthy life year saved (DALY*)
Condom distribution	yes	1–99
Blood safety	yes	1–43
Peer education of sex-workers	yes	4–7
Stop mother to child transmission	no	1–731
Control of STIs	yes	12
Voluntary counselling and testing	yes?	18–22
Short course TB therapy	no	2–68
Co-trimoxazol prophylaxis	no	6
Home care of AIDS patients	no	77–1230
TB preventive therapy	no	169–288
Anti retroviral therapy	no?	1,100–1,800

* Varies depending on the HIV prevalence and whether a well functioning health service exists or not.

Source: Creese 2002.

5.2.1 The HIV infection

The human immune system consists of an antibody-mediated defence and a cell-mediated defence by the type of blood cells called lymphocytes. Simplistically it can be said that the antibodies kill bacteria whereas the lymphocytes are more important to overcome viral infections, tuberculosis, fungal infections and parasites. As viruses infect cells, the cell-mediated defence attacks by killing the infected cells to clear the infection. The white blood cell called "CD4 T-lymphocyte" has a central role in the immune system. It is the co-ordinator of the system, like an officer directing soldiers. The cell-mediated defence depends on the good functioning of the CD4 cells and it is this leading cell in the immune system the HIV viruses infect and destroy.

The HIV virus consists of an outer envelope with buds made of a glycoprotein that is called gp120. Inside the envelope there is a core with the genetic code in the form of RNA as well as three enzymes called 1) reverse transcriptase, 2) integrase and 3) protease.

It is important to remember that the HIV virus has a very low infectivity. It can only transmit from one human to another through some special mechanism that helps

it to get 'under the skin'. Blood transfusion is such a mechanism, and sexual relations is another. Outside the human body HIV is rapidly killed by soap, sun or some other desinfectant.

If the HIV virus gets into the human body, it will infect many of the body's cells. However, the gp120 buds on the virus envelope fit especially well onto a receptor on the CD4 T-lymphocytes, and the CD4 cells therefore become the prime target of HIV infection. The presence of so-called chemokine-receptors is also needed for HIV to attach to the lymphocyte and to fuse with the cell membrane. Thereafter HIV will enter to the inside of the cell where the contents of the virus are released. The reverse transcriptase will now start to make a DNA copy of the virus RNA. This is the reverse of the usual procedure, which is to make RNA 'working copies' of the DNA 'original' stored in the cell nucleus. This is why this group of viruses are called retroviruses. Once the virus has produced DNA copies of its genetic code, the integrase enzyme will introduce this DNA code into the genes of the cell, in other words into the chromosomes of the lymphocyte. When the genetic code of the virus is included in the chromosomes, the body can no longer eliminate the infection, because the genetic code of HIV can no longer be identified as an infection. Instead, the genetic code of the virus resembles a part of the genes of the infected individual.

When the virus gene is activated, it takes command of the CD4 cell and converts the cell into a virus production unit. When it does so, it will be targeted by the cell-mediated immune defence system, and the infected CD4 cell will rapidly be killed. The body will compensate for the loss of CD4 cells by increasing production of this type of lymphocytes, but with time the capacity to do this will be exhausted and the number of CD4 cells /ml of blood will decrease. When the number of CD4 cells decreases from the normal 800–1,500 cells/ml of blood to below 200 cells/ml, the body's cell-mediated defence system becomes weakened and the body is easily infected with viruses such as Herpes zoster, with funguses such as Candida causing thrush in the mouth and by bacteria such as tuberculosis. The control of transformed cells is also affected, and cancers appear more readily. The number of CD4 cells /ml of blood is thus an important measurement in the assessment of an HIV infected person. The CD4 count can predict when a HIV infected person begins to suffer from the immune deficiency, in other words when the HIV infected individual develops the disease AIDS (acquired immuno deficiency syndrome). At this point in time the weakened immune defence can no longer stop the HIV virus from multiplying, and disease progression speeds up. Without antiretroviral treatment AIDS is a deadly disease, even if treatment is available for the opportunistic infections. However, cost-effective treatment of opportunistic infections can prolong life for many years.

5.2.2 The AIDS disease

The HIV infection has three phases: the primary HIV infection, an asymptomatic phase and the symptomatic phase called AIDS. During the primary infection (first 4–12

weeks), the virus replicates rapidly and the viral load is high. During this first period blood and body fluids from the infected person are highly infective. In the second, asymptomatic phase, the immune system gains control over viral replication and keeps the viral load low. This also means that infectivity is lower than during the initial phase. The CD4 count is almost normal and the infected person has no symptoms. However, the CD4 count gradually declines, and after some years the number of CD4 lymphocytes has become so low that the person will start to get more infections and other symptoms of AIDS. In this third phase viral replication will also escape the host's immune defences, the viral load increases and the person becomes more infective again. If HIV infection is not counteracted with anti-HIV drugs, a number of disease symptoms will emerge as the patient develops AIDS. The most common clinical presentations of AIDS in adults in sub-Saharan Africa are as follows:

- Severe weight loss ('slim disease')
- Enlarged lymph nodes known as lymphadenopathy
- Chronic diarrhoea
- Persistent cough

The human immunodeficiency virus (HIV) is genetically closely related to the simian immunodeficiency viruses (SIV) that are found among monkeys in Africa. Scientifically, there is little doubt that HIV and SIV have a common origin. HIV probably originated as a zoonosis, an infection that passed from animal to man (Zhu 1998). This is the same as happened with the human influenza virus, which is closely related to similar viruses found in domestic birds in China. But how did this cross-infection happen? There is evidence that HIV has existed for several decades before it was discovered. Because monkeys are hunted for meat in Central Africa, it is not improbable that the virus spread through blood contact during slaughter. Just as with the influenza virus, a mutation of the 'foreign' virus is needed for it to be able to survive in humans. Two other proposed hypotheses should be considered. The first one suggests that the virus originated from polio vaccine obtained from cultures on monkey kidney cells. This vaccine was used in campaigns in Central Africa in the 1950s. The main argument against this hypothesis is that neither SIV nor HIV viruses grow in kidney cells; they both need lymphocytes to grow. A third hypothesis suggests that the virus was produced in laboratories as part of biological warfare research. The plausibility of the last hypothesis should be considered in the light of the difficulties present-day virologists have in incorporating new genes into viruses for 'gene therapy'. The knowledge needed to make a new virus was not there 30–40 years ago. As with the other major viruses that have passed from animals to humans we do not yet understand the mechanisms by which this occurred.

5.2.3 The HIV tests

There are two main types of tests for HIV. Both tests are made on blood. The direct tests detect the RNA or DNA of the virus. The indirect tests detect the body's antibodies against the virus. The best known of the direct tests is called PCR (polymerase chain reaction). This test method can detect small amounts of the virus in the blood and it can establish for sure whether the person is infected or not. The disadvantage with the PCR method is that it is expensive. It costs 50–100 USD per test which is ten times more than the total amount of money that is annually available per person for health services in the majority of HIV affected low-income countries in Africa. The PCR method is costly because it requires sophisticated laboratory facilities and well-trained staff. The advantage with the PCR test is the estimate of how many virus particles there are per unit of blood. This is referred to as the 'viral load'. A viral load of less than 10 000 particles/ml is low, indicating that the infection is under control and that the person is not so infective. A high viral load of several million of particles/ml blood indicates that the person is either newly infected or is starting to get AIDS. Such persons are usually highly infective.

There are many indirect, 'rapid' tests, which involve different so called ELISA or Western Blot techniques. The rapid tests are relatively cheap (USD 4 per test) and they are easy to perform. The major problem with the indirect tests is that they do not become positive until the body has started producing antibodies against the virus. This usually takes 1–3 months from the time of infection. In this first period after infection, an indirect test may be negative in spite of the person being infected. Somebody who is testing negative should therefore come back after 3 months for re-testing. An alternative is a direct test, which will give the correct result to those that can afford it.

Another disadvantage with indirect tests is that they cannot be used in children born to HIV-positive mothers. The reason is that most mothers transfer their antibodies to the child, but often not the virus. Many of these children will be positive in an indirect test without being infected. Indirect tests in children cannot be used reliably until the age of 15 months. To know if a child is infected before this age, a direct test must be performed.

5.2.4 The HIV transmission

The four modes of transmission of the HIV virus are through (1) sexual intercourse, (2) blood transfusion, (3) intravenous drug use, or (4) from mother to baby during pregnancy, delivery or breastfeeding. The risk of transmission between sexual partners is considerably increased when there is a simultaneous infection with gonorrhoea or other sexually transmitted infections (STIs). In general, susceptibility to HIV is enhanced when the genital mucosa is damaged or infected, presumably both by facilitating the entry of the virus into the bloodstream and

150

through the recruitment to mucosal surfaces of the cells of the immune system that are targets for HIV invasion.

A number of infections can be transmitted from mother to foetus or infant during pregnancy, delivery or infancy. This is called vertical transmission, with one generation infecting the next, as opposed to horizontal transmission, where persons of the same generation infect each other. HIV is only one of the infections that can be transmitted vertically. It may be transmitted to the foetus during pregnancy, during delivery or through breastfeeding after birth. If no special measures are taken about 30–40 % of HIV positive mothers in Sub-Saharan Africa, will transmit HIV to their babies. Although this is a high proportion it means that almost two-thirds of these babies born to HIV positive mothers in Sub-Saharan Africa will not be infected! Up to 10 % of the babies are infected before birth. Most of this transmission takes place in the last month of pregnancy, when the placenta may leak blood from mother to child. Most of the children that get infected, about 10–20 % of all children born to HIV infected women, get the infection during labour. This is thought to take place through exposure to maternal blood in the birth canal. It is noteworthy that the first twin is infected twice as often as the second twin, indicating that much of the transmission occurs in the birth canal, where the first twin spends more time. Mucosal damage due to other sexually transmitted infections (STIs) or vitamin A deficiency is associated with higher rates of transmission to the child during birth. Transmission after birth almost exclusively occurs through breastmilk. Up to 10 % of newborns may be infected through this route. Newly infected women have a very high level of virus in their blood, and the risk of transmission through breastmilk to their foetuses is therefore higher. A peculiar feature of HIV-2 is that it is transmitted from mother to offspring at a much lower rate, around 5 % or less.

The fact that transmission of HIV through breastfeeding has been confirmed in several epidemiological studies constitutes a big dilemma for health authorities and infected women in low-income countries. If the Ministries of Health advise HIV infected women against breastfeeding and if they follow such an advice, more children would most probably die from diarrhoea and malnutrition than are saved from reduced HIV transmission. The reason is that most mothers cannot afford to buy enough breastmilk substitutes, and even if these were distributed free the women are not in a position to prepare them hygienically enough. Therefore, the poorest countries and the poorest HIV infected women must accept the risk of transmission through breastfeeding, as the alternative is even more risky for the health of the child. Needless to say, the will to breastfeed is enormously strong among many of these mothers. At the same time, high and middle-income countries are strongly advising against breastfeeding, and a few countries, such as Sweden, are even forbidding HIV infected mothers to breastfeed. This ethical dilemma has become even more dramatic now that drugs are available to reduce the risk of transmission, as this treatment is not affordable to those populations that have the highest prevalence.

The risk of postnatal transmission rises if the mother is sick or if she has breast problems such as cracked nipples or mastitis. Recent studies also indicate that mixed feeding, with a combination of breastmilk and other feeds, may increase transmission. So, at present, it is advised that the mother should either exclusively breastfeed or replace the breastmilk completely with other forms of feeding. Exclusive replacement feeding should only be used if it is 'AFASS': acceptable, feasible, affordable, sustainable and safe. It is judged that this is not the case in many African settings, and exclusive breastfeeding therefore remains the wisest recommendation in these areas today.

5.2.5 Antiretroviral therapy

Antiretroviral (ARV) drugs have dramatically changed the future for HIV infected persons in high-income countries. With a combination of several drugs it is now possible to give a highly active antiretroviral therapy (HAART). HAART has increased the expected lifespan of HIV infected persons from one to several decades. But the drugs have many side effects, and experience shows that it is not easy to comply with such extensive life long medication. To reduce compliance problems, the tendency has therefore been to delay the introduction of ARVs to a point where the CD4 count has fallen to 200 cells/ml of blood.

There are currently four groups of ARV:

- Nucleoside reverse transcriptase inhibitors (NRTI).
- Non-nucleoside reverse transcriptase inhibitors (NNRTI)
- Protease inhibitors (PI)
- Fusion inhibitors (FI)

Several others are in the pipeline but are not yet in routine clinical use. A minimum of three drugs are needed for HAART. For a long time, one PI was combined with two NRTI. Today there are several combinations used without any PI, as the protease inhibitors cause most side effects. During treatment with HAART the patients are followed up with CD4 counts and viral load assessments four times a year. Ideally, the CD4 count should return virtually to normal, and the viral load should be less than 50 particles/ml. Adherence to the prescribed drugs seems to be the single most important factor for sustainable effect of the therapy.

Antiretroviral therapy is already in wide use in some middle-income countries. It has been very successfully supplied through the public system in Brazil. The authorities in Thailand have started to supply treatment for some thousands of the more than one million infected persons in the country. In 2002, the Vietnamese government provided treatment for only 50 of the more than 300 000 infected persons in the country. The treatments were given to those that had probably been infected during their work in the health service. ARV is also slowly being made available to some of the infected persons in low-income countries, both to those that can afford to pay, and in some projects also free of charge to those that cannot afford. The cost of the drugs has dropped sharply but a three-drug combination still costs 300 USD per year in the capital of Uganda. Leaving drug cost aside, many other costs must be covered such as medical consultations for patient follow-up and management of side effects, and laboratory analysis as well as for treatment of other infections.

As a welcome and rational new response to the challenge to finance basic health services in low and middle-income countries The Global Fund to Fight AIDS, Tuberculosis and Malaria was created in 2002 on the initiative of the Secretary General of the UN.[1] The aim of the fund is "To attract and disburse additional resources to prevent and treat AIDS, tuberculosis and malaria. As a partnership between governments, civil society, the private sector and affected communities, the Global Fund represents a new approach to international health financing. The Fund works in close collaboration with other bilateral and multilateral organisations, supporting their work through substantially increased funding."

In spite of the low cost effectiveness of the provision of ARV in low-income countries the fund is contributing a part of the grants to purchase such drugs (Table 5.2). Of the commissioned 3.5 billion USD for the first four rounds of applications the fund uses 56 % for HIV/AIDS and a part of that for drugs. The outcome of the provision of free anti retroviral drugs in low-income countries will only be judged after some years. It may prove to be a way to achive more openness about HIV and thereby more effective prevention. It may also prove to have a low direct effect due to low compliance and the

[1]   www.globalfundatm.org

effect on prevention may be doubtful as the political focus may remain on the medical aspects of the epidemic. Readers are strongly suggested to look for recent studies on the impact of provision of free anti-retro viral drugs in the most affected low-income countries.

5.2.6 ARVs to prevent mother-to-child transmission

It has been shown that short-course, single-drug or two-drug regimens can reduce HIV transmission from mother to infant at relatively low cost. Cheapest, at only USD 4 per pregnancy, is a single oral dose (200mg) of the non-nucleoside reverse transcriptase inhibitor, Nevirapine, to the mother at onset of labour and a follow-up dose to the infant (2mg/kg) within the first 72 hours of life. Such treatment cuts intrapartal transmission by more than 50 %. Functionally, this is a prophylaxis to the infant at the time when risk of transmission is greatest per time unit. Alternatives where the mother is treated in the last trimester to cut down the viral load (= infectivity) before delivery has also been attempted, but these treatment regimes are more expensive. Most programmes to cut vertical transmission have built on antenatal voluntary counselling and testing (VCT), followed by treatment of positive mothers. The total cost of transmission avoidance depends very much on the acceptability of the screening component; with low acceptance rates and low coverage, the cost is high. The introduction of ARVs for the prevention of vertical transmission raises several ethical questions. For instance: is it right to focus on identifying women as HIV-positive and letting them be the messengers of bad news in the family? And will subsequent treatment with ARVs be less effective, due to brief exposure to ARVs at delivery?

However, despite measures to prevent the spread of HIV and advances in the treatment of AIDS, the incidence of HIV infection and the number of AIDS deaths and AIDS orphans will continue to increase

alarmingly in several low and middle-income countries during the years to come. Endurance is the main character needed for those that want to contribute to stop the HIV pandemic.

5.3 Diarrhoea (4%)

Diarrhoea is usually a harmless condition of short duration, but severe acute diarrhoea can lead to the loss of large amounts of fluids, dehydration and death. Diarrhoeal diseases caused the fifth largest number of DALYs lost in the world in 2002 (Table 4.4). Although the vast majority of the estimated 1.8 million deaths due to diarrhoea occurred in low and middle-income countries, diarrhoea remains a common disease all over the world. In health statistics, diarrhoea is often listed as one disease entity, but it is in reality just a symptom that can be caused by a number of different viruses (of which Rotavirus is the most common), bacteria or protozoa. These microorganisms are generally spread from the faeces of one person to the mouth of another via food, water or unwashed hands. Improved hygiene decreases the occurrence of diarrhoea due to all types of microorganisms. It is also justified to regard diarrhoea as a single clinical entity because the treatment is relatively similar, independently of the cause. Diarrhoea is clinically defined as having loose stools at least four times per day. Depending on duration of illness, character of the stools and whether other symptoms occur simultaneously, diarrhoeal diseases are divided into three major types: acute watery diarrhoea; dysentery and persistent diarrhoea, respectively (Table 5.3).

One of the most important medical advances in the second half of the 20th century was the introduction of oral rehydration therapy (ORT) for the treatment of life-threatening dehydration from diarrhoea. Following the introduction of ORT in 1972, there has been a worldwide decrease in the mortality due to diarrhoea, and much of

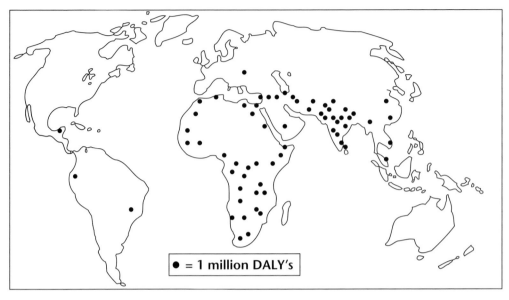

Map 5:3 Diarrhoeal disease cause 63 million disability adjusted life years (DALY) lost per year.
Source: WHO, 2002.

this decrease can be attributed to ORT. This treatment is given by mouth instead of intravenous drip directly into the blood stream. It is based on the finding that a solution containing the right mixture of water, salt and sugar allows for a very effective absorption of water through the mucous membrane of the gut. This absorption takes place through transport of glucose accompanied by sodium and water. It was first used in practice to treat large numbers of refugees from Bangladesh who suffered extensive epidemics of cholera while living in camps in India in 1972. It was shown that giving patients water mixed with salt, some bicarbonate and glucose to drink was almost as effective as intravenous infusions. The treatment with ORT was also found to be effective in children with dehydration from other types of diarrhoea. Hence, ORT was soon widely promoted for better treatment of dehydration in children with all types of diarrhoea, through extensive international programmes led by UNICEF and WHO. These programmes have been relatively successful in recent decades, because they have included a willingness to reformulate policy and adapt it to conditions in different countries on the basis of the results of evaluations and operational research.

Table 5.3 The three main types of diarrhoea.

Type of diarrhoea	% of all childhood diarrhoea	% of all childhood deaths due to diarrhoea	% of deaths preventable by standard case management
Acute watery	80	50	100
Dysentery	10	15	80
Persistent	10	35	80
Total	100	100	90

Source: IMCI: the integrated approach. WHO/CHD/97.12 rev 1.

The initial exclusive emphasis on ORT was found to have no effect or even to aggravate the malnutrition that follows in children after frequent, prolonged diarrhoeal episodes. Hence, the importance of feeding children and of continued breastfeeding during diarrhoeal episodes was included in the WHO guidelines. Furthermore, it was found very difficult to make the ready-made package in aluminium foil, containing the right proportion of salt, bicarbonate and glucose to prepare one litre of ORT, available at all times to the mothers in low-income countries who needed to prevent dehydration in their children. This was due to both the cost of such packages and the poor functioning or unavailability of health facilities in many parts of low-income countries. Hence, it was found that the promotion of home-based ORT could be included in the treatment recommendations for less severe forms of dehydration, to complement the use of industrially produced ORT packages for more severe forms. The last change in the policy for reducing deaths in diarrhoea has been to include this activity into a programme for Integrated Management of Childhood Illnesses. This is mainly because the focus has changed from simply providing the treatment to increasing the skills of peripheral health workers in assessing the level of dehydration of sick children.

ORT remains the basic treatment for dehydration from acute watery diarrhoea, and intravenous fluids are only recommended for the most severe cases. Box 5.2 illustrates the recommended treatment according to the degree of dehydration.

It was also realised that persistent diarrhoea contributes to proportionally more deaths than diarrhoeal episodes, and that concomitant malnutrition is a very significant contributing factor in many child deaths from diarrhoea. The incidence of persistent diarrhoea is also increasing because of the HIV epidemic. For persistent diarrhoea, which is the most difficult of all the different types of diarrhoea to treat, the focus is therefore on combating malnutrition. A combination of dietary therapy, zinc and vitamin supplementation, and treatment of co-existing infections is the basis for the management of this type of diarrhoea.

Dysentery is a type of diarrhoea that is combined with other signs of infection such as fever and/or bloody stools. Bacteria such as Shigella and Campylobacter, or protozoa such as Entamoeba histolytica and Giardia lamblia are the main causes. This type of diarrhoea is treated with antimicrobial drugs. As with antibiotics for lower respiratory tract infections, national guidelines may differ, and the rapid development of resistance

---

Box 5.2

Treatment of diarrhoeal disease

A. If the child is not dehydrated:
Oral rehydration therapy (ORT) at home
ORT = 4 table spoons of sugar (20g) + 1/2 table spoon of salt (3.5g) + 1 litre of water
Food + BREASTFEED

B. If the child is dehydrated but can drink:
ORT at the health facility until he child is rehydrated and the mother understands the message.
BREASTFEED

C. If the child has severe dehydration and can not drink:
Hospitalisation for treatment with intravenous fluids
BREASTFEED

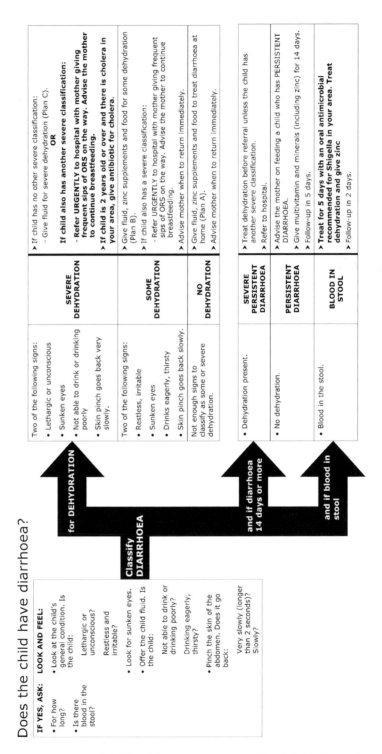

Figure 5.2 Integrated management of childhood illnesses. Assessment of level of dehydration in a child with diarrhoea.

Source: IMCI programme at WHO.

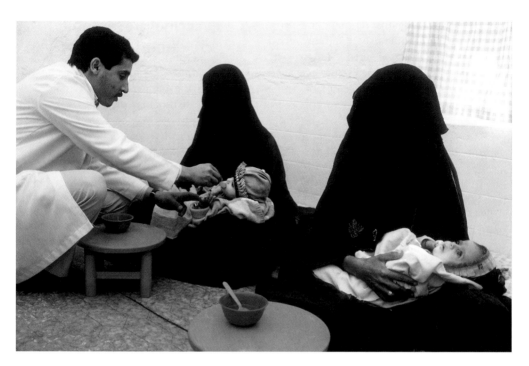

YEMEN, Taiz. Nurse at the children´s hospital is showing a mother how to spoonfeed her dehydrated child with oral rehydration salts.
© Heldur Netocny/PHOENIX.

against many of the cheaper antibiotics is a major global problem. Ciprofloxacin or norfloxacin for five days is an effective choice against Shigella, and cotrimoxazole, ampicillin or chloramphenicol may be a cheaper alternative if the resistance pattern permits. Campylobacter does not always require antibiotics, but if necessary ciprofloxacin can be used. Metronidazole is used to treat dysentery caused by protozoa. This type of diarrhoea thus requires quite advanced diagnostic resources to choose effective treatment, and thus it is difficult to cure all cases in countries with scarce resources. A central part of the global policy for treatment of diarrhoea is that non-dysenteric diarrhoeas should not be treated with antibiotics, since this does not help. The main way to reduce the global burden of diarrhoeal diseases remains prevention through improved hygiene, reduced malnutrition and treatment of acute dehydration with ORT.

The prevention of diarrhoea includes the promotion of safe drinking water supplies and latrines that interrupt faecal-oral transmission. It also includes improvements in personal hygiene and clean cooking practices, which depend on knowledge, attitudes and cultural practices, but above all on economic factors. Good nutrition starts with exclusive breastfeeding during the first six months of life, which reduces the risk of infection for the young child. Continued breastfeeding during the first two years and intensive feeding during and after an episode of diarrhoea prevent it from developing into persistent diarrhoea and malnutrition. Breastfeeding has been shown to lower the mortality rate and severity of cholera and Shigella infection by a factor of 2.5 to 4.0 (WHO 1998).

Vaccines are still of limited significance in reducing the global burden of diarrhoeal diseases. A relatively new vaccine provides good protection against cholera for three years, and simultaneously relatively good protection (70 %) against enterotoxic Escherichia coli diarrhoea (the so-called "tourist diarrhoea"), but only for three months. Several new vaccine candidates are now being tested and there is a high expectation that a new and safer rotavirus vaccine will become available. A vaccine against rotavirus would reduce mortality due to diarrhoea in the world, but the question is whether it can be made available at a sufficiently low cost to the countries and families in greatest need. From a conventional public health point of view, it can be argued that the best use of resources in these countries is to permanently improve water supply, handling of excreta and personal hygiene. However, this is so costly that the cheaper treatment offered by ORT is preferable. Using resources for vaccination against one of the main causes of diarrhoea can only be justified if this saves more lives than using these resources for improved hygiene or better treatment. The idea expressed here may seem a bit strange, as the opposite is usually stated. Most readers would probably prefer to apply a preventive approach rather than first contracting a disease and then applying a cure, even if the cure may be cheaper.

5.4 Vaccine-preventable childhood diseases (3 %)

Edward Jenner took material from a pustular lesion on the hand of the milkmaid Sarah Nelmes and inoculated it into the skin of James Phipps on 14 May 1796. This was the first scientifically developed vaccine (from Latin *vacca* = cow), and the only one to be developed in the 18th century. In the 19th century another four vaccines were developed, starting with rabies in 1885 (Pasteur), and in the 20th century around 30 new vaccines, including different combinations, followed.

The world experienced the last case of smallpox in 1977. The last patient was a cook at the hospital in the town of Mecca, south of Mogadishu, in Somalia. The World Health Organization declared smallpox to be eradicated in 1979, following decades of very determined vaccination campaigns against this devastating viral disease. This success provided a hope of eradicating other diseases, such as measles and poliomyelitis, for which effective vaccines now existed.

A worldwide Expanded Programme on Immunisation (EPI) was started by WHO and UNICEF in 1974, with the goal that all countries should start national programmes to immunise all children according to a proposed schedule (Table 5.4). Latterly, hepatitis B has been added to the programme in countries with a high prevalence of infec-

Table 5.4 WHO recommendations for standard routine immunization schedule for infants.

Disease	Vaccine	Time of Vaccination
Tuberculosis	BCG	at birth
Poliomyelitis	OPV	at birth, 6, 10 and 14 weeks
Diphtheria	DTP	6, 10 and 14 weeks
Pertussis	DTP	6, 10 and 14 weeks
Tetanus	DTP	6, 10 and 14 weeks
Measles		9 months
Yellow Fever		9 months —if relevant
Hepatitis A+B		at birth —if relevant
Tetanus in pregnancy		2 injections during pregnancy to avoid neonatal tetanus

tion with this virus. Haemophilus Influensae and other immunisations are recommended.

Immunisation is one of the most cost-effective interventions to lower the under-five mortality rate. The cost of DTP (diphtheria-tetanus-pertussis), measles, polio, and BCG (Bacille Calmette-Guérin) vaccines for a fully immunised child (FIC) is now no more than USD 1.5. This is due to a very effective international purchase system initiated by UNICEF and WHO. However, the total cost of these immunisations, including labour, transport and logistics, health facilities, planning and the training of staff and management, as well as provision of refrigerators and other cold chain equipments can be estimated at around USD 17 per child. In other words, the cost of the vaccines is only 10 % of the cost of the vaccination. This is an average across different countries. In individual countries this cost may vary from USD 6 to over USD 20. The cost increases for example in nomadic populations. When coverage rises above 80 % the marginal cost for reaching additional children also tends to rise steeply in most countries. With the newer and more expensive vaccines, the costs of the vaccines will inevitably rise. However, a vaccine tends to become less and less costly over time. The first recombinant hepatitis B vaccine in the mid-1980s, for example, cost USD 50 a dose, while the latest price is now down to USD 0.3 per dose. In contrast the cost of delivering the vaccine remains more or less the same. It is important to realise that the cost of the vaccine is a minor part of the cost of vaccination.

A multitude of immunisation strategies has been tried over the years. The basic strategy, however, remains to provide the basic routine immunisations in fixed health facilities, supplemented by outreach strategies of various kinds, especially in low-density populated areas. Although many of the present vaccines were developed, overall global immunisation coverage of children in the early 1970s was less than 5 %. This was the time when the WHO established its

Expanded Programme on Immunisation (EPI).

In a 15-year period up to 1990, immunisation rates rose to around 80 %, under the slogan of 'Universal Childhood Immunisation'. This was largely a result of the successful guidance provided by the organisations of the United Nations, especially the practical approach of UNICEF. They developed new material for transporting and storing vaccines at the lowest cost possible. Special credits should go to the dynamic leader of UNICEF, James Grant.

Unfortunately, these achievements are difficult to sustain. Under the impact of economic crises, and with global support decreasing, coverage rates stagnated or even began to decline. By 1999, the coverage rate (as measured by DTP3) stood at 76 %. Many countries today, particularly in Africa, have coverage levels below 50 %. Among countries in crisis or at war, rates are less than 30 %. An exception has been polio, where eradication efforts have been focused on National Immunisation Days, on which all children are expected to receive Oral Polio Vaccine (OPV). As this oral vaccine does not require an injection, the advantage is that health service staff is not required to give the immunisation. This has frequently led to OPV coverage levels above 90 or 95 %. Unfortunately, all other vaccines in the EPI programme need to be injected.

A particular problem is that all injections are not given in a safe manner. Unsterilised needles may be used. One problem may be that disposable syringes are not successfully destroyed after use. Informal health practitioners may reuse such needles again without proper sterilisation. This could result in the spread of blood-borne infections, particularly hepatitis B, hepatitis C and HIV. Up to one-third of the estimated 12 billion injections given every year are not safe. Of these 12 billion, an estimated one billion are immunisation injections, while the rest are injections for curative purposes. Great efforts have been made to develop systems that diminish the risk of unsafe injections in the

---

Box 5.3

Combination vaccines, with several antigens in the same injection, are especially important for low-income countries. The most common of these is the DTP (diphtheria-tetanus-pertussis) vaccine. MMR (measles-mumps-rubella) and MR vaccines are mainly used in high-income countries. Industry has now developed a tetravalent vaccine including hepatitis B (DTP-HBV) and even a pentavalent DTP-HBV-Haemophilus type B. Obviously combination vaccines have a great potential in countries with fragile health systems, even if the cost of the actual vaccines becomes higher. These new combination vaccines are still costly and in short supply but may become much more used in a few years.

The development of new vaccines is costly, and somebody has to pay. If this cost is to be covered by the 'market', through high prices, most children in low and middle-income countries will not benefit from these scientific achievements. Put more bluntly, the new vaccines will not be used to save millions of lives, but only to reduce the incidence of illness among children who already have access to adequate treatment if they get pneumonia. The development of rational and adequate financing mechanisms for the development, purchase and provision of new vaccines to all the children in the world is obviously as great a challenge.

Vaccines that are not in sufficient demand on the market are called 'orphan vaccines'.

Manufacturers do not feel that there is sufficient incentive to spend around USD 200 million to develop such a vaccine without the assurance of a market that will make it possible to recover the research investments. It must be realised that the objective of commercial pharmaceutical companies is to make profit on invested capital. The market mechanisms will not provide the vaccines that the world needs. Therefore there has been little research into vaccines for malaria and tuberculosis. A 'pull' mechanism in the form of an artificial market has been suggested to encourage the pharmaceutical industry to step up research efforts for orphan vaccines (Sachs 2001). This requires a system whereby the public sector, through donor agencies or multilateral organisations, guarantees the purchase of a specified quantity of malaria vaccine at an agreed price, e.g. USD 10 per dose. If manufacturers succeed in producing such a vaccine, they will know what the return will be, and if they do not, they take on the risk of losing their investment themselves. Traditional 'push' mechanisms are also possible; but this implies that the public sector or philanthropic billionaires pays for research to be conducted and take the risk of loosing the money if the research fails. The currently promising vaccine candidates to meet the needs of low-income countries are those against rotavirus and the common bacteria causing pneumonia and meningitis (NIH 2000).

---

vaccination programmes. Disposable (one-time) syringes were once thought to do so, although it has been found that they actually entail increased risk, as they are in practice often reused without sterilisation. The simplistic idea that disposable needles could solve the problem of unsafe injections in poor countries is but one of many strange suggestions originating from high income countries that are contra-productive because they completely fail to understand the character of poverty. It is very difficult to introduce the practice of throwing things away in poor countries. The most promising development is the invention of the auto-destruct (AD) syringe, which cannot be reused once the plunger has been depressed. WHO-UNICEF and UNFPA have adopted a policy by which only these AD syringes are provided, and countries are to make a scheduled switch to them within a few years. Pending the switch, sterilisable syringes should be used in preference to disposable ones in many settings.

160

One of the most important and controversial recommendations by WHO was that the primary health care services in low and middle-income countries should also use the opportunities to vaccinate sick children. These children are in fact a special priority group for immunisation. The success of this policy has also undoubtedly contributed to the falling under-five mortality rate in the world.

Estimates indicate that 3 million children are saved annually by vaccinations. Another 4 million lives could be saved by immunisation utilising all existing vaccines and extending coverage (WHO 1998). In the following sections we will describe one by one the diseases, that can be prevented by immunisation.

5.4.1 Measles (1.4 %)

Measles is a very contagious viral infection that spreads by direct contact or by droplets in the air. It is a severe febrile disease, affecting mainly children. The peak incidence is at 2–3 years of age in an unimmunised population. An estimated 40 million children contract measles each year. This corresponds to about 30 % of all children born; the remaining 70 % do not get the disease because they are protected by vaccination. About 600 000 children still die of this disease each year, and measles remains one of the five most common causes of death in children on a global scale. It is noteworthy that this is the case even though an effective and safe vaccine has been available for almost 30 years. The fact that measles still ranks as number 14 among diseases causing most loss of healthy years of life in the world indicates that the provision of vaccination for those who need it seems to be more difficult than many would think. The vast majority of DALYs lost due to measles are in Sub-Saharan Africa, where the combination of low immunisation coverage and widespread malnutrition render children susceptible to severe forms of measles. In middle and high-income countries, the disease has become rare, due to high immunisation rates.

Measles is always a severe disease, but it has an extremely low mortality among well-nourished children. In contrast, measles is a devastating disease for a malnourished child without access to health care. It has a 3 to 5 % case fatality rate in low-income countries. In refugee camps and other high risk populations the percentage of children dying from measles is commonly 10 to 30 %.

The disease starts with a cough and fever. After a few days, the fever reaches a peak and a skin rash appears. The measles virus infects all of the mucous membranes of the body. The body needs vitamin A to repair mucous membranes, and thus measles easily depletes stores of vitamin A, especially if they are already low. The disease increases the risk of the most severe complications of vitamin A deficiency: blindness due to destruction of the cornea and death from secondary infections due to a compromised immune system. In children that survive the measles infection severe malnutrition is a common complication that may take months to recover from. The child is prone to get complicating infections in the eyes, mouth or ears, as well as diarrhoea and respiratory tract infections, including reactivation of primary tuberculosis. Following an episode of measles, the immune system becomes weakened, both during the acute illness and for months afterwards. A higher energy intake than usual is necessary to fight the infection, but the child with measles has difficulty eating enough to secure even basic energy needs due to fever, diarrhoea and infection in the mouth. It is very demanding and resource consuming to care for a child with measles.

There exists no treatment for the viral disease itself, but malnutrition and secondary bacterial infections can be successfully treated. Vitamin A supplementation is crucial for survival. Since measles appears in association with pneumonia, diarrhoea and malnutrition, the Integrated Management of Childhood Illnesses approach is particu-

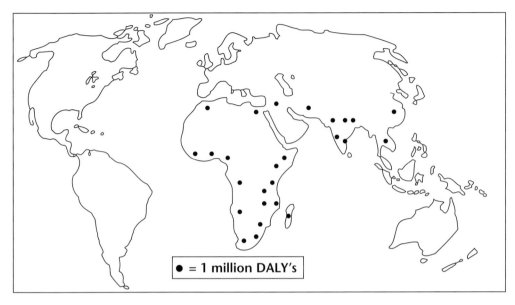

Map 5:4 Measles cause 26 million disability adjusted life years (DALY) lost per year.
Source: WHO, 2002.

larly appropriate for this disease. Good nutrition, including continued breastfeeding during and after the disease, is essential for the survival of children with measles.

It is sad that so many resources must be used to treat measles, since it is a very easily preventable disease. A live attenuated vaccine, which provides good protection, is safe and today also cheap. It is estimated that more than 70 % of all children in the world currently are vaccinated, and this has already saved many lives. But hopes of eradicating measles through vaccination have been tuned down, since immunisation coverage of more than 95 % is required to stop the transmission and thus eradicate the virus. WHO recommends one dose of vaccine at the age of 9 months, although in special situations two doses may be needed.

Although new stabilisers have made the freeze-dried vaccine less heat-sensitive, the present vaccine still requires a well-functioning 'cold chain'. This expression refers to the need to store and transport the vaccine at a temperature below 4°C from its site of production, through storage and during distribution to the final child health clinic, where the vaccine is finally to be injected under the skin of the child. This may seem easy, but in practice it is an enormous obstacle in countries with scarce and irregular energy supplies. The need to maintain sterility at immunisation also places high technical demands on both equipment and the knowledge and skills of the staff. The cost of the vaccine itself is only about 10 cents per dose. In fact the cost of the vaccine is a negligible part of the cost of vaccination. The success entirely depends on the coverage and quality of the health service in each country.

The coverage of immunisation against measles and DTP (diphtheria-tetanus-pertussis), is a good indicator of how well the health service system functions in a country. National immunisation rates vary from 90–100 % in high or middle-income countries to only 30–35 % in a few low-income countries, or even lower in some of the most war-torn countries. In all of Sub-Saharan Africa, it is estimated that about 50 % of the children are immunised. Further improvement of the coverage of measles immunisation thus remains one of the most cost-effective health interventions in the world.

5.4.2 Pertussis (0.8%)

Whooping cough is the lay term for pertussis. This disease caused an estimated 300 000 child deaths in 2002, almost all in low and middle-income countries. Pertussis was, after measles, the vaccine-preventable childhood disease that caused the most DALYs lost globally in 2002.

It is an infection of the airways by bacteria of the Bordetella pertussis species. The disease starts with a nasal discharge, cough and fever. After ten to fifteen days, the cough gradually worsens and each coughing attack is followed by a peculiar airway spasm resulting in the whooping that has given the disease its name in many languages. In Chinese, the disease is called '100-day cough' because the cough generally lasts more than three months, but the disease is eventually self-limiting. The child often vomits at the end of the coughing attacks, and is therefore prone to becoming malnourished during the period of illness. The disease can be especially life threatening if the affected child is less than one year of age and if the child is already malnourished at the start of the disease.

Pertussis is special in that, although bacteria cause it, it cannot be cured with antibiotics. Antibiotics only have effect if given before the convulsive cough starts, but at that early stage the disease is very difficult to diagnose. In small children, pertussis may be complicated by a bacterial pneumonia that can be treated with antibiotics. Otherwise, treatment is symptomatic. Above all, parents need great patience to wait for the disease to pass and frequent small feeds as long as the cough lasts. The only prevention is immunisation with the low cost vaccine (Table 5.4).

5.4.3 Tetanus (0.5%)

Although the bacteria that cause tetanus are present worldwide, this disease causes DALYs to be lost almost exclusively in low and middle-income countries. The main reason is that the populations of high-income countries are protected from tetanus through a very effective immunisation. The few cases occurring in high-income countries occur in elderly people or immigrants with inadequate or absent immunisation. An estimated 210 000 deaths due to tetanus occur in the world every year, which represents a decrease from about 1 000 000 in the early 1980s. This decrease is mainly due to more or less successful national immunisation programmes in most countries.

The bacteria causing tetanus, Clostridium tetani, is abundantly present in soil and may be introduced into the body through wounds. The use of unclean instruments to cut the umbilical cord after delivery can also cause tetanus in the newborn, known as neonatal tetanus.

After an incubation period of 1–2 weeks, the bacteria produce a neurotoxin that causes generalised muscular spasms. The muscle rigidity and spasm start in the face, spread within days to involve the whole body, and continue for two to four weeks. These generalised spasms cause the death of 10 to 90% of the patients affected by tetanus. The death rate is highest in newborns and the elderly, but the prognosis largely depends on whether ventilator care is available. Modern high-technological intensive care can save almost all cases of tetanus, but there is no low-cost treatment that can achieve this.

However, a very cheap, safe and effective vaccine is available against tetanus. The disease can be prevented in the newborn baby if the pregnant woman is given at least two doses of tetanus vaccine during pregnancy, if she has not already been immunised. The antibodies formed in the mother following vaccination are transferred to the child and protect it during the first months of life. Prevention also includes clean care of the umbilical cord after birth. Vaccination with the diphtheria-pertussis-tetanus (DTP) vaccine should be carried out three times during the first year of life, starting from the age of six weeks (Table 5.4). Health education is important to prevent tetanus. People must come early for treatment of severe wounds by cleaning and booster-vaccination, and must understand the importance of vaccination and clean birth practices.

5.4.4 Poliomyelitis (< 0.5 %)

Before the development of the vaccines against polio in the 1950s, it was a worldwide disease. In the year 1988, when the decision to eradicate polio was taken, there were 350 000 cases per year around the world. Polio has been eradicated in Europe, the Western Pacific region and the entire American hemisphere. Following the successful eradication of smallpox 20 years ago, the poliovirus may be the second major microorganism to be eradicated from the world. Due to high coverage of vaccination, polio is also on the verge of eradication in North Africa, Middle East and East Asia. The majority of cases now occur in India, and Pakistan, and to a lesser extent in western and central Africa. Particularly vulnerable populations are: refugees, victims of war and the urban poor in countries whose infrastructure and preventive health services have been destroyed. To finally eradicate polio, these pockets of populations at high risk need to be reached with vaccination.

Poliomyelitis is a diarrhoeal disease caused by a very contagious virus, which spreads from faeces to the mouth, like other diarrhoeas do. More than 90 % of all subjects infected by the virus show no sign of disease or only a slight fever, headache or diarrhoea for a few days, and yet they gain immunity for the rest of their lives. However, in about 1 % of persons infected with the poliovirus, the disease progresses to destroy the anterior horn cells in the spinal cord, transmitting signals to the muscles. Various forms of flaccid paralysis may result, often permanent. The paralysis is usually asymmetrical, i.e. it affects only one arm or leg. Before WHO and UNICEF launched the worldwide vaccination programme, polio caused about half of the walking disabilities in the world. Most of the healthy life years lost from polio are due to permanent paralysis. Only if the respiratory muscles are affected may the disease be fatal.

As late as the 1950s, epidemics of polio occurred in all high-income countries, but in the 1960s the vaccine ended polio as a public health problem in high-income countries. In the last epidemic in Sweden in 1953 a total of 5 000 victims suffered from various degrees of paralysis. The last case in the Americas was reported in Peru in 1991. This was after six years of joint international work towards eradication, using routine vaccinations, national vaccination days and 'mop-up' operations to control outbreaks, as well as building up a surveillance network. The success in the American hemisphere indicates that it should be possible to eradicate polio throughout the world and WHO has formed a special organisation for this eradication. In the year 2002 less than 2 000 cases occurred in the 7 countries where polio is yet to be eradicated. These countries are India, Pakistan, Afghanistan, Somalia, Egypt, Niger and Nigeria. It is interesting that economic calculations show that the cost of the extra effort needed is less than the cost of the ongoing vaccinations in the world. But with very few cases in some areas, there is a false sense of security and the motivation to keep up massive national campaigns may decline. It is feasible but by no mean clear that polio eradication will succeed in the near future. The readers are suggested to follow the outcome of this important effort through the web site.[1]

5.4.5 Diphtheria (< 0.5 %)

Around 100 000 new cases of diphtheria occur every year, leading to around 5 000 annual deaths worldwide at the turn of the

---

[1] www.polioeradication.org

21st century. Diphtheria was one of the leading causes of childhood mortality in the world until the introduction of the vaccine and antibiotics 50 years ago. The reason for including it in this review of global health problems is that vaccination against diphtheria is part of the EPI programme. It is also interesting to note that the socio-economic decline in the former Soviet Union after 1990, resulted in an epidemic of diphtheria that spread to 15 countries and caused as many as 25 000 (WHO 1996). Thus the importance to keep up the vaccination efforts.

Diphtheria is a bacterial infection that causes a severe respiratory tract infection with fever and severe damage to the mucous membranes of the nose, throat and larynx. The bacteria also produce a toxin that spreads through the blood and can affect the heart and nerves. Death may occur due to obstruction of the larynx or to effects on the heart. The case fatality rate is 5 to 10 %. Penicillin and erythromycin are both effective against the diphtheria bacteria. However, diphtheria can be fully prevented by immunisation with the diphtheria-pertussis-tetanus (DTP) vaccine three times from the age of six weeks. To avoid epidemics, it is essential to maintain immunisation coverage in all countries. Surveillance and rapid management of cases of diphtheria, as well as the detection and prevention of close contacts, are necessary to further hinder the spread of epidemics.

5.5 Malaria (3%)

Worldwide the malaria parasite is estimated to be the direct cause of about 1.3 million deaths and an estimated 300 to 500 million clinical cases annually. More than 90 % of all parasite carriers live in Africa (WHO 2001), and currently 5 % of all children born in Africa are expected to die of malaria. Two-fifths of the world's population live in areas of risk for malaria infection in Sub-Saharan Africa, Asia and Central and South America. The disease is among the top ten causes of healthy life years lost in the world. In high transmission areas malaria affects mainly children and pregnant women. The cost of malaria is enormous, both in lost productivity through death and disease and in treatment costs. In Africa alone the direct costs are estimated to be more than USD 2 billion per year (Sachs 2001).

Four types of malaria parasites can infect humans. These four types are known as Plasmodium falciparum, P. ovale, P. vivax and P. malariae. These parasites are all transmitted from one person to another via the Anopheles mosquito. When a mosquito sucks blood, it infects the person with parasites that are present in the saliva that the mosquito injects before sucking. Plasmodium falciparum is the most dangerous type of malaria, since it causes the severe and potentially fatal form of cerebral malaria. This species of the parasite multiplies most rapidly in the blood, but cannot remain dormant in the liver like the other types.

An attack of malaria typically has a sudden onset, with fever, muscle stiffness and headache. Other general symptoms, such as diarrhoea and vomiting, are also common. When an attack of falciparum malaria involves the brain, the disease may suddenly be aggravated with convulsions, unconsciousness and death. The most terrifying aspect of the falciparum type of malaria is the speed with which the disease can develop. Respiratory distress and acidosis are severe symptoms. Particularly in children the disease can progress from chills and fever to death in the course of one to two days, if treatment is not commenced in time. A single episode of malaria lasts 1–14 days. Anaemia is a common complication of malaria attacks, especially in populations with co-existent malnutrition.

Malaria attacks are more frequent in pregnant women than in other adults. The reason is that pregnancy decreases the immunity they have earlier acquired against the disease. Malaria is a major cause of maternal mortality, abortion and low birth weight. Mothers transmit a passive immunity via

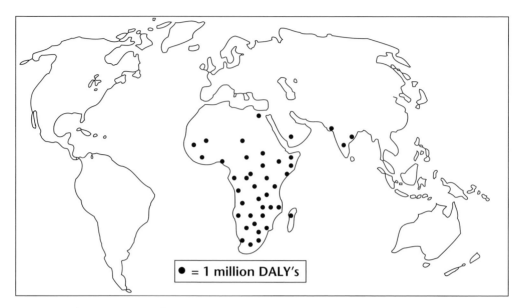

Map 5:5 Malaria causes 41 million disability adjusted life years (DALY) lost per year.
Source: WHO, 2002.

the placenta, and these antibodies protect the infant for the first four to six months in life. In areas with intensive malaria transmission, young children are the main victims. Children who survive the attacks of the disease gradually develop immunity. However, immunity against malaria is transient. If a previously immune individual spends a year outside areas with malaria-transmitting mosquitoes, she again becomes susceptible to the parasite and may suffer a fatal attack of the disease on return.

Treatment of simple malaria is fairly easy if it is diagnosed early and the parasites are not resistant to the anti-malarial drugs used in the area. Most attacks of malaria can be cured through home treatment prescribed by briefly trained staff at primary health care facilities or by the parents of the sick child. In contrast, successful treatment of very severe forms of cerebral malaria requires the most sophisticated form of intensive care. Children in heavily affected areas often die from anaemia, resulting from repeated malaria infections. It is in the absence of early diagnosis and proper treat-

ment, as well as due to increasing drug resistance that so many children in Africa die of malaria.

During recent decades, the drug most commonly used to treat malaria was chloroquine. This drug was developed in the 1940s. It replaced quinine, because it was as effective and much safer. For this reason chloroquine became very widely used. The malaria parasites began to become resistant to chloroquine in South-East Asia and Latin America in the 1960s, and this resistance spread to Africa in the 1970s. In large parts of Sub-Saharan Africa, the resistance levels are now as high as 60% or higher. In the areas in East and Central Africa with the highest percentage of resistance to chloroquine, this drug is no longer an efficient treatment. Despite this chloroquine is still the drug of choice for uncomplicated malaria in many countries. This is due to its low cost, lack of political will and slow procedures to change national treatment policy.

A major alternative to chloroquine has been sulfadoxine-pyrimethamine (Fansidar®), but this drug produces more side effects. Resistance to it is also spreading in South-East Asia, Latin America and East Africa. Mefloquine is used in multi-resistant strains, but resistance is also developing rapidly against this drug in South-East Asia. Artemisin has been developed and used in China for hundreds of years. It is obtained from plant extracts and is now being tried with success in the treatment of severe, multi-resistant malaria. The malaria treatment of the future in which most researchers believe today is a combination of artemisin with one or two other drugs. The combination therapy is due to a rapidly developing resistance to the first and second-line drugs, chloroquine as well as sulfadoxine-pyrimethamine, and to avoid future resistance to artemisin. These combinations are currently being used in Asia and are under trial in Africa. The problem is the increasing costs of these combination drugs, which is why many Ministries of Health still recommend outdated malaria treatment.

The fact that quinine after 300 years of wide use still remains the most important treatment for severe malaria reflects the appallingly limited investment in research into new drugs for this disease. Quinine is a naturally occurring compound, initially found in a traditional herbal drug in South America that has been used against malaria for centuries. It has a very good effect against severe forms of falciparum malaria. Resistance to quinine has only been documented in some parts of Latin America, and in South-East Asia, but not yet in Africa. The disadvantage with quinine is that it is very toxic and an overdose may cause lethal cardiac effects.

It is very easy to foresee a great need for more drugs against malaria in the near future. The advances in molecular biology and pharmacology make it scientifically highly possible that such drugs can be developed. The obstacle is on the financing side. Since the disease affects almost exclusively the poorest populations of the world, the research required is not a high priority for the multinational pharmaceutical industry.

Multinational pharmaceutical companies have the scientific expertise and capacity required, but they have no economical reason to invest in a project that will not provide sufficient profit. The world is waiting for the innovative financial solution that can enable medical research to solve this major global health need.

Global strategies to prevent malaria have changed several times during the last half-century. Given the spread of resistance and the occurrence of toxic side effects, chemoprophylaxis for populations in endemic areas is today out of the question. After the Second World War, the aim was to eradicate malaria by a two-pronged attack. The new pesticide DDT, was sprayed in large campaigns to reduce the number of mosquitoes, and chloroquine was given widely to eradicate the parasite from humans. It was gradually realised that DDT itself might be dangerous to humans and that it caused side effects in the environment. The mosquitoes soon developed resistance to the pesticide, just as the malaria parasite developed resistance to chloroquine. The large-scale eradication campaigns were stopped, because positive results were not sustainable with this approach. In India malaria was almost eradicated in the 1970s, but the disease has been recurring during the last decades of the 20th century. India is now estimated to have 11 to 15 million cases of malaria per year. WHO had to adopt the more modest goal of controlling mortality by providing treatment for those contracting malaria rather than to try to eradicate the disease.

The latest preventive option is to promote insecticide-impregnated bed nets. These have been widely tested as an ecologically sound, large-scale intervention. The distribution of impregnated bed nets in rural villages in Gambia has achieved a 70 % reduction in mortality among children (Alonso 1991). Unfortunately, the cost of bed nets is still too high in relation to the resources available to the Ministries of Health and the average families in the most affected African countries. The cost per healthy life year saved is about USD 25. The problem of preventing malaria is thus economic, organisational and scientific. The scientific challenge is not to find effective methods—they already exist. The challenge is to find methods cheap enough to be sustainable among the poor in the low-income countries where malaria mainly occurs, or to find increased external funding. In November 2002, the Global Fund against AIDS, TB and Malaria (GFATM) signed an agreement with the government of Tanzania to provide millions of impregnated bed nets for the children of Tanzania. The drainage of mosquito-breeding wetlands is also a potentially simple and effective measure in areas where the breeding sites are well defined, but it appears to be a feasible intervention in only a few areas.

Extensive research efforts to find a vaccine against malaria are being made, but so far the few candidate vaccines tested have not been sufficiently protective. Only one vaccine candidate has shown some protective effects in adults, which increases the hope of finding a vaccine that is sufficiently effective for children. The progress in molecular biology, including the revelation of the whole genome of both the malaria parasite and the Anopheles mosquito in September 2002, makes vaccine development a more hopeful goal. However, it remains very difficult to predict how much more research is needed to produce an effective vaccine. Estimates are that an effective vaccine will not be available within the next decade.

At present there is no doubt that the burden of malaria is increasing in the world, although the disease occurs almost exclusively in low-income countries. WHO has responded with a programme called 'Roll Back Malaria', which presents a joint strategy to co-ordinate existing resources in a better way.[1] In the short term, the focus is to improve the use of existing drugs and to improve the use of health services by the affected populations. The best long-term re-

search strategy remains unclear. Some priority issues include allocating more scientific resources to developing new drugs, investigating how malaria is treated in affected communities, improving the way bed nets are made available and the development of a vaccine, which may take years or decades, if at all possible.

5.6 Tuberculosis (3 %)

Infection with the tubercle bacteria causes about 7 million new clinical cases of tuberculosis annually, and half a century after the discovery of life-saving treatment, it is still estimated to kill around 1.6 million people per year (WHO 2004). The majority of cases occur in South and East Asia and Sub-Saharan Africa. Tuberculosis is, after HIV/AIDS, the leading killer of adults among the communicable diseases. 99 % of all DALYs lost due to tuberculosis occurred in low and middle-income countries. The economic burden of the disease is extensive, since it mainly affects economically productive young adults.

At the end of the 19th century and during the first half of the 20th century tuberculosis was a major public health problem in Europe and North America. Overcrowded housing and poor sanitary conditions gave rise to the spread of the disease. The fact that the incidence of tuberculosis was higher in Scandinavia a hundred years ago than it is in Africa today may be because transmission is higher under poor living conditions in a cold climate. The reason being that indoor crowding is worse when poor people have to stay warm during the winter. In the climatic sense of the term, tuberculosis is definitely not a tropical disease, although the incidence today is highest in the tropics. The disease incidence decreases with socio-economic development and was under control in all high-income countries by the 1970s or 1980s. The decrease of tuberculosis in the richest countries occurred mainly before the discovery of tuberculo-

[1]   http://mosquito.who.int

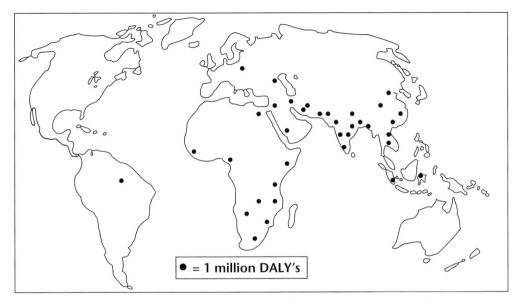

Map 5:6 Tuberculosis causes 36 million disability adjusted life years (DALY) lost per year.
Source: WHO, 2002.

static drugs around 1950. The decrease in TB before the drugs has been attributed to better nutrition, better housing, better symptomatic care of the sick and early isolation of contagious cases as correct diagnosis became available at the end of the 19th century. However, there has been a resurgence of tuberculosis in the world, including many of the high-income countries, since the mid-1980s. This is because HIV infection increases the risk of contracting tuberculosis and, more importantly, of reactivating dormant TB. Other reasons are that many tuberculosis strains have developed resistance to the drugs used against the disease, and that control programmes have missed many socially deprived cases even in some high-income countries.

The bacteria causing tuberculosis, Mycobacterium tuberculosis, is transmitted via droplets from coughing persons with pulmonary tuberculosis. The bacteria can be directly diagnosed by microscopy after staining of sputum. This is a low-cost test, while diagnosis through cultivation of the bacteria requires advanced and costly laborato-

ries. The PPD test involves injecting a protein from the bacterium into the skin, which develops a red swelling in people infected with the bacteria. Unfortunately, the result is also positive in those vaccinated against tuberculosis, and so this test is not of much use in the fight against tuberculosis. Only in countries where immunisation against TB is rare does this test have good diagnostic value.

A special feature of Mycobacterium tuberculosis is that only 10 % of newly infected persons have any signs of disease. Although the primary infection passes unnoticed in most persons, the bacteria spreads via the blood and may remain dormant in many body organs. The dormant bacteria may wake up and cause disease many decades later in life. In fact most forms of tuberculosis, especially pulmonary tuberculosis is a result of reactivation of an infection that was acquired many years or decades earlier. Malnutrition, diabetes, alcoholism and HIV infection are predisposing factors for reactivation. Most reactivations occur in the lungs. We will restrict the discussion about tuber-

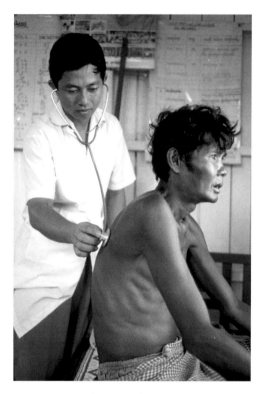

CAMBODIA, Tonle Sap. A doctor examining a man suffering from tuberculosis.

© Sean Sprague / PHOENIX.

velopment of resistance. Second, the drugs must be taken regularly for a period of 6 to 8 months, although most symptoms will disappear after a few months. The drugs used are combinations of isoniazid, rifampicin, streptomycin, pyrazinamide, and ethambutol. Because of the long treatment and unpleasant side effects of some drugs, the risk of interruption of treatment is high. Drug resistance is worse in Asia, but is now becoming a problem all over the world. For many decades WHO has promoted non-hospitalised treatment for TB patients. Compliance to treatment has remained low in most countries. WHO's strategy is known as 'directly observed treatment short-course' (DOTS). This strategy implies that patients must swallow their tablets daily in front of a trained health worker or specially designated 'controller' in their local community. There should be a good, regular supply of anti-tuberculosis drugs to health facilities. The case detection is based on self-reporting at health centres and on the use of sputum-smear microscopy. The collection of a representative sputum sample is quite demanding. So is the correct staining and examination in the microscope. It thus requires well-trained laboratory staff. In special intervention studies, the DOTS strategy has been found to produce about 95 % cure rate among TB patients. However, when implemented countrywide the cure rate has been found to be lower.

culosis to this form that should be called post-primary pulmonary tuberculosis, but it is often only called lung TB. Pulmonary tuberculosis is especially important as it both constitutes the majority of cases and is responsible for almost all transmission. The most common symptoms are prolonged cough, shortness of breath, fever, weight loss and fatigue. A particular feature of tuberculosis is that treatment of patients is the best way to prevent the spread of the infection.

Effective drugs against tuberculosis have been available for the last 50 years. There are many reasons why the control of tuberculosis has failed in many middle and low-income countries in spite of the existence of effective drugs. First, it is necessary to treat with a combination of drugs to avoid the de-

Besides improved treatment of pulmonary tuberculosis, the main options to prevent the disease are of general character, i.e. improved housing and nutrition. The BCG (Bacille Calmette-Guérin) vaccine against tuberculosis is given at birth. Unfortunately the vaccine provides protection mainly against severe forms of primary tuberculosis infection in young children. The vaccine does not protect well against the secondary pulmonary forms of TB. Health education programmes dealing with the mode of transmission, methods of control and the importance of early detection and treatment are important. Delayed diagnosis or ineffective treatment of tuberculosis often cause long-term dysfunction of the lungs, loss of job, economic hardship for families and impaired national economic development.

5.7 Sexually transmitted infections (excluding HIV) (1 %)

It is estimated that 330 million cases of curable sexually transmitted infections (STIs) occur in the world every year, most of them in low-income countries. Excluding HIV infection, the STIs jointly caused 0.8 % of the world's DALYs lost in 2002. Syphilis infection caused most of those DALYs lost, followed by chlamydial infections and gonorrhoea. For many decades STIs have ranked among the top five conditions for which adults in many low and middle-income countries seek health care services. Signs of genital infection are common in several Sub-Saharan African countries. STIs are often the third most frequent diagnosis, after malaria and diarrhoea, in primary health care facilities. After tuberculosis and pregnancy-related disorders, STIs are reported to represent the third greatest burden of disease in women between 15 and 45 years of age.

The occurrence of STIs does not seem to be diminishing in the world. However, few domains of ill health show such a pronounced global variation in occurrence as STIs. This is obviously related to cultural and social norms related to sexuality and reproduction. Syphilis and gonorrhoea are two illustrative examples. In various parts of Sub-Saharan Africa, the prevalence of seropositive syphilis is 15 %, and prevalence rates for gonorrhoea may reach up to 10 % in the sexually active part of the population. During recent decades, prevalence figures for these two classic STIs have fallen to very low levels in high-income countries, while simultaneously rising rapidly in some middle-income countries, especially in the coun-

tries formally belonging to the Soviet Union. Other middle-income countries, such as Cuba, China and Costa Rica, are known to have implemented successful strategies to counteract the spread of STIs. Chlamydia trachomatis infection remains a widespread problem in middle and high-income countries alike, but the contribution of Chlamydia infection to the panorama of STIs in low-income countries is largely unknown.

During pregnancy the STIs may cause foetal diseases and low birth weight. They may also cause pre-term birth and postpartum infections in the mother and newborn, including eye infections in the newborn. It is estimated that up to 80 million women in the world are infertile. The vast majority having lost their fertility due to pelvic inflammatory disease resulting from various STIs. The pelvic inflammatory diseases also increase the incidence of ectopic pregnancy, leading to severe maternal morbidity and even mortality. The burden of disease from STIs is aggravated not only by the high rate of complications but also by an increasing problem of antimicrobial resistance.

Conventionally, the three most important aims of STI control are: (1) interrupting transmission by promoting safer sexual practices; (2) rapidly curing those infected; and (3) preventing the development of complications and sequelae by screening for the diseases in high-risk groups. However, only a few countries have national health programmes dealing specifically with STI control. Where they exist, such programmes are often fragmented, with a focus either on a particular disease, such as HIV/AIDS, or on a general aspect, such as fertility control or maternal and child health. Different disease-oriented programmes often overlap and may be interrelated in terms of the problems each programme attempts to address. An integrated approach has many advantages. STI programmes generally need to improve access to and quality of services, be more responsive to clients' needs, more cost-effective and more likely to reach groups currently poorly served, such as women and young people. In low-income countries, with budgetary constraints, the need for integrated services is even more urgent. Countries are presently advised to deliver more broadly based reproductive health care interventions, preferably integrated into basic health care, maternal and child health care and family planning services. There is a general consensus in the world today that most countries need to develop a more comprehensive approach to STI control. In practice, however, programme development always requires selection of activities and interventions on the basis of countries' current needs and available resources.

Primary prevention activities consist of the promotion of safer sexual behaviour and the provision of condoms at affordable prices. Secondary prevention activities consist of the promotion of rational health care seeking behaviour directed particularly towards those at increased risk of acquiring STI and HIV infections. It also encompasses the provision of accessible, effective and acceptable services, which offer diagnoses and effective treatment for both symptomatic and asymptomatic STI patients and their partners.

Globally speaking, there is no single strategy for the control of sexually transmitted infections. There are, however, guiding principles that apply almost everywhere. Strategies for the attainment of reproductive health and the prevention and care of reproductive tract infections including STIs must be based on the underlying principles of human rights. The improvement of prevention and care for STI requires a careful adaptation to local realities.

5.8 Other parasite infections and intestinal worms (1 %)

This group of diseases consists of parasitic diseases that all have a particular geographic distribution that is determined by the occurrence of the transmitting vector, most often

an insect, and mostly also occurrence of a low level of socio-economic development (Cock 2002). However, it should be noted that the burden of most of these diseases could be greatly reduced by cost-effective control programmes making use of the knowledge of the life cycle of the parasite. The interventions are based on breaking this cycle at one or several points. Altogether, these parasitic diseases caused about 1 % of the global burden of DALYs lost and about 140 000 deaths in 2002, almost all in low and middle-income countries. Leishmaniasis and trypanosomiasis cause most of these deaths, but lymphatic filariasis alone causes by far the greatest number of DALYs lost in this group of diseases. One or the other of these diseases may be very important in some local areas.

Lymphatic filariasis (0.4 %) (mainly Wuchereria bancrofti) is caused by parasites that are transmitted by mosquitoes. The parasite causes inflammation of lymphatic vessels and lymph nodes, mainly in the axilla and groins. This sometimes results in lymphatic obstruction, leading to elephantiasis, i.e. a monstrous swelling of the scrotum or the legs. It is treated with diethylcarbamazine citrate, and controlled with treatment and insecticide campaigns. Filariasis occurs in countries with hot and humid areas, both urban and rural, in Africa, Asia, the Pacific, South America and the Caribbean.

Schistosomiasis (0.1 %) (S. japonicum, S. mansoni) also known as bilharzia, is caused by a parasite with a very special life cycle. The parasite is passed through human urine into fresh water in lakes and rivers. There it infects special types of snails and transforms into a form that returns to the water and can penetrate the skin of other humans when they take a bath or expose their skin to the water for other reasons. Having passed the skin the parasite travels through the blood stream to the blood vessels of the guts and urinary bladder. There the male and female parasites mate and produce eggs that are released into the bladder and gut to be passed into water by urine and faeces. The most common sign is blood in the urine. The disease is seldom lethal but causes a lot of weakness and discomfort. The resulting chronic inflammations may lead to cancer in the urinary bladder. Drugs can cure the parasite infection and the disease can be controlled if people, especially children, use latrines and if the amount of snails can be reduced. This has been achieved in large parts of China, but still 700 000 are infected in that country.

Leishmaniasis (0.1%) is a parasite transmitted by sandflies. It causes skin ulcers and inflammation of liver and spleen that can be fatal if untreated. Treatment with drugs such as pentavalent antimony is very expensive. In Sudan and Ethiopia leishmaniasis poses a severe health problem. Social unrest is a risk factor for its spread. In Afghanistan thousands of cases have been reported yearly due to war and population displacement. Co-infection with HIV and leishmaniasis is especially problematic, since the immune defence against leishmaniasis is dependent on cellular immunity. A vaccine against leishmaniasis would be the best control measure and this may become available in the near future.

Sleeping sickness (0.1%), or African trypanosomiasis, is a severe public health problem in some tropical parts of Sub-Saharan Africa. Trypanosoma gambiense and rhodesiense are transmitted by tsetse flies. The disease starts with fever, headache, joint pain, enlarged spleen and lymph nodes. It may progress to a severe and life threatening neurological disorders. The drugs that are available (melarsoprol, pentamidine and suramin) often cause severe side effects. Production of a very effective drug with few side effects, called eflornithine, was discontinued because of the limited market. After massive lobbying from MSF and other NGO's, the drug company has now guaranteed the supply of eflornithine for five years from May 2001, and Bayer has followed with the same measure for their two drugs. It helped that it was recently discovered that eflornithine is useful against excess facial

hair in women—a potentially huge and profitable market in rich populations. Insecticide-impregnated traps and screens are used to control the tsetse fly. An additional problem is that the tsetse fly also uses cattle as a host, and therefore large areas must be free of cattle, which reduce access to animal protein.

Roundworm (0.1%) (mainly Ascaria lumbricoides) is transmitted by ingestion of eggs on vegetables. The adult worm causes digestive disorders and malnutrition, and a large worm mass can cause death by obstruction of the gut. Children are most affected by worms. This is also a health problem that can be eradicated through the use of latrines. Meanwhile, drugs are effective and cheap enough to be able to reduce the burden of this disease in affected populations.

River blindness (<0.1%), or onchocercosis, occurs in parts of Africa and Central and South America. A fly called Simulium, which lives beside rivers, transmits the parasite. The parasite infects the skin and eyes, causing severe itching and possibly also blindness. In some endemic areas, it is one of the most common causes of blindness. The drugs ivermectin and diethylcarbamazine kill the microfilariae. Ivermectin is dispensed free by Merck, which has also made 40 million USD/year available for distribution. Using these drugs, the disease is being subjected to extensive and quite successful eradication campaigns in West Africa. However, sustainable eradication requires a functioning health care system.

Chagas disease (<0.1%) is the Central and South American type of trypanosomiasis, which is spread by an insect that lives in the walls of poorly built houses. A WHO-led campaign against the vector has dramatically decreased the incidence of the disease, but the fear is that the insect will develop resistance against the insecticides used in the same way as the malaria mosquito did with DDT. Infection with the parasite may cause a severe disease of the heart and brain of young children. Decades after the initial infection, adults may slowly develop a severe chronic disease of the heart, gut and brain. Drugs are available to treat the acute but not the chronic form of the disease.

Hookworm (<0.1 %) (Anchylostoma duodenale and Nector americanus) is globally the most important of the intestinal worms, also known as nematodes. The microscopic larvae of the hookworm live in the soil and can penetrate the skin or be ingested with unboiled vegetables. The larvae pass via the blood system to reach the wall and mucous membrane of the small intestine, where they mature and survive by sucking blood. This causes no pain or discomfort other than a gradual development of severe anaemia as the host loses blood to the worm. The worm's eggs are passed with the faeces to hatch in the soil, from where the larvae can infect other humans. This disease disappears with the use of latrines. Hookworms are very difficult to control without the use of latrines, even though effective and cheap drugs are available. If children, who are the most exposed group in the affected communities, are successfully treated, they will soon be reinfected unless the whole community begins to use latrines.

The global burden of these parasitic diseases may appear limited. However all mainly affect very poor populations and each disease may be a very severe public health problem in a special area. In such areas one of these diseases may be the main obstacle for poverty alleviation. Cost-effective interventions are thus needed for all of these diseases if the millennium development goals are to be achieved.

5.9 Other major infections (0.6 %)

Bacterial meningitis (0.4 %) is estimated to have caused around 170 000 deaths worldwide in 2002. This severe bacterial infection affects the membranes that surround the brain and spinal cord. It exists all over the world and in all climates. The heaviest bur-

den of disease is in Africa, India, and the Eastern Mediterranean region. Outside the neonatal period, the most common bacteria causing meningitis are Streptococcus pneumoniae, Haemophilus influenzae and Neisseria meningitidis. Epidemics of the latter bacteria, also known as the meningococci bacteria, are common in the so-called 'meningitis belt' in Africa. This belt stretches in a semi-arid area from Sudan to Senegal just south of the Sahara. The transmission is by droplets or saliva and it is probable that a combination of the hot and dry climate and poor living conditions in this dusty landscape explains the distribution of the meningitis belt.

Meningitis in the newborn is hard to distinguish from other severe bacterial infections, because the typical signs are uncommon in very young children. Meningitis outside of the neonatal period starts with fever, proceeding to vomiting, headache and the characteristic sign of neck stiffness. Meningitis can, within hours, very rapidly progress to unconsciousness and death. Diagnosis can generally be made by clinical examination and is verified by a test for a turbid cerebrospinal fluid (CSF) in the patient. The diagnosis can be confirmed if laboratory examination of the CSF is possible to do. The normally clear CSF-liquid can be obtained through a needle inserted between the vertebrae of the spinal cord, a demanding procedure that may be dangerous to perform at primary health care level. Severe meningitis can easily be confirmed by just observing if the drops are turbid. Examination of CSF under a microscope by specially trained technicians, or preferably by cultivation in bacteriological laboratories, may provide information about the specific bacteria that caused the meningitis. If advanced diagnostic services and treatment are not available, the mortality rate varies between 15 and 60 %, and severe life-long neurological sequelae may occur in half of surviving patients. If advanced intensive care is provided, the mortality is still 5 % for Haemophilus meningitis and 20 % for pneumococcal meningitis, and again there is a high incidence of sequelae among the survivors.

Intravenous treatment of bacterial meningitis with antibiotics needs to be applied rapidly. An infusion of benzylpenicillin, the original substance discovered by Alexander Fleming, can still be used, but more and more of the bacteria involved, including pneumococci, are becoming resistant. Chloramphenicol is cheap and effective and is therefore often used in low-income countries, but not much in other parts of the world because it sometimes causes severe side effects. A single dose of intramuscular chloramphenicol may reduce mortality considerably during epidemics. New forms of cephalosporin antibiotics are generally used if they can be afforded.

Several vaccines can now be used to reduce the burden of meningitis. The new vaccine against Haemophilus influenzae, which offers about 75 % protection against this kind of childhood meningitis, is still used mostly in high-income counties, due to its high cost. A polysaccharide vaccine incorporating 23 of the 84 types of pneumococci is used mainly to treat elderly people and those who have undergone splenectomy in high-income countries. A new conjugated vaccine against pneumococci is on the market but is too expensive for low and middle-income countries. Vaccines against meningococcus types A and C are effective and useful in the control of meningococcus epidemics, even in poor countries. However, recent outbreaks in Africa are caused by meningococcus type W, which requires a more expensive vaccine.

Hepatitis viruses (0.2 %) were estimated to cause only 0.2 % of the global burden of disease and about 160 000 deaths in 2002. Chronic infection with hepatitis virus types B and C causes chronic inflammation and scarring of the liver, known as cirrhosis. This may induce liver cancer. About 70 % of the cases of liver cancer worldwide are caused by the hepatitis B virus infections in East and South-East Asia, the Pacific Basin and Sub-Saharan Africa. In these regions, the carrier rate of Hepatitis B may be as high as 7 %, and transmission occurs mainly from mother to child. In Western Europe, North America and Latin America with the exception of the Amazon Basin, the carrier rate of hepatitis B is less than 1 %, and sexual transmission between adults is the most common form of transmission. South- and East Europe and South Asia have intermediate rates of carriers, i.e. 2 to 7 %, and a mixed adult and child type of transmission. At present 350 million persons are chronic carriers of the hepatitis B virus, and 90 % of women who are carriers transmit the virus to their children at the time of birth. Children aged 2 to 5 years are at high risk as they come in contact with small sores and saliva of other children during play. Other risks include intravenous drug use and sexual transmission in adulthood. The hepatitis virus is up to 100 times more contagious than HIV. The earlier an individual gets infected, the more likely it is that the individual will become a chronic carrier, with a risk of developing complications later in life.

Hepatitis C is transmitted mainly by blood transfusions and contaminated needles, but it is considerably less infective than hepatitis B. It is therefore not easily transmitted sexually or from mother to child. Hepatitis C is widespread in the world, with prevalence rates of 0.3 to 2 % in most countries.

There is a good vaccine against hepatitis B, but the vaccine is expensive in comparison with other vaccines in the Expanded Programme of Immunisation (EPI). Ninety countries have integrated the vaccine into their national immunisation programmes. Unfortunately, there is no simple cure for hepatitis B. Nor is there any simple cure, or even a vaccine against hepatitis C. One preventive measure against the transmission of hepatitis virus is blood donor screening.

The long-term effect of hepatitis B and C is the possible development of cancer many decades after the infection has occurred. Likewise, Helicobacter has been shown to cause stomach ulcers, with a subsequently increased risk of stomach cancer, and the human papilloma virus has been shown to cause cervical cancer. Thus, recent scientific advances point out the blurred demarcation between communicable and non-communicable diseases (see further chapter 7).

References and suggested further reading

Alonso PL et al. The effect of insecticide-treated bed nets on mortality in Gambian children. Lancet 1991;337:1499–1502.

Benenson S. (ed.) Control of Communicable Diseases. Sixteenth edition. APHA; 1995.

Bygbjerg IC. AIDS in a Danish surgeon (Zaire, 1976), Lancet 1983;1:925.

Cook GC, Zumla A. (ed.) Manson's Tropical Diseases. 21st edition. London: Saunders; 2002.

Creese A, Floyd K, Alban A, Guinness L. Cost-effectiveness of HIV interventions in Africa: systematic review of the evidence. Lancet 2002;359:1635–43.

Kwesigabo G, Killewo JZ, Urassa W, Mbena E, Mhalu F, Lugalla JL, Godoy C, Biberfeld G, Emmelin M, Wall S, Sandstrom A. Monitoring of HIV-1 infection prevalence and trends in the general population using pregnant women as a sentinel population: 9 years experience from the Kagera region of Tanzania. J Acquir Immune Defic Syndr. 2000;23:410–7.

Lambrechts T, Bryce J, Orinda V. Integrated management of childhood illnesses: a summary of first experiences. Bulletin of the World Health Organisation 1999; 77(7).

NIH, (National Institutes of Health) The Jordan Report 2000.

Nuwaha F. The challenge of chloroquine-resistant malaria in Sub-Saharan Africa. Health Policy and Planning 2001;16:1–12.

Sachs J. Report of the Commission on Macroeconomics and Health. Macroeconomics and Health: Investing in Health for Economic Development, World Health Organisation, Geneva, 2001. page 31 and 84 ff.

UNAIDS report on the global HIV/AIDS epidemic 2003 and 2004. (www.unaids.org/barcelona/presskit/report.html).

Walker

WHO, Global burden of disease estimates 2001. (www.who.int/whosis).

WHO, World Health Reports 1996–2004. (www.who.int/whr/en/).

WHO, State of the World's Vaccines and Immunisation. 2002.

Zhu T, Korber BT, Nahmias AJ, et al. An African HIV-1 sequence from 1959 and implications for the origin of the epidemic. Nature 1998;391:594.

6 Nutritional disorders (2%)*

> *Let hunger be ranked first because if you are hungry you cannot work. No, health is number one because if you are ill you cannot work.*
>
> Discussion group, Zambia

A nutrition transition is taking place along with the demographic and disease transitions (see chapter 4). This is the shift from a diet dominated by starchy low-fat, high-fibre food items, combined with a labour-intensive daily life, to a diet high in fat and sugar combined with a sedentary daily life. In other words the nutritional transition is the change from hunger to obesity. For the first time in the history of mankind the number of overweight people today rivals the number of underweight people. About 1.1 billion in each group, is equal to 20% of the world's population. Both the overweight and the underweight suffer from malnutrition, a deficiency or excess in a person's intake of nutrients needed for healthy living. The hungry and the overweight both have high levels of sickness, shortened life expectancies and lowered productivity. Only about 60% of humans have a healthy weight.

This escalating global epidemic of overweight and obesity—'globesity'—is also affecting part of the population in the low-income countries and a substantial part in middle-income countries. This creates a 'double burden of disease', from both under- and over-nutrition. In the urban slums in South Asia and Africa it is not rare that an obese mother with type-2 diabetes has children with malnutrition.

The human body is biologically prepared for periodic food scarcity, but not for a continuous abundance of food. This means that when life conditions in a population improve and sufficient food becomes available

every day, there is no physiological regulation to avoid over-consumption. Therefore, all people exposed to permanent abundance of food must learn new behaviours to voluntary restrict fat and sugar intake, to increase fruit and vegetable intake, and also to increase physical activity. In this way the second nutritional obstacle on the road to a long and healthy life can be reduced by new dietary practices. This is necessary for 'successful ageing', that is, postponing infirmity and increasing the years of healthy life expectancy. The WHO response has been first to ring the alarm bell, then to initiate public awareness campaigns and to develop strategies that can 'make healthy choices easy choices'.

Whether these new behaviours will constitute a large-scale transition in diet and body shape, with the anticipated health benefits, remains to be seen. It seems that the last generation born in scarcity remains psychologically more prone to over-consumption than later generations. It seems as if the second nutritional transition, from over-consumption to adequate intake, will not take place in the generation that personally benefited from the transition from scarcity to over-consumption.

The number of DALYs lost due to nutritional under- or over-consumption is difficult to estimate. The reason is that under and over-nutrition are causes of diseases rather than diseases *per se*. A high body mass index will never appear as the cause of death, not even in extreme cases. A person weighing 200kg will always die of something

* % of global disease burden is small, but the indirect effects are enormous

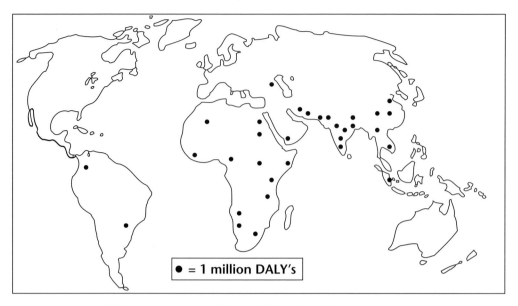

Map 6:1 *Nutritional deficiencies cause 32 million disability adjusted life years (DALY) lost per year.*
Source: WHO, 2002.

other than obesity, such as a cardiovascular event, even if the overweight condition contributed to the death. Similarly, a severely wasted and malnourished child will more likely die from diarrhoea or pneumonia than

Table 6.1 *The contribution in % of different risk factors to the global burden of disease.*

Rank	Risk factors	% of global DALY
1	Underweight	9
2	Unsafe sex	6
3	High blood pressure	4
4	Tobacco	4
5	Alcohol	4
6	Unsafe water and hygiene	4
7	High cholesterol	3
8	Indoor smoke	3
9	Iron deficiency	2
10	High BMI	2
11	Zinc deficiency	2
12	Low fruit and vegetable intake	2
13	Vitamin A deficiency	2
14	Physical inactivity	1

Source: Ezzati et al. Lancet 2002.

from malnutrition itself. But again the child's low weight and malnutrition will have largely contributed to the death from those infectious diseases. Only during famines and starvation will malnutrition appear as a direct cause of death. Although the different aspects of malnutrition cannot easily be quantified as causes of death and diseases, malnutrition is a major cause of disability and death in the world. The best available estimate of how nutritional factors contribute to the burden of disease in the world is summarised in Table 6.1 based on the study presented in World Health Report 2002 (WHO 2002) and later published in Lancet (Ezzati 2002). The number of overweight people in the world is approaching the number of underweight. However, the impact on health differs as shown in table 6.1. Under-nutrition causes 9% whereas overweight only causes 2% of the global burden of disease. The reason being that under-nutrition mainly affects young children and leads to high death risk in infections whereas overnutrition mainly affect an older age group with less immediate death risk.

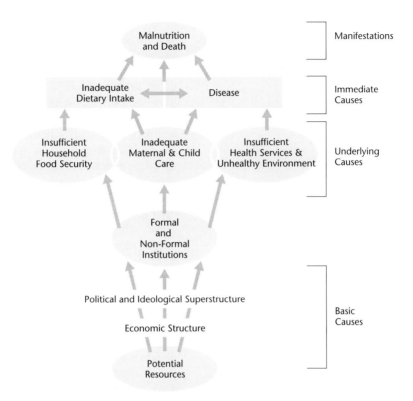

Figure 6.1 Causes of malnutrition.
Source: Urban Johansson, UNICEF 1997.

Under-nutrition is very closely related to poverty. Note in table 1.5 that the first of the United Nation's Millennium Development Goals is "*Eradicate extreme poverty and hunger*". A person living in absolute poverty will use most of the resources available to acquire food. Therefore poverty can often be better measured as lack of food and low weight rather than as a daily income below a certain cut off limit in US dollar per day. Poverty can thus be measured in the adult population as the proportion of persons with a Body Mass Index below 18.5 (Chapter 3.11.1).

In contrast to adults, malnutrition among children is only partly due to a lack of appropriate food. Other causes of child malnutrition are ignorance about optimal feeding practices or lack of access to specific micronutrients, such as iodine or vitamin A. However, the most important causes of malnutri-

tion in children are infectious diseases that increase the nutritional demand or decrease the ability to eat and absorb nutrients from the gut. Paradoxically vaccination against measles is one of the best preventions against child malnutrition. Use of hygienic latrines is another way to prevent malnutrition, as it will reduce the burden of diarrhoea and hookworm among children. A complex web of contributing factors, from socio-economic conditions to more immediate causes such as feeding practices and infectious diseases (Figure 6.1), determines the amount of child malnutrition in a community. This chapter focuses on the immediate causes, since the underlying causes are dealt with in Chapter 2 about health determinants.

The burden of nutritional disorders is not visible as direct causes of DALYs lost, but it has been estimated that under-nutrition

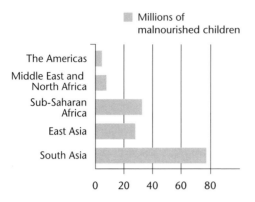

Figure 6.2 Millions of underweight children by region, 2001.

Source: UNICEF, 2002.

contributed to more than half of the childhood deaths in low-income countries (Black 2003) (Figure 3.3). The World Health Report 2002 identified the following childhood and maternal under-nutrition factors as those mostly contributing to childhood deaths:

- Underweight
- Iron deficiency
- Vitamin A deficiency
- Zinc deficiency
- Iodine deficiency

At the other end of the income range the following were the nutrition-related risks, along with high blood pressure and physical inactivity, that most contributed to the DALYs lost in the world:

- High cholesterol
- High body mass index
- Low fruit and vegetable intake

The key role of malnutrition for the global health status is illustrated by the fact that about 15 % of the global disease burden can be attributed to the joint effects of childhood and maternal underweight or micronutrient deficiencies. Underweight is estimated to cause 9 % of the global disease burden. Iron deficiency, vitamin A deficiency, and zinc deficiency are estimated to cause

2 % each. The relative contributions of each of these factors are shown in Table 6.1. Additionally, almost as much can be attributed to risk factors that have substantial dietary determinants—high blood pressure 4 %, high cholesterol 3 %, high BMI 2 %, low fruit and vegetable intake 2 % as well as low physical activity 1 %. The patterns are not uniform within regions. In some countries the nutrition transition has reached a healthier stage than in others.

One third (150 million) of the world's children are classified as underweight (UNICEF 2004). The highest proportion of underweight children are found in Southern Asia; India, Pakistan and Bangladesh (Figure 6.2). In these three countries almost half of the children weigh less than 2 standard deviations below the mean for children with optimal growth as shown in Table 3.7.

The main effect of poor nutrition is the negative impact on the immune system. In this chapter we first describe the interaction between nutrition and the immune defences. Secondly, we will describe general under-nutrition first in adults and then in children. Thereafter the four major micronutrient deficiencies in the world: iron, vitamin-A, zinc and iodine will be presented. Finally, we review other major nutrition-related risks. Three UN web-sites are useful sources for information about nutrition: the United Nations System Standing Committee on Nutrition[1], the nutrition section at WHO[2] and FAO's division of nutrition[3].

6.1 Nutritionally Acquired Immune Deficiency Syndrome (NAIDS)

There is a natural priority among the different body functions. Some are more vital than others and therefore given highest priority. Top priority is given to breathing and

[1] www.unsystem.org/scn
[2] www.who.int/nut
[3] www.fao.org

blood circulation. When the dietary intake is insufficient to run all the body functions, some functions are given low priority by the body metabolism and will receive fewer nutrients. The first priority to be lowered is physical activity. If a person does not get enough dietary energy, the physical activity will be kept to a minimum. But there will also be a priority inside the body. A starving woman will lose her menstruation periods and her fertility, as survival is more important than procreation. A child with malnutrition will stop growing. When the child later gets sufficient food and is less at risk from infection it can grow faster than normal to "catch up". In periods of scarcity the immune system will not have top priority to nutrients. During hunger the body mass is being consumed and the body becomes thin. This will cause cell turnover to be slowed down and cells with rapid turnover like the immune cells will replicate slower and their activity will be decreased. A consequence is that the body becomes more susceptible to infections. Such adverse consequences of malnutrition have been designated "Nutritionally Acquired Immune Deficiency Syndrome" or NAIDS. This emphasises the close relationship between nutritional status and immune function.

NAIDS impairs both the general host defences and the more specific immune system functions. The general defences include the protective anatomic barriers such as the skin, the mucosal surfaces and the products these surfaces produce, e.g. gastric acid. Some micronutrients are especially important for the immune system, and are called immuno-micronutrients. These are: vitamin A, zinc (see sections 6.4.2–3), vitamin E and, to some extent, selenium and vitamin C. This means that if these micronutrients are deficient in addition to a general lack of food, then the immune deficiency becomes even worse.

The most devastating forms of NAIDS are associated with a severe atrophy (shrinking) of all lymphoid (immuno-competent) tissues. Functionally, the immune system is divided into two systems; one based on cells, known as the cellular system, and one based on the immuno-globulins, called the humoral (liquid) system (see section 5.2.1 on HIV). Nutritionally induced atrophy of lymphoid tissues predominantly affects the cell-mediated immune defence, while the humoral system tends to be spared. This is similar to what happens in HIV infection, and therefore malnutrition and HIV are synergistic in reducing the capacity of the immune system.

NAIDS explains why the malnourished child becomes so susceptible to infections. In the extreme case of under-nutrition, the child may have bacteria in the blood (septicaemia) without developing fever or an increase in the white blood cell count, which is generally used as a clinical sign of an infection.

The wonderful thing about NAIDS, compared with AIDS, is that it is curable. If the child is properly treated and fed, all signs of immune deficiency disappear.

6.2 Underweight

6.2.1 Adult underweight

Adults with a Body Mass Index (BMI) below 18.5 kg/m^2 are by definition underweight. They are thin in relation to their length. This means that their immune system is tuned down due to a small energy and micronutrient budget. Physical activity is compromised, which affects working capacity.

6.2.2 Hunger

Inadequate food intake does not only contribute to diseases and specific nutritional conditions. Hunger has severe direct effects on the well being of humans, as well as on their capacity for physical and intellectual work. The effect of food insecurity, i.e. insufficient food to eat, is both loss of weight and reduced physical activity. Hunger is so closely related to absolute poverty that it is almost the same thing. As mentioned when the United Nations made the eradication of poverty the first Millennium Development Goal, indicators that measure hunger and malnutrition were chosen as the measure of whether poverty is being reduced. The reason for this is that a person who lives in absolute poverty uses most of her or his resources, time or money, to acquire the basic 1,500 kcal/day a person needs to survive.

6.2.3 Famine

Famine may be defined as hunger that has become so severe that it has started to kill. The Nobel Prize laureate in economics, Amartya Sen, has advanced the understanding of famines. Firstly, by noting that famine is not primarily a matter of a lack of food, but rather of a lack of food entitlement, i.e. ability to acquire food. When a rural area is hit by a drought that destroys all the crops, there will be no famine if the farmers have sufficient cash, savings and assets which they can use to purchase food. Food will be transported to the area if they have something to pay with. When a drought causes famine, it is thus not directly because the crop has been lost but because the value of an agricultural year's work has been lost and that the farmers are destitute and lack savings that can be converted to food through trade or barter. If this happens the whole society will start to break down. This can be stopped if government, as well as voluntary or international organisations make food available to those who cannot buy food. Famine is an extremely severe form of social collapse due to insufficient political leadership. An interesting observation is that a famine has never occurred in a country with a free press in a time of peace.

The World Food Programme is a specialised UN organisation that has acquired good competence in supporting countries with food if there should be a threat of famine somewhere in the country. This means that famine today only occurs when rulers do not care and suppress freedom of speech.

The famines seen in Somalia, Afghanistan and other places in recent years have all been associated with severe civil wars.

Persons who have suffered malnutrition as children or severe hunger during adolescence run an increased risk to suffer from cardio-vascular disease much later in life as recently shown in males 50 years after their survival of the siege of Leningrad during the second world war (Sparén 2004).

6.3 Child malnutrition

Malnutrition among young children is still a very common disorder of children in the world. The usual way to divide child malnutrition is into three types, namely *wasting* (weight-for-height below –2 standard deviations), *stunting* (height-for-age below –2 standard deviations) and *underweight* (weight-for-age below –2 standard deviations). These measures constitute so-called anthropometrical measurements, i.e. body weight and length (see chapter 3.11). In 2002, 10% of the world's children were wasted, 31% stunted and 27% underweight (UNICEF 2004). Wasted children are to a varying degree affected by NAIDS, and it is in the group of wasted children that many of the child deaths occur. It should be noted that malnutrition among children are largely caused by infectious diseases, and not only by diet deficiencies.

6.3.1 Under-nutrition is often 'over-diseasing'

Under-nutrition and *malnutrition* make us think about food. These words do not indicate any involvement of diseases. But the conceptual framework in Figure 6.1 shows that both 'inadequate dietary intake' and 'diseases' jointly contribute to under-nutrition. The phrase 'malnutrition-infection complex' has thus been proposed to avoid the linguistic problem of using a term that only addresses one of the causes of the

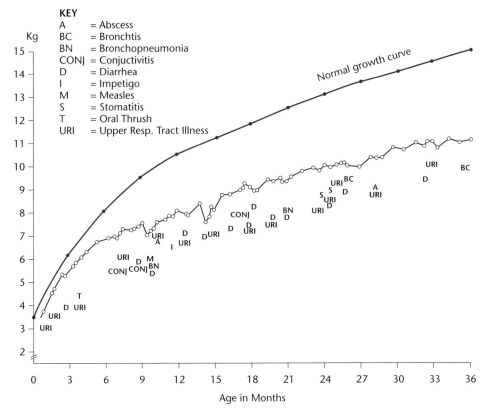

Figure 6.3 Illnesses and weight curve of a child from birth to 3 years of age. The weight loss during a period of measles and one of diarrhoea illustrates the close link between malnutrition and infection.

Source: Mata et al. 1977.

abnormal nutritional condition. Another suggested term is 'under-nutrition—overdiseasing'. Infections thus cause under-nutrition and under-nutrition causes infections. It is estimated that half the deaths in malaria, pneumonia, diarrhoea and neonatal disorders are due to under nutrition (Black 2003).

Figure 6.3 shows the weight development during the life of a malnourished boy. This child became stunted and was periodically even wasted. He suffered from under nutrition. The cause was partly that his feeding patterns were sub-optimal. However, another cause was the large number of infections that he was subjected to. The infections contributed to his under-nutrition. The under-nutrition in turn gave him

NAIDS, which made him more susceptible to new infections. In this vicious circle of infections and dietary insufficiencies he could not grow in an optimal way.

Diseases cause deterioration of the nutritional status through several mechanisms. The most important are:

- anorexia (loss of appetite), which decreases the food intake in the child;
- fever, which increases the nutritional needs of the child;
- catabolic effects, tissue degradation due to tissue damage;
- production of immunological proteins, which increases nutritional needs;
- decreased intestinal function, producing malabsorption;

- decreased availability of micronutrients. For instance measles consumes much of the vitamin A that is present and diarrhoea increases the loss of zinc.

The predominant causes of under-nutrition in children vary with their age. During the first six months the main cause is failure to breastfeed. In the period 6 to 12 months the main cause is infections, but the nature of how complementary foods are given is also critical. In the period between 1 to 3 years of age malnutrition most commonly manifests itself clinically. This is the time when oedematous under-nutrition is most common. Inadequate care and poverty in the household are the main underlying causes. Above 3 years of age specific diseases such as tuberculosis and HIV/AIDS are the main causes of malnutrition. However, in times of famine or disaster, the lack of food may become the main cause at any age. At all ages, and particularly in marginal groups, heavy intestinal worm infestation may tip the balance towards under-nutrition.

6.3.2 Occurrence of wasting and stunting

The World Health Organization has established a Global Database on Child Growth in which all major surveys of child anthropometry are compiled. This makes it possible to get a global view of the occurrence of wasting and stunting (Table 3.7). The database is accessible online.[1]

Different kinds of emergencies may rapidly raise the proportion of wasted children in affected areas. Wasting among children is an important measure of the degree of a humanitarian emergency in underprivileged populations. Wasted children should be an important target group for any kind of nutritional intervention undertaken in humanitarian assistance.

In contrast to wasting, stunting is widespread among children in low-income countries even in non-emergency periods. Almost half of the children in India and Bangladesh are stunted. The global average for stunting among children in low-income countries is 32 %. The proportion is less in middle-income countries. Increasing evidence shows that stunting is associated with poor developmental achievement in young children and poor school achievement or intelligence levels in older children. The causes of this growth retardation are deeply rooted in poverty and lack of education. Economic development in any significant long-term sense will be faster if optimal child growth and development are ensured for all children.

6.3.3 Long-term effects of malnutrition

There may be long-term adverse effects on the intellectual capacity of previously malnourished children. However, it is difficult to differentiate the biological effects of malnutrition and those of the deprived environment on children's cognitive abilities. Iodine deficiency during pregnancy and iron deficiency in childhood cause both mental and physical impairments. Malnourished children lack energy and become less curious and playful, and communicate less with the people around them, which impairs their physical, mental and cognitive development (UNICEF 1998).

Stunting in childhood has a specific long-term effect in girls. Because of insufficient growth, the birth canal will also be narrower, with all the subsequent risks of obstructed labour. The children of a woman who has suffered stunting are also going to be stunted in the uterus; an adaptation of the child. This means that stunting is partly carried over to the next generation. Malnutrition in early life also seems to increase the risk of developing coronary heart disease, diabetes and high blood pressure later in life.

---

[1]   www.who.int/nutgrowthdb

6.3.4 Treatment of severe under-nutrition

If a child becomes seriously wasted, this in itself is a life-threatening condition. Even if the child is taken to hospital, the risk of dying still remains very high unless sufficiently good care is available. WHO has issued a manual for the management of severe under-nutrition (WHO, 1999). It may be downloaded from the Internet.[1]

Imagine a car going downhill at a considerable speed and the steering wheel is not working. So when the road makes a small bend the driver cannot follow the road. But not only the steering wheel but also the brakes and the accelerator are not working. So the driver has very little opportunity to influence the direction or the speed of the car. This situation is similar to the one you face when you treat a child with severe malnutrition. The child's body has lost its normal capacity to compensate for external influences. The body of a healthy child is able to accommodate for a lot of external changes; for instance, if it is getting hot outside, the body will start to sweat in order to keep the body temperature constant inside. When food enters the body, insulin is produced to keep the blood sugar normal, and if there is a prolonged period of fasting, the body will start to produce glucose to keep the blood sugar up. So a healthy body is able to maintain the internal balance; to continue the metaphor it has a steering wheel, brakes and an accelerator. Each of the three phases in the treatment of severe under-nutrition has a specific aim:

- Initial treatment: Prevent the car from getting further off the road = Help the child to survive any life-threatening problems, reverse metabolic abnormalities and commence feeding.
- Rehabilitation: Repair the car = intensive feeding is given to regain lost weight, emotional and physical stimulation are increased, the mother is trained to con-

tinue care at home, and preparations are made for the child to be discharged.
- Follow-up: Get the car back on the road = after discharge, the child and his family are followed to prevent relapse and assure continued physical, mental and emotional development of the child.

The *initial treatment* is needed for about one week. When the compensatory mechanisms are lost due to severe under-nutrition, the undernourished body is fragile and should be protected from powerful external influences that might put the life of the child at risk. The child with wasting, anorexia (loss of appetite) and infections needs to be treated in a hospital, which the parents can rarely afford if the hospital care is not provided free of charge. Successful initial management requires frequent, careful clinical evaluations (Figure 6.4). The hospital treatment is needed until the child's condition is stable and his or her appetite has returned, which usually occurs after 2–7 days. The principal tasks during initial treatment are:

- to treat or prevent low blood sugar with oral sugar solution via a tube that is passed through the nose down into the child's stomach;
- to treat or prevent low body temperature with adequate warmth;
- to treat or prevent dehydration and restore electrolyte balance;
- to treat infection routine antibiotics should be administered;
- to treat possible shock due to infection;
- to start to feed the child, usually with a milk mixture. While the anorexia is severe, this may have to be performed by tube feeding;
- to identify and treat any other complication, including vitamin deficiency, severe anaemia and heart failure.

The *rehabilitation* starts when the child's appetite has returned after about one week. The principal tasks during the rehabilitation phase are:

[1] www.who.int/nut Click on <publications and documents> and scroll down.

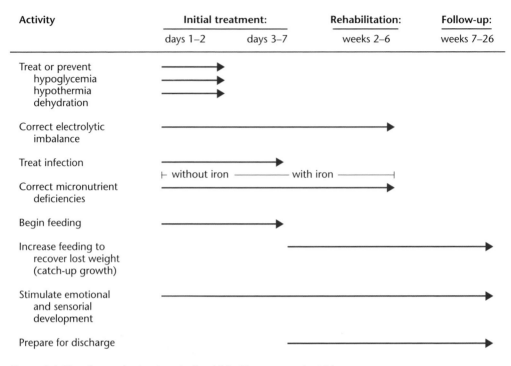

Activity	Initial treatment:		Rehabilitation:	Follow-up:
	days 1–2	days 3–7	weeks 2–6	weeks 7–26

Figure 6.4 *Time frames for treatment of a child with severe malnutrition.*
Source: WHO, 1999.

- to encourage the child to eat as much as possible, using food with high energy density;
- to re-initiate and/or encourage breast-feeding;
- to stimulate emotional and physical development through comfort, affection and mental stimulation for the child, support and sympathy for the family, assistance with the family's social problems, counselling for AIDS if necessary;
- to prepare the mother or any other care giver to continue to look after the child after discharge, by showing the family how to feed the child, talking with the family about the child's food needs, and encouraging mothers to learn from each other on the ward.

Follow-up is important even if the child is much improved at the time of discharge. The child usually remains stunted, and mental development is delayed. Managing these conditions and preventing the recurrence of severe malnutrition requires a sustained improvement in the feeding of the child and in other parenting skills. Planned follow-up of the child at regular intervals after discharge is essential. Most severely malnourished children come from poor families and poverty alleviation is the only adequate long-term prevention.

6.3.5 Marasmus and kwashiorkor

Two main clinical patterns have been distinguished in severe under-nutrition: marasmus and kwashiorkor. Marasmus is Greek for 'slim disease', and today it is more often called wasting. Kwashiorkor is a clinical syndrome whose main clinical sign is swelling of the legs (oedema), today mostly called 'oedematous under-nutrition'.

Marasmus is thus the same as extreme wasting. The affected child is often less than two years of age, but if the cause is failure to

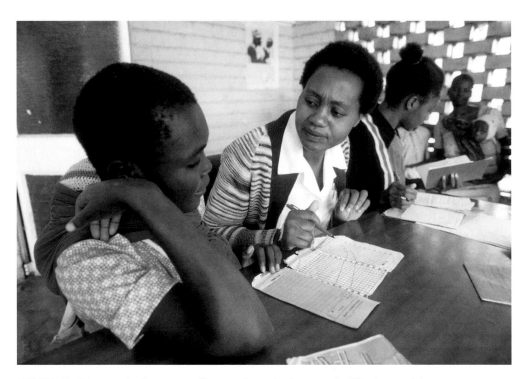

ZAMBIA. Health centre in the country. The growth monitoring curve is difficult to explain.
© *Trygve Bølstad / PHOENIX.*

breastfeed, the child may be less than one year old. The child usually has an extremely low weight for age, under 60 % of the standard, with evidence of extreme wasting of the arms, legs and buttocks. Growth has ceased and the child consumes subcutaneous fat, and ultimately its own muscles, to release energy. The child's body often consists of only 'skin-and-bone' with the typical 'old man's face' because of wasted muscles in the face, but the abdomen is often distended, a so called potbelly. The child may be irritable and fretful, but is often alert and hungry, if not infected. The child is often dehydrated because of diarrhoea or other infections. It is not uncommon that the state of marasmus is explained by underlying infections such as tuberculosis or HIV. Marasmic children without incurable infections who receive appropriate treatment recover within a few weeks. Marasmus usually starts after a long period of underweight, and a marasmic

child may develop kwashiorkor after an episode of acute illness such as measles or diarrhoea.

Kwashiorkor is the same as oedematous under-nutrition. The affected child is usually 1 to 3 years old. There is oedema of the face, legs and arms, causing a deceptive increase in weight. There is often a moon face, and the child usually has a moderately low weight for age, at around 60 to 80 % of the standard. There is muscle wasting, especially over the shoulders and upper arms. There is often a potbelly, with an enlarged liver and diarrhoea is common. The child is often pale and thin, with peeling skin, where dark 'flaky paint' contrasts against pale 'milk chocolate'-coloured skin. The hair is often sparse and thin, with a lighter colour and poor roots, so that it can easily be pulled out. Mental disturbance is shown in the form of misery and apathy, with poor appetite. The child is often not crying, but whines and resists examination and feeding. Vitamin A deficiency is often so severe that it may cause permanent destruction of the corneas, resulting in blindness. Associated infections are almost the rule. Pneumonia may cause sudden death, without previous signs of cough or fever, since the immune system is not functioning adequately.

Children with marasmus and kwashiorkor are intensive-care patients and unless properly treated they are at high risk of dying. In the first phase of treatment, the oedema disappears and the weight therefore decreases during the first week. Blood transfusions are given according to need. In the second phase weight increases first to regain what has been lost, and then to gain normal weight for height. This second phase may take two to three months. Kwashiorkor and marasmus are a reflection of absolute poverty or severe social neglect of children's needs.

6.3.6 Growth monitoring

The growth chart is a simple instrument for assessing the growth of children. The weight of the child in kilograms to one decimal is plotted against the age in months on a curve. The plotted weight is compared with the WHO standard line for average child growth, as well as a line for—2 standard deviations of the average weight for age (Figure 6.3). The growths of all pre-school children with good nutrition follow the international growth standard. Genetic differences between population groups in growth are negligible during the children's first five years. There may be significant genetic variation within populations, but the differences in averages between countries are not big enough to justify differences in growth standards.

The growth chart is used all over the world at the primary health care level in all types of countries. It was designed to be the method of screening for dangers of growth failure so that correct advice about feeding practices and care could be given early. If correctly used in a resource-strong health service, the growth chart may be a very sensitive instrument for detection of a number of diseases that affects the growth of young children.

But several studies indicate that the growth chart is not really cost-effective as a public health intervention in countries where more than half of the children have abnormal growth and most mothers know the reason why, but are unable to do much about it. Notably, the state of Kerala in southern India has had a child health card without the growth chart during the period when their child health status became the best of all low-income countries in the world. The correct use of the growth chart requires competent health staff, firstly to measure the weight, secondly to be able to plot the weight correctly on the chart, and thirdly to interpret whether the growth pattern is normal or not. Fourthly, they need to interview the mother to find out the underlying causes. Fifthly, they should suggest or prescribe possible actions to improve the child's situation that are available within the resources in the home and health service. On the receiving end the parents of the children should also understand the interpretation of the weight curve, and the fifth step is possibly the most difficult, i.e. for the mother and father to comply with the advice given. Hence, there are many links in the chain that may be weak, before the growth chart can be applied in an effective way.

Equipment consisting of weighing scales and a growth chart for each child must also be available, affordable and in good condition. This has been a major priority for UNICEF for many decades. Growth monitoring is a typical example of a technology that has been deemed appropriate and widely promoted before any solid community based research had provided evidence for its cost-effectiveness. After being in the top position for UNICEF's strategy in the early 1980s, growth monitoring has quietly been tuned down during the last decade.

It is food for thought that the image most commonly used in rich countries to illustrate development co-operation and aid is a photograph of a child being weighed during a growth monitoring session. Yet this intervention is probably the least effective of the four high priorities that UNICEF launched for the children of the world 20 years ago. Oral rehydration, promotion of breastfeeding, vaccination against measles and polio have all proven to have much greater impact than growth monitoring. This is not to say that growth monitoring is not a useful tool in screening for children's health and nutritional needs, but it appears that it is a better tool for finding a few children in need in populations where most children are healthy. As an intervention in low income countries growth monitoring and growth promotion for children does not appear to have the capacity to break the vicious circle of poverty and disease.

6.4 Micronutrient deficiency

'Micronutrients' is the term used for those essential nutrients that are needed in small amounts for human growth and functioning. They are used in the body as co-factors for enzymes engaged in various biochemical reactions. They comprise fat and water soluble vitamins, as well as trace elements (minerals). Iron, vitamin A, zinc and iodine are estimated to be the most important, but other important micronutrients are vitamin C and the B-vitamin complex. Diets that supply adequate energy and have an acceptable nutrient density will usually also cover the needs for micronutrients. However, when the diet is otherwise monotonous, it is recommended to supplement it with micronutrient-rich foods. Food preservation methods, high temperature and exposure to sunlight can reduce the activity of many vitamins, particularly vitamins A and C. Most of the micronutrient deficiencies are strongly linked to poverty and human deprivation. However, four of these conditions are much more significant with regard to their global occurrence than are the other micronutrient deficiencies. We will therefore leave out descriptions of scurvy (vitamin C deficiency), beriberi (vitamin B1 thiamine), pellagra (vitamin B6 nicotinic acid) and rickets (vitamin D deficiency). These nutritional diseases still occur in deprived populations that survive on different types of monotonous diets. In humanitarian emergencies these specific dietary deficiencies may present as epidemic outbreaks that are often mistaken to be infectious diseases. In this chapter we only focus on the four micronutrient deficiencies that are most prevalent in the world.

6.4.1 Iron—necessary for blood and enzymes

Iron is a necessary component of haemoglobin that carries oxygen in the red blood cells. Iron is also necessary for many other body functions. Iron deficiency anaemia (IDA) affects almost half of the world population, making it the most frequent micronutrient deficiency. Iron deficiency seems to be the only micronutrient deficiency that occurs across high, middle and low-income countries. Of the total burden of disease in DALY over 2 % is lost due to anaemia. Iron deficiency causes anaemia because iron is necessary for the production of red blood cells. Anaemia leads to tiredness, breathlessness, decreased immune function and impaired learning in children. The most affected populations are children in their preschool years and pregnant women in low and middle-income countries. In these populations, deficiencies of dietary iron are aggravated by loss of iron due to repeated episodes of parasitic diseases such as malaria, hookworm infestation or schistosomiasis. Women also lose iron by menstruation or repeated pregnancies with blood loss at delivery. A low dietary intake of iron and the influence of factors affecting absorption also contribute to iron deficiency. About 40 % of the women in low and middle-income countries suffer from anaemia, and up to 15 % in high-income countries.

Better nutrition, iron supplementation or fortification, child spacing and the prevention and treatment of malaria and hookworms can all prevent iron deficiency. Iron is found naturally in meat, fish, liver and breastmilk. Vitamin C increases iron absorption. Correction of iron deficiency anaemia with iron tablets is very cheap. However, a functioning health service is needed to promote the appropriate use of iron tablets among the most vulnerable groups. Perhaps one of the worst inadequacies of the health service of the world is that so many pregnant women still lack sufficient advice and the cheapest of drugs, iron tablets, to prevent anaemia during pregnancy.

An international expert group called International Nutritional Anaemia Consultative Group (INACG) organises regular international meetings to discuss the scientific and programmatic challenges around iron deficiency anaemia.[1]

6.4.2 Vitamin A—protecting life and vision

Vitamin A assumes both important systemic functions in the whole body and local functions in the eye. The systemic functions of vitamin A were identified about 100 years ago. At that time, it was found that animals fed on a diet with vitamin A as the limiting nutrient suffered a sharp increase in mortality, a clear increase in the number and severity of infectious episodes, and growth retardation. In the later stages, these animals also developed signs of an eye disease. This illustrates the two types of function of vitamin A: systemic and local functions.

For a long time, the knowledge of the systemic functions of vitamin A in protecting against death and severe, prolonged infectious diseases was overlooked in humans. The reason was possibly the discovery of antibiotics, which led to a neglect of the preventive role of nutrition in most infections.

[1] http://inacg.ilsi.org

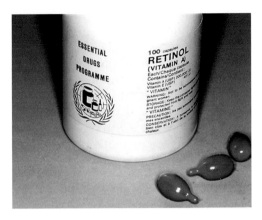

Vitamin A capsules.

Vitamin A deficiency was thought to cause mainly eye problems and blindness. But over the last decades, the full role of vitamin A has been rediscovered and this has had important implications for promotion of child health and survival (Sommer 1998).

Vitamin A is very important for the mucous membranes. These are the linings of the mouth and gastrointestinal tract, the lungs and the eye. Here, vitamin A is needed for the proper production of mucopolysaccharides, which keep mucous membranes in good shape to protect against infections. If vitamin A is deficient, the wetness of the mucous membranes will decrease and the membranes will become more like skin than mucous membranes. This can be seen in the eye as xerophthalmia ('dry eye' in Greek). Inside the eye, vitamin A is used in the rods (the receptors for low intensities of light). If there is too little vitamin A, the person will not be able to see in low light intensity, she or he will become night-blind. Vitamin A deficiency has long been identified as the major cause of nutritional blindness. This is still an important problem around the world. It is estimated that 250 000 to 500 000 children suffer blindness each year by an eye damage brought about by severe vitamin A deficiency. The resulting eye damage, known as xerophthalmia (dry eyes), is composed of several components. The first

190

is night blindness, dryness of the conjunctiva (the white parts of the eye), spots on the eyeball called Bitot's spots, and dryness of the transparent part of the eyeball. The dry cornea is susceptible to wounds that easily get infected. This may lead to a rupture of the cornea and hence the eyeball may be emptied through the cornea, creating a blind eye.

Vitamin A deficiency does not only cause eye damage. In 1983, Sommer published a study in Indonesia, which showed that mild and moderate vitamin A deficiency increases mortality due to increased vulnerability, especially to diarrhoeal diseases and measles. Vitamin A deficiency can also develop quite quickly in children with measles, as this infection makes the body consume its vitamin A stores much quicker. Vitamin A supplements in severely affected communities can reduce childhood mortality by as much as one-third. Data from Ghana, Sudan and India have indicated that vitamin A supplementation in cases of measles and diarrhoea has a particularly dramatic effect.

Children between six months and four years old are most vulnerable to vitamin A deficiency.

This finding led to a new intervention that has been included in immunisation programmes in certain countries. Children are given vitamin A capsules every 6 months when they visit health centres for their immunisations. The cost of the capsule is low (US 5 cents) and through immunisation programmes it is hoped to reach the majority of those in need (Sommer 1997).

An estimated 100 million pre-school children globally are estimated to have vitamin A deficiency (Figure 6.5). Vitamin A is the single most important cause of blindness in low and middle-income countries (UNICEF 1998). Also for vitamin A, there is an international expert group organising regular meetings about vitamin A. It is called the International Vitamin A Consultative Group (IVACG), and their informative Web site has the following address.[1]

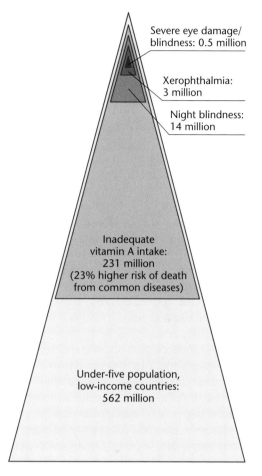

Figure 6.5 Estimated impact of vitamin A deficiency on children under five in low income countries.

Source: State of the World's Childern. UNICEF, 1995.

Severe eye damage/blindness: 0.5 million

Xerophthalmia: 3 million

Night blindness: 14 million

Inadequate vitamin A intake: 231 million (23% higher risk of death from common diseases)

Under-five population, low-income countries: 562 million

6.4.3 Zinc—a potent immuno-micronutrient

The adult human body contains 1–2 grams of zinc which is distributed to every cell of the body. It is crucial for the function of over 150 different enzymes in the body. Zinc is therefore important in numerous metabolic processes, including the synthesis of DNA, RNA and protein. Zinc is useful in the enzyme because it is like a 'gentle hand' with which the enzyme can hold, for exam-

[1]   www.ivacg.ilsi.org.

ple, nucleotides for manufacturing DNA without destroying them by oxidation. The fact that zinc is important for the synthesis of DNA, RNA and protein means that rapidly growing cells, such as the immune cells, will be affected earlier if the zinc containing enzymes are scarce. Zinc is, together with vitamin A, one of the important 'immuno-micronutrients'.

The other important fact about zinc is that there is no storage of zinc in the body. Deficiency develops rapidly in animals on a zinc-free diet. The daily requirement of 10 to 20mg of zinc has to be taken every day. Meat is the best source of zinc in the diet. A high content of plant material with phytates in the diet may lower the absorption.

A deficiency of zinc, which occurs in, for instance, a congenital zinc malabsorption syndrome called acrodermatitis enteropathica, causes retarded growth, depressed immune function, skin disorders, delayed sexual maturation and lowered fertility. The T-lymphocytes are more affected than other immune cells, and the cell-mediated immune response is therefore affected.

There is no good laboratory test for the zinc status of the body. The blood concentration varies little and does not reflect the situation well. In addition, progressive degrees of zinc deficiency probably produce a graded response in the severity of effects. Mild chronic zinc deficiency may be indicated by impaired immune function and reduced growth in children. The lack of obvious clinical signs and reliable tests of human zinc deficiency has delayed the recognition of its importance for child survival and child growth in resource-poor settings.

It is estimated that zinc deficiency affects about one-third of the world's population, mostly as mild-to-moderate deficiency. The main consequence of this deficiency is an increase in infections. Zinc deficiency is estimated to be responsible for approximately 16% of lower respiratory tract infections, 18% of malaria and 10% of diarrhoeal disease.

It has been demonstrated that zinc supplementation improves the immune status of children in low-income countries, with decreased morbidity as a consequence. But several clinical trials are also inconclusive, possibly indicating that zinc is not the only limiting nutrient in many places. In many programmes, multiple micronutrients are now being administered to eliminate deficiencies of these micronutrients as limiting factors for child survival, growth and development. The International Zinc Nutrition Consultative Group (IZINCG) was recently founded, and hosts regular meetings with a focus on zinc.[1]

6.4.4 Iodine—essential for the main metabolic hormones

At the World Summit for Children in 1990, the world's politicians promised to try to end iodine deficiency disorders by the year 2000. At that time the scale and severity of the iodine problem was only just being realised. Since then several surveys have shown even more severe damage from this deficiency in many regions of the world.

Iodine is a very peculiar chemical element. At room temperature, it exists as a shiny, grey-black substance. When exposed to the air, it turns into a violet-coloured gas and will have disappeared after some days. This property of iodine explains why the distribution of this element is so uneven in the world. Long ago iodine was more evenly distributed. But with time the iodine on the surface of the earth has evaporated into the air, and it is also easily dissolved in water. Therefore mountainous areas and areas subject to flooding are now deficient in iodine. On the other hand, iodine has accumulated in the oceans, and everything growing in the ocean or close to the ocean is rich in iodine. The atmosphere absorbs iodine from the sea and brings it back to the soil through the rain. In this way, there will be enough iodine in areas close to the sea, while land-

---

[1]   www.izincg.org

locked, remote areas will lack iodine. In these iodine-deficient areas, everything will lack iodine, the soil, the water, the plants, the animals and the humans.

The body uses iodine for only one single function. It is as a part of the thyroid hormones produced in the thyroid gland. The thyroid gland is a small butterfly-shaped gland located on the front of the neck, just below the Adam's apple. The thyroid hormones, tri-iodothyronine (T3) and tetra-iodothyronine, or thyroxine (T4), both assume a similar role in the body, namely to regulate the basic metabolic rate in the body, just as you might regulate the heat of an electric stove. If there is too much of the hormone, the body will become overheated, and if there is too little, the basic metabolic rate will slow down. The thyroid gland will trap the iodine passing through the bloodstream and incorporate it into the hormones. The hormones can then be stored in the gland until needed. The thyroid hormones are also crucial to the early development of the foetus and child. A lack of hormone will have serious repercussions on both the growth of the child and the development of the brain.

The pituitary gland which is located below the brain, controls the thyroid gland by production of a thyroid-stimulating hormone (TSH). When there is too little iodine in the diet, the pituitary gland will stimulate the thyroid gland to produce more thyroid hormones by increasing the levels of TSH.

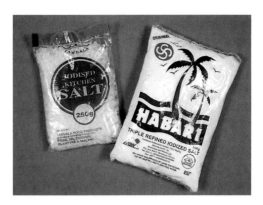

A package of iodized salt.

This results in an increase in the activity and size of the thyroid gland. The gland will better trap the little iodine that passes through it in the blood. This increase in size can reach extreme proportion. The enlarged thyroid gland can be seen as a hump in the front of the neck, known as goitre. The enlargement of the thyroid may be enough to compensate for the scarcity of iodine. But if the iodine deficiency is severe, there will still not be enough iodine to keep up the production of hormones. Such iodine deficiency does not cause one single disease, but several disturbances in the body. These are denoted by the term 'iodine deficiency disorders' (IDD).

IDD range from increased mortality of foetuses and children to constrained mental development. Its worst form is called cretinism that designates a form of severe mental

---

Box 6.1

Iodine Deficiency Disorders (IDD)

Goitre	Enlargement of the thyroid gland
Hypothyroidism	Decreased production of thyroid hormones
Miscarriages	Early death of foetuses in the womb
Stillbirths	Late death of foetuses (the child is dead at birth)
Perinatal mortality	Stillbirths and deaths in newborn children (to seventh day of life)
Congenital abnormalities	Birth defects of the newborn child
Cretinism	Mental and growth retardation, deaf-mutes and physical disability
Decrease in IQ	Reduced mental capacity

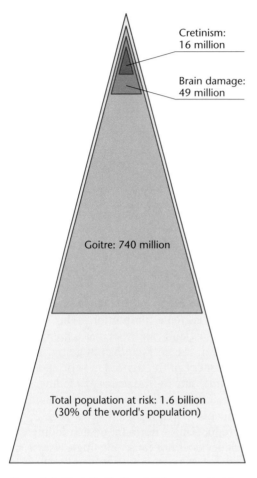

Cretinism:
16 million

Brain damage:
49 million

Goitre: 740 million

Total population at risk: 1.6 billion
(30% of the world's population)

Figure 6.6 The toll of iodine deficiency worldwide.
Source: Adapted from State of the World's Children.
UNICEF, 1995.

retardation. IDD results in impaired school performance and impaired socio-economic development.

WHO has estimated that 1.6 billion people in a total of 130 countries live in areas where they are at risk of becoming iodine-deficient. Goitre is present in 700 million people, and some 300 million suffer from lowered mental ability as a result of a lack of iodine (Fig 6.6). IDD today constitutes the single greatest cause of preventable brain damage in the foetus and infant, and of retarded psychomotor development in young children. At least 120 000 children are born

every year with mental retardation as a result of iodine deficiency (cretinism). In addition, an estimated annual total of at least 60 000 miscarriages, stillbirths and neonatal deaths stem from severe iodine deficiency in early pregnancy.

The simple way of assessing whether an area suffers from iodine deficiency is to perform a survey for goitre among school-aged children by straightforward palpation based on strict criteria (Peterson 2000). If 10 % or more of school-aged children have goitre, IDD is a public health problem that calls for action. In Sweden, a similar survey was carried out in the 1920s among 16 to 18-year old men undergoing check-ups for military service. It was found that in some areas up to one-third of the population suffered from goitre. Based on this survey, it was decided to eliminate this micronutrient deficiency in the population by fortifying salt with iodine. Today, 70 years after the introduction of 'universal salt iodisation' iodine deficiency has been eliminated as a public health problem in Sweden. This intervention must be maintained; the problem would re-occur if salt iodisation were to be stopped in Sweden.

At the World Summit for Children in 1990, IDD was highlighted and a strong political will to eliminate IDD was demonstrated. The main intervention strategy for control of IDD has become Universal Salt Iodisation (USI). Salt was chosen for a number of reasons: it is widely consumed in fairly equal amounts by most people in a population. It is usually produced centrally or at a few production sites, and the cost of iodising is relatively low, about US 5 cents per person per year. Over the last decade, extraordinary progress has been made in increasing the number of people consuming iodised salt. In 1998, more than 90 countries had salt iodisation programmes. Now, more than two-thirds of households living in IDD-affected countries consume iodised salt. Because of active programmes of salt fortification, iodine deficiency disorders are rapidly declining in the world. In 1990 it was estimated that 40 million children were born with

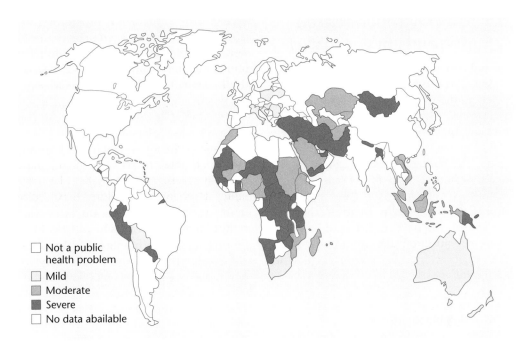

Figure 6.7 Iodine deficiency disorders, 1996.
Source: The World Health Report, WHO, 1997.

mental impairment due to iodine deficiency. This number dropped substantially in just seven years. WHO has estimated that the number of people with goitre will decrease to 350 million by the year 2025, due to iodine enrichment and supplementation programmes. A challenge is to enforce the legislation that has been passed in most countries of the world that have a recognised iodine-deficiency problem. All salt producers, from large industries to small-scale producers, need to be encouraged to use the more expensive procedure to fortify their salt production, and the consumers also need to be informed. The difficulty in many low income countries is that the salt is sold in a very coarse form that is more difficult to iodise compared to the fine granular forms of salt sold in richer countries. Another problem is that salt is often sold in poorer countries from open sacks; the purchaser takes it in small quantities wrapped in paper or banana leaves and therefore the iodine

will evaporate in varying degrees. The actual process of iodisation also requires a well functioning spraying machine that many salt producers in low-income countries do not manage to maintain. The iodine solution is often sprayed on the salt with very simple spraying devices that cannot guarantee the right concentrations. Quality control and monitoring of the salt iodisation procedures is therefore a continuous task related to the world's most widespread preventable cause of mental impairment (UNICEF 1998).

An international NGO called the International Council for the Control of Iodine Deficiency Disorders (ICCIDD) is constantly pushing for a sustainable elimination of IDD. The organisation has several Web sites, one of which is www.indorgs.virginia.edu/iccidd/.

6.5 Other nutrition-related risks and physical inactivity

As pointed out in the beginning of this chapter, new nutritional disorders emerge when under-nutrition decreases. The new nutritional risks are obesity, high blood pressure, high cholesterol, low fruit and vegetable intake, and increased physical inactivity. The burden of disease caused by the over-nutrition is today of the same order of magnitude as the diseases caused by under-nutrition. The present trend is that the world soon will have more health problems from over-nutrition than from under-nutrition. WHO even speaks of a global epidemic of obesity.

6.5.1 High blood pressure

More than 4 percent of the losses of DALYs in the world are due to high blood pressure. High blood pressure results in an increased risk of vascular disease, including myocardial infarction and stroke. Recent studies demonstrate that it is possible to reduce the mean blood pressure in a population through a reduction in salt intake. It is important to note that high blood pressure occurs across different types of countries and it is not a disorder limited to affluent populations. Haemorrhages in the brain due to high blood pressure occur in populations in rural Africa and the advice on limited salt intake applies across all socio-economic levels. This applies both for the most common form of hypertension without underlying diseases as well as for those forms of hypertensions that are secondary to kidney diseases.

Here, again, our physiology is prepared for scarcity but not for abundance. For land-based life forms, the regulatory control (homeostasis) of the salt balance in the body is crucial. If salt is scarce, the kidney will, on hormonal command, begin to recycle the little salt there is and not let any salt leave the body. Even the sweat glands will start saving salt, if sweating is profuse and the diet low in salt. This is very useful; otherwise

we might run into water intoxication. Because salt is relatively scarce for life forms that do not live in the ocean, all land-living animals, including humans, like salt. So our physiology will not prevent us from eating too much salt, and salty food is palatable. Processed food is typically high in salt content to increase palatability.

But what happens when we consume more salt than we need? More sodium in the diet will increase the sodium content in the blood, which is automatically balanced by more water in the bloodstream. More water in the bloodstream results in a higher blood pressure, and this is the signal to the kidney to increase salt excretion. The kidney will excrete the salt excess over 12 days, and the blood pressure will return to normal. But what happens if too much salt is consumed every day? The blood pressure will then be slightly elevated every day, keeping the kidney informed of the need to excrete the extra salt.

A recent US randomised cross-over trial (Sacks 2001) demonstrates that, in a group of 400 persons equally distributed between males/females, blacks/whites, with/without hypertension, it was possible to demonstrate a significant reduction in blood pressure through a reduction in salt intake. This was true irrespective of whether the subject operated around the level of 9, 6 or 3 grams of salt per day. So a reduction of salt intake to below 6 grams per day could reduce the need for medication of high blood pressure by half in the population of the United States.

WHO has looked at the cost-effectiveness of different interventions to counteract high blood pressure. These have been grouped into non-personal interventions, personal interventions and combined interventions with different amount of input. They conclude that non-personal health interventions, including government action to stimulate a reduction in the salt content of processed foods, are a cost-effective way to limit cardiovascular disease and could avert the loss of over 20 million DALYs per year worldwide. Combination treatment for people whose risk of a cardiovascular event over the next 10 years is above 35 % is also cost-effective, leading to substantial additional health benefits by averting an additional 63 million DALYs lost per year worldwide.

6.5.2 High cholesterol

WHO has calculated that high concentrations of blood lipids, of which cholesterol is one, contribute to 2.8 % of DALYs lost annually. A total blood cholesterol above 3.8 mmol/1 accounts for about 18 % of strokes and 55 % of cases of ischaemic heart disease. This risk factor acts in synergy with high blood pressure.

Cholesterol is a molecule used in the body as a precursor for hormones; it is involved in fat metabolism and is a precursor for bile salts. The body is able to produce cholesterol, but also uses the cholesterol that comes from the diet. An elevation in blood cholesterol indicates an increase in unhealthy blood lipids. An increase in polyunsaturated fat fraction in the diet has been shown to lower the blood cholesterol level, as does a reduction in overall fat intake. Intervention may increase the fraction of polyunsaturated fat in the diet, and multi-factor interventions with intensive health education may include support to stop smoking and increase in physical activity.

The nutrition transition from high-fat diet to reduced fat, to increased consumption of fruits and vegetables, and increased physical activity is advisable but not an easy task to achieve, not even in countries with well-educated populations.

6.5.3 Obesity

The current rate of global overweight contributes over 2 % of the world's DALYs lost. The frightening thing is the speed of change, where the percentage of overweight and obese people in all countries and on all continents is increasing steeply, especially in the cities.

Overweight and obesity lead to adverse metabolic effects on blood pressure, cholesterol and insulin resistance. The risks of coronary heart disease, ischaemic stroke and type 2 diabetes increase steadily with increasing BMI.

Nutrition education and an increase in physical activity have been suggested as the main actions to decrease the risk. Avoiding hidden calories from sources such as soft drinks and fatty sauces, and replacing high-fat products with low-fat products is logical. But country-specific campaigns needs to be designed.

Several web sites focus on the global epidemic of overweight and obesity. On the web site of the International Food Policy Research Institute[1], a search for the word 'obesity' brings up PDF files of books and papers that deal with obesity in low-income countries. The Center for Disease Control and Prevention in the US has a site on nutrition and physical activity.[2] WHO's nutrition unit[3] provides relevant documents, as does the International Obesity Task Force[4]. Easy-to-use calculators for body mass index and menu planners are available at the National Health, Lung and Blood Institute Obesity Education Initiative.[5]

6.5.4 Low fruit and vegetable intake

A low intake of fruits and vegetables contributes 1.8 % of DALYs lost. Fruits and vegetables are important components of a healthy diet, which seem to protect against cardiovascular diseases and cancers of the gastrointestinal tract. A fruit contains several substances that prevent it—for some time at least—from decomposing. These are mainly compounds known as antioxidants and are also capable of preventing oxidative DNA damage. Together with many other substances, these may prevent cellular dam-

[1] www.ifpri.org
[2] www.cdc.gov/nccdphp
[3] www.who.int/nut
[4] www.iotf.org (and go to 'about obesity')
[5] www.nhlbi.nih.gov/about/oei

age. The other advantage of increasing the intake of fruits and vegetables in the diet is that they are usually not so energy-dense, so they are beneficial for the cholesterol concentration and body mass index.

6.5.5 Physical inactivity

Opportunities for people to be physically active exist in the four major domains of the daily life: at work, transport, domestic duties and leisure time. There is no agreed definition or measurement of physical activity, but less than 2.5 hours of moderate activity per week has been suggested as a cut-off for physical inactivity. Due to this lack of agreement, the estimates are uncertain, but approximately 1.3 % of DALYs lost are attributed to low physical activity.

Physical activity reduces the risk of cardiovascular disease and type 2 diabetes. Furthermore, it may improve musculoskeletal health and control body weight. Physical activity in childhood and adolescence increases the peak bone mass (the maximum bone mass), which is beneficial for the prevention of fractures in old age.

References and suggested further readings

Antonsson-Ogle B, Gustafsson O, Hambraeus L, Holmgren G, Tylleskär T. Nutrition, agriculture and health when resources are scarce. 2nd ed. Uppsala: Swedish University of Agricultural Sciences & Uppsala University; 2000.

Black RE, Morris SS, Bryce J. Where and why are 10 million children dying every year? Lancet 2003;361:2226–34.

Caballero B, Popkin BM (eds). The nutrition transistion. Diet and disease in the developing world. Amsterdam: Academic Press; 2002.

Ezzati M, Lopez AD, Rodgers A, Vander Hoorn S, Murray CJ. Comparative Risk Assessment Collaborating Group: Selected major risk factors and global and regional burden of disease. Lancet 2002;360:1347–60.

Ghana VAST Study Team. Vitamin A supplementation in northern Ghana. Lancet 1993;345:7–12.

Gibson RS. Principles of Nutritional Assessment. Oxford University Press; 1990.

Greiner T. The concept of weaning: definitions and their implications. Hum Lact 1996;12:123–8.

King M, King F, Martodipoero S. Primary child care: A manual for health workers. Oxford University Press 1978.

Mata LJ, Kromal RA, Urrutia JJ, Garcia B. Effect of infection on food intake and the nutritional state: perspectives as viewed from the village. Am J Clin Nutr. 1977;8:1215–27.

Murray CJL, Lopez A. Alternative projections of mortality and disability by cause 1990–2020: Global Burden of Disease Study. Lancet 1997;349:1498–1504.

Peterson S, Sanga AB, Bunga B, Eklof H, Taube A, Gebre-Medhin M, Rosling H. Estimation of thyroid size with ultrasound and palpation in field surveys. Lancet 2000;355:106–10.

Sacks M, et al. Effects on Blood Pressure of Reduced Dietary Sodium and the Dietary Approaches to Stop Hypertension (DASH) Diet. New Engl J Med 2001;344:53–55.

Sommer A. Vitamin A prophylaxis. Arch Dis Child 1997;77:191–4.

Sommer A. Moving from science to public health programs: lessons from vitamin A. Am J Clin Nutr 1998;68(2 Suppl):5135–5165.

Sparén P, Vågerö D, Shestov DB, Plavinskaja S, Parfenova N, Hoptiar V, Paturot D, Galanti MR. Long term mortality after severe starvation during the siege of Leningrad: prospective cohort study. BMJ 2004;328:11–4.

UNICEF. Progress of Nations. 1998.

UNICEF. State of the World's Children. 2001 and 2004.

WHO. Management of severe malnutrition: a manual for physicians and other senior health workers. 1999.

WHO. World Health Report. 1998, 2002, 2004.

7 Non-communicable diseases (47%)*

> *We are not allowed to get sick anymore because we have to pay for medication… what with?*
>
> An older man, Bosnia Herzegovina

Diseases that are not caused by infectious agents are jointly referred to as non-communicable diseases. This group of diseases has also been called chronic disease or degenerative diseases. But this division is a simplification of a quite complex reality. The boundary between diseases caused by infectious agents and those caused by other factors is unclear and keeps moving as research advances. All forms of cancer are by convention classified as non-communicable diseases, but today we know that both liver cancer and cervical cancer are mainly caused by chronic infections with the hepatitis and papilloma viruses respectively. Realising that the classification is far from perfect, it can still be used to provide an overview of the pattern of diseases.

Non-communicable diseases cause about 47% of the global burden of disability and premature death. In high-income countries up to 80% of all DALYs lost are from non-communicable diseases. Successful reduction of malnutrition and infections will inevitably increase the relative importance of non-communicable diseases. Although the populations of low-income countries still mainly suffer from malnutrition and infections, the non-communicable diseases now cause more than 40% of their total burden of disease. In many middle income countries the non-communicable diseases are already a bigger burden than are malnutrition and infections. This is the situation in most of the Middle East and Latin America. Some non-communicable diseases like hypertension and cancer are quite common causes of human suffering also in rural areas of Africa. Stroke is not a rare disease among poor people in rural Africa. Out of all healthy years of life (DALYs) lost in the world due to non-communicable diseases, the vast majority are in fact lost in the low and middle-income countries. The absolute number of DALYs lost per 1 000 population through non-communicable diseases is at the same level in Africa and in high income countries. Most DALYs are lost in the low-and middle income countries in Europe reflecting the health transition (Figure 7.1). It is in relative terms that the non-communicable diseases are of lesser significance in poor countries. The risk of a person developing cancer and/or a psychiatric disease is more or less the same throughout the whole world if they do not die at younger age from some other disease!

Estimates point at the increased importance of the non-communicable diseases in all countries, in other words, the world population will see more of lung cancer, diabetes, depression and heart attacks. By 2020 it is estimated that the burden of non-communicable diseases will have risen to three-quarters of the total burden of disease in the world. This is partly due to the fact that the population of the world is ageing. It is also due to the decreasing mortality of communicable diseases and to increased tobacco smoking in some parts of the world, as well as increasing overweight and alcohol consumption. To avoid human suffering and to

---

* % in parentheses is estimated share of global burden of disease.

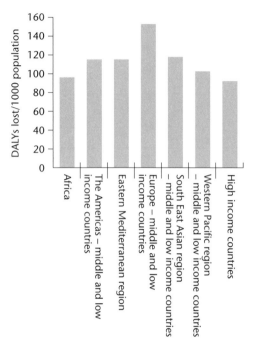

DALYs lost/1000 population

- Africa
- The Americas – middle and low income countries
- Eastern Mediterranean region
- Europe – middle and low income countries
- South East Asian region – middle and low income countries
- Western Pacific region – middle and low income countries
- High income countries

Figure 7.1 DALYs lost per 1 000 population due to non communicable diseases by region in 1998.

Source: The World Health Report, WHO, 1999.

spare economic resources in caring for the costly non-communicable diseases, WHO has started a campaign against tobacco and obesity throughout the world. However, it is difficult for individuals, families, communities and countries to pay attention to upcoming health problems when they are fully occupied avoiding hunger and deadly infections (Box 7.1)

The major contributors to the global burden of disease among the non-communicable diseases are: neuropsychiatric disorders (13 %), cardiovascular diseases (10 %), cancers (5 %) and respiratory diseases (4 %). In this chapter, we briefly review the occurrence, causes, symptoms, diagnosis, treatment and possible preventive measures for the major non-communicable diseases.

7.1 Neuropsychiatric disorders (13 %)

Mental and neurological diseases caused about 10 % of the global burden of disease

---

Box 7.1

Father and son discuss disease transition

A West African musician made a career in Europe and became a Swedish citizen. He regularly sent money to relatives in his home village in Africa like most Africans resident in Europe do. On his first return visit home to Africa his father was keen to show him how he had used the money. The proud father led his son to the rice field. He wanted to show off his new pesticide-spraying machine; he was the first farmer in the village to own one. With it strapped on his back he proudly walked across the field leaving a cloud of nasty smelling chemicals that drifted in the evening breeze into the face of his son.

"But father," shouted the son, "stop spraying, those chemical can be dangerous."

"On the contrary my son these poisons keep the pests away from our crop so that

the family can eat good food every day and thereby stay healthy."

"No! The chemicals are dangerous, you need to wear protection clothing, otherwise you will die from cancer," shouted the son.

The father was saddened by his son's unforeseen reaction. He stopped the machine, put it on the ground and responded with anger:

"That is precisely what we want to do, die from cancer! In our village we struggle to get enough food to keep hunger away and to avoid dying from malaria. If we succeed we will live to old age and die from cancer like the rich people do. What's the problem?"

---

in 1990, 13 % in 2002 and is estimated to rise to 15 % by the year 2020. Psychiatric diseases such as schizophrenia and depression cause several times more DALYs lost than do classic neurological diseases such as Parkinson's disease and multiple sclerosis. Neuropsychiatric disorders are observed in all societies of the world. Contrary to popular belief, all research indicates that the occurrence of schizophrenia and bipolar affective disorders (manic-depressive illness) is about the same in all countries. Often persons with such severe psychiatric diseases do not survive for long in poor communities and therefore the percentage in the whole population may be lower although the the incidence is the same in both poor and rich countries. In each age group the occurrence of dementia also seems to be about the same around the world. Countries with an ageing population and long life expectancy will exhibit a much greater prevalence of Alzheimer's dementia because this disease is so common in old age, and affected persons will die early from complications if they do not have access to advanced care. In contrast to dementia, Parkinson's disease is more common in high-income countries, but the reason for this remains to be discovered.

It is estimated that a total of 450 million people in the world suffer from neuropsychiatric conditions. These include unipolar depressive disorders, bipolar affective disorders, schizophrenia, epilepsy, alcohol and selective drug use disorders, Alzheimer's and other dementia, post-traumatic stress disorder, obsessive-compulsive disorder, panic disorder and primary insomnia. This constitutes a heavy burden of human suffering for both the individuals and their families. Neuropsychiatric disorders cause both a high indirect and direct cost for the individual and for society. But even if neuropsychiatric disorders cause 13 % of all DALYs lost, most countries dedicate less than 1 % of their health budgets to mental disorders.

There are effective neuropsychiatric drugs and successful psychological treatments that have the potential to relieve much human suffering. Unfortunately, these treatments are usually affordable only to the rich populations of the world. In low-income countries there are fewer chances of employment and survival for neuropsychiatric patients, because of a lack of medical treatment. The only relief may be for psychiatric patients to seek traditional practitioners. They have to rely heavily on their families and social networks for daily support.

Europe and the Americas are the regions with the highest proportion of DALYs lost due to neuropsychiatric disorders, 20 and 25 % respectively. Is the burden of being a 'modern' human being too heavy? Is depression the price for being socio-economically developed and physically healthy? Or do individuals vulnerable to psychiatric disorders have a higher survival rate in rich countries, resulting in a greater prevalence of these disorders in the population? It seems as if, when we prevent and cure the other diseases, we will be left with an increased relative importance of psychiatric diseases. Much more research is needed to understand the worrying trend of increased occurrence of neuropsychiatric disorders throughout the world. WHO dedicated its entire 2001 yearbook to mental health (WHO 2001).

7.1.1 Unipolar depression (4 %)

Unipolar depression, i.e. depression without any manic periods, was ranked as the fourth most significant disease in the world in terms of DALYs lost in 2002, causing 4 % of the healthy years lost. Depression is expected to be the second most significant disease in the world by the year 2020. In low and middle-income countries, depression is projected to be the most significant cause of DALYs lost by the year 2020 (Murray and Lopez 1997). Already depression is the second most important disease in the world among those aged 15–44 years. It is difficult to rejoice in the victory over malnutrition and infections when the outcome is such a

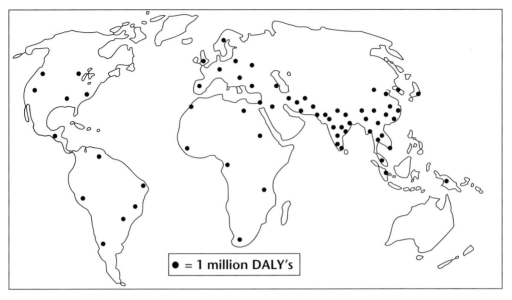

Map 7:1 Depression causes 65 million disability adjusted life years (DALY) lost per year.
Source: WHO, 2002.

high prevalence of depression. Urbanisation in middle-income countries consists mainly of young people who have attended school. They have avoided hunger and death from infection, but instead they find themselves unemployed in an urban slum with weak social identification and a high risk for drug abuse or depression.

Unipolar depression may be regarded as 'reactive', i.e. caused by sad events in a person's life, or as 'endogenous', meaning without apparent external cause, or a mixture of the two. The exact cause of the endogenous type of depression is not known, but there is a decreased level of the neurotransmitter serotonin in all types of depression, and this is therefore utilised in pharmacological treatment.

Symptoms are feelings of sadness and hopelessness, with thoughts of guilt and suicidal ideas. Patients develop psychomotor retardation, and facial expressions become minimised. Sleeping disturbances, anorexia, weight loss and psychosomatic pain are also common symptoms. The majority of people who commit suicide are depressed.

Unipolar depression may present differently in different cultures. The symptoms of depression tend to be more somatic and less psychological in many low and middle-income countries compared with in high-income countries. Patients with depression often present at health facilities complaining of sleeping difficulties or somatic pain instead of saying that they are feeling sad. In the short time available patients are often not given the correct diagnosis and treatment.

The use of new, effective anti-depressant drugs has been widespread in high-income countries. Selective Seretonine Reuptake Inhibitors (SSRI) the 'happy pill', is being prescribed and used in increasing amounts but this costly treatment is out of reach for most of those who suffer from depression in the world. The reason is that drugs are expensive and require long treatment periods as well as considerable amounts of professional consultations. Cognitive behavioural therapy has been found to be almost as effective as treatment with drugs. As this therapy can be given in groups it may offer a more cost-effective option for treatment of depression.

Individual prevention of depression is difficult, since it has multi-factorial causes. Improved social security and social networks, and early detection of cases for social and medical support are just some of the possible paths. The prevention and treatment of depression will constitute an enormous challenge to world health in the coming decades.

7.1.2 Anxiety disorders (2 %)

Anxiety disorders give rise to varying degrees of disability and exist in many forms. This group of diseases can be divided into generalised anxiety, obsessive-compulsive, phobias, panic, acute stress, post-traumatic stress disorder (PTSD) and psychosomatic disorders.

Many patients with anxiety disorders seek help for somatic reasons, and it may be difficult for them to accept that their symptoms have psychiatric causes. Anxiety may start due to a tragic 'life event', or as a reaction to stress. Obsessive-compulsive disorder involves an excessive and unnecessary repetition of thoughts or actions, for example washing hands for many hours each day. A phobia is a strong fear that disrupts normal behaviour. A panic disorder is characterised by bouts of a fast heartbeat, with sudden fear for life, sometimes coupled with a feeling of breathing difficulty.

The treatment of anxiety disorders has improved considerably over the last decades with psychiatric drugs, psychotherapy and psychosocial interventions. Benzodiazepines (e.g. Valium) are useful only for short periods, because they induce dependence. Antidepressants are useful in obsessive and compulsive disorders, as well as panic disorders and PTSD. Phobias can be successfully treated with behavioural therapy. Even in high income countries only a portion of patients with anxiety disorders seek and get the help they need from modern health care. Many all over the world turn to traditional medicine, where they may get good help and support for these types of conditions. The effective behavioural treatment of phobias is almost exclusively accessible to patients in high-income countries and to the rich in the rest of the world. This may become more accessible if provided as group therapy.

7.1.3 Bipolar disorders (1 %)

The occurrence of bipolar disease, or manic-depressive illness, is remarkably similar all over the world. It is an integrated aspect of human life across cultures and economic resources. Bipolar disorders account for the same proportion of healthy years lost per population on every continent. The clinical features and the treatment are also similar worldwide. The disease is characterised by periods of mania and periods of depression, which explains the name bipolar. The periods of mania tend to be self-limiting, ceasing after weeks or months, even without treatment. Between periods of illness, the person can mostly live a normal social life. There is a strong genetic factor in bipolar disorders.

Treatment may be given in the acute periods: tranquillisers against mania and antidepressants during depressions. Long term treatment with the cheap drug lithium effectively prevents acute episodes. Unfortunately, lithium has a narrow therapeutic window, which means that the difference between effective and toxic concentrations is small. This implies that, even if the drug is very cheap, it requires costly care and regular laboratory analysis to avoid side effects. Therefore, this therapy is still not available for most patients in middle and low-income countries.

7.1.4 Schizophrenia (1 %)

Schizophrenia caused about 1 % of the total DALYs lost in 2002. It is the most common form of psychosis, i.e. severe psychiatric disease. The incidence of psychosis is similar all over the world. Psychosis can be caused by schizophrenia, mania, depression, acute organic mental disorders or drug or alcohol intoxication.

Schizophrenia usually starts when the person is between 15 and 30 years old. It is probably caused by a complex combination of genetic, biological and social factors. The symptoms are the same all over the world. The most prominent symptom is delusions and disturbed thinking, hearing of voices, and inability to participate in social life. The patient may experience that an outside person or organisation is controlling them. Paranoid thoughts or megalomania may be combined with other odd and inappropriate behaviour. One-third of cases recover completely from the first psychotic episode, but schizophrenia most often becomes a lifelong disease.

Pharmacological treatment may help an individual to integrate into the social life of the community, but in most countries the health service cannot afford the life long supply of medicines, and the consultations with psychiatrists that is needed. Social acceptance of patients with this disease varies across nations. An understanding and socially supportive network is important for recovery and for prevention of new episodes of psychosis. Traditional healers can in many cultures provide important support to patients with schizophrenia.

7.1.5 Dementia (1 %)

Dementia will invariably increase with the transition to an older population. The two most common types of dementia, Alzheimer's disease and cerebrovascular dementia, are leading causes of disability among the oldest age groups in all countries. Dementia is estimated to have caused almost 1 % of the total DALYs lost in the whole world. However, in high-income countries as much as 6 % of the DALYs lost were due to dementia in 2003.

Dementia slowly manifests itself with loss of memory. First recent events are forgotten, and later events further back in the history of the individual. Thereafter dementia affects the person's ability to take care of themselves and dressing as well as washing become difficult. Finally, all aspects of consciousness, emotion, intellect and behaviour deteriorate. In Alzheimer's disease the progress of the disease is earlier in onset and the progress much more rapid than in the vascular dementia of old age. The cause of Alzheimer's dementia is not known, but an increased deposition of amyloid is seen in the brain tissue of an Alzheimer patient. Cerebrovascular dementia is thought to be caused by small, repeated microemboli that cause infarctions in the brain.

Cerebrovascular dementia could be prevented to some extent by life-style choices and treatment of hypertension, but so far Alzheimer's disease cannot be prevented. Research efforts focusing on the aetiology and new pharmacological treatment for Alzheimer's disease are intense, but the current treatment slows the progress of the disease only slightly, without providing any effective cure. All countries that manage to reduce the prevalence of other diseases are prone to experience more dementia. Dementia is a very costly disorder, as the patients are very sick and need a lot of care and surveillance for many years before they die.

A paradoxical effect of successful prevention of diseases is thus that the health service gets more expensive. Economic arguments are often used to mobilize resources for prevention of cancer and hypertension. Although such preventive programmes have enormous benefits by avoiding deaths in upper middle age they will not reduce the cost for health services. Few diseases are as costly as Alzheimer and osteoporosis. Caring for the old is becoming a more and more central part of human life and of the political debate. It takes a larger and larger part of the economy in post-industrial high-income countries. Many middle-income countries with a good health policy are now rapidly approaching the same demographic and health care situation without having the economic means to provide care for a growing proportion of chronically ill old people. Cuba is rapidly getting into this situation and many of the former communist countries are already in this situation. The disease panorama of these countries is similar to that of Sweden, the demographic profile is similar and is becoming the same, but the countries have less than one tenth of the resources for health and social service for the elderly.

7.1.6 Alcohol and substance dependence (2 %)

Alcohol dependence is a very serious medical and public health problem in most parts of the world. However, the severity and extent of alcohol dependence varies with cultural, religious and socio-economic factors. The occurrence of dependency on narcotic drugs varies even more between and within countries. The consequences of alcohol abuse range from direct toxicological effects to injury and violence, as well as psychological and behavioural problems.

The gender differences are considerable. Globally the direct burden of disability from alcohol is about eight times higher in men than in women. Alcohol abuse is the leading cause of disability for adult men in high-income countries, and number four in low and middle-income countries. In high-income countries, alcohol caused 4 % of all DALYs lost, whereas in low and middle-income countries it only caused 1 % of the DALYs lost. The trends for the last forty years have been a steady increase in alcohol consumption almost all over the world.

Estimates of the prevalence of alcohol dependence range from 2 to 19 % of the total male population of the world and from 1 to 9 % among women in different countries (Beaglehole 2003). The highest rate of alcohol dependence in the world is in the Americas. The middle-income countries in Latin America have the highest burden of alcohol

abuse in the world. The Arab countries have low rates of alcohol use and dependence but some have increasing problems with abuse of narcotic substances.

Alcohol dependence leads to both acute and chronic diseases of the liver and nervous system. Another important health effect is that alcohol and substance abuse also lead to an increased occurrence of injury, suicide and violent behaviour, as well as adverse pregnancy outcomes. Most of these conditions will be discussed further elsewhere in the book.

The prevention of alcohol dependence includes a range of interventions. These may include economic restrictions, with increased taxation on alcohol and control of accessibility through placing limitations in time and location on the selling alcohol to the public, as well as awareness campaigns about the adverse effects of alcohol use. The same can be said for most types of substance abuse. The early detection and treatment of an individual who abuses alcohol or narcotic drugs appear to be effective in preventing dependence. Preventive actions could be implemented within the health service, but community-based actions involving families, work places and religious and non-governmental organisations seem to be more effective. The pattern of alcohol and substance abuse varies a great deal. Preventive measures need to be broad in scope and yet adapted to each context. It is important to note that substance abuse is already a very severe and rapidly growing problem in many Asian and Middle East countries, such as Vietnam and Iran, partly due to the opium and heroin trade through these two densely populated countries. A number of narcotic drugs are also becoming a public health problem in low-income countries in Africa.

The global alcohol policy alliance is one of the international organisations that try to reduce the adverse effects of alcohol.[1] Such actions work against enormous economic

[1]   www.alcohol-alliance.org

interest both in the legal alcohol trade and in the illegal drug trade. Sweden is a major exporter of alcohol in the world and the aggressive marketing of "Absolute Vodka" in countries like India is a prominent example of the negative health effects of globalisation. The multinational companies trading in alcohol often try to follow regulations to protect the health of especially vulnerable groups like young people. But with their unfortunately effective marketing they counteract such preventive efforts many times over. A pathetic example can be seen on the web page[1] where the web user is told "You must be of legal drinking age to use this Site". WHO has a special programme against substance dependency[2] but the commercial alcohol promotion has not been pursued with the same vigour as WHO has tried to stop promotion of tobacco smoking.

7.2 Cardiovascular diseases (10%)

Cardiovascular diseases (CVD) are estimated to cause one third of all deaths in the world, but only one tenth of all the healthy life years lost. The reason for this discrepancy is that the diseases of the heart and blood vessels mainly kill late in life. In high-income countries a high percentage of the population dies from CVD, but it is important to know that the low and middle-income countries contribute to about 80% of the total number of deaths due to cardiovascular disease in the world. Even in Sub-Saharan Africa, it is estimated that 10% of all deaths are due to CVD. Hypertension, cigarette smoking, high-fat diet, diabetes and lack of physical activity are the main risk factors for CVD.

The mortality from cardiovascular diseases is increasing fast in middle-income countries, while it has been falling in high-income countries since the 1960s. Cerebrov-

[1] http://absolut.com/
[2] www.who.int/substance_abuse

ascular disease mortality has shown an even sharper decline than coronary heart mortality in high-income countries. The reason for this decline is an increased knowledge of the risk factors in the population. The health services in rich countries are capable of tracing high-risk individuals to offer treatment for hypertension and other predisposing factors. This has also contributed to the decline in deaths from CVD. In Eastern Europe the trend is the opposite, an increasing mortality. CVD strikes at a younger age in low and middle-income countries, where half the victims dying of CVD are under 70 years of age. In contrast only a quarter of the CVD victims in high-income countries occur under 70 years of age (Reddy 1998). The main cardiovascular diseases in the world are ischaemic heart disease and cerebrovascular disease, leading to deaths in myocardial infarction and stroke, respectively.

7.2.1 Ischaemic heart disease (4%)

Ischaemic heart disease causes most deaths in the CVD group, about 7 million out of the 57 million people who die in the world each year. In high-income countries ischaemic heart disease causes nearly a quarter of all deaths, and in low and middle-income countries it causes an estimated one eighth of all deaths. Even if it mainly kills late in life, ischaemic heart disease causes about 4% of the DALYs lost, thus ranking sixth among the major diseases in the world according to the number of healthy life years lost.

The burden of ischaemic heart disease varies between countries according to people's habits and diet. The middle-income countries of Europe, i.e. the former Soviet Union and Eastern Europe, have by far the heaviest burden of ischaemic heart disease in the whole world. Africa and the Western pacific region have the lowest burden (Figure 7.2).

The main symptom of ischaemic heart disease is cardiac pain caused by impaired blood flow to the heart, due to arteriosclerosis in the arteries of the heart. Depending on severity the pain may be reversible or develop

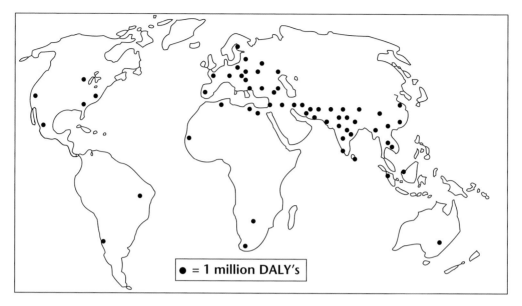

Map 7:2 Ischaemic heart disease causes 58 million disability adjusted life years (DALY) lost per year.
Source: WHO, 2002.

into an acute cardiac infarction, when the blood flow to the heart muscle is blocked, resulting in permanent damage to the heart. Death may be sudden, due to disturbances of heart rhythm. Complications can also occur later or after the patient has suffered a second or third heart infarction. The emergency care of acute infarction has improved considerably over the last decades, but it involves very costly ambulance and intensive care services. Acute heart infarction can be treated at great cost in ways that decrease mortality and damage to the heart, for instance through the use of fibrinolytic drugs.

Preventive treatment against ischaemic heart disease ranges from lifestyle changes to pharmacological or surgical interventions. Cessation of smoking, weight loss and increased physical activity may lower the risk of ischaemic heart disease. Pharmacological control of hypertension, high blood lipids and diabetes mellitus are crucial. Surgical interventions such as "coronary by-pass" operations are even more expensive. There is already a high demand for advanced prevention and treatment of acute heart attacks in

Asia, Middle East and Latin America. This advanced care is mainly provided by private hospitals, and is definitely not accessible to the majority of the population in these countries. Even the Ministers of Health in the poorest low-income countries in Africa are faced with a political demand for the provision of advanced care for heart attacks at the same time as they are trying to provide vaccination to all children. The availability of intensive care for heart diseases may however be of importance for the development of the tourist sector, as well as other forms of international investment and collaboration. Poor countries are faced with a truly difficult policy dilemma, whether to provide advanced care for the few while still hot providing basic care for the many.

7.2.2 Cerebrovascular diseases (3 %)

Cerebrovascular disease causes stroke, including both vascular occlusion and vascular rupture leading to brain haemorrhage. The most common cause of stroke is due to vascular occlusion. The neurological signs

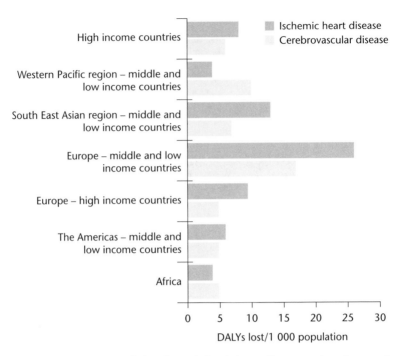

Figure 7.2 DALYs lost per 1 000 population due to ischemic heart diseases and cerebrovascular diseases by region in 1998.

Source: The World Health Report, WHO, 1999.

and symptoms depend on which part and how much of the brain has been affected by the stop in blood circulation. The most common effects are complete or partial paralysis of one half of the body.

Second to ischaemic heart disease, cerebrovascular diseases cause most deaths in the world, about 5 million per year or 10 % of all deaths. The heaviest burden of cerebrovascular disease is found in middle-income countries in East Europe and in China. It may come as a surprise to some readers that the risk of death due to a cerebro-vascular disease is greater for a middle-aged person living in a poor country in Africa than it is for a person living in a rich countries in Europe or North America. The main reason is that the risk of cerebrovascular disease is related to high blood pressure, a disease that does not spare the poor. However, poor people have almost no access to diagnosis and treatment for high blood pressure. They

cannot afford the costly life-long treatment that has reduced the number of deaths from cerebrovascular diseases in the high-income countries.

Besides hypertension, the main risk factors for stroke are diabetes mellitus, high fat intake, obesity, smoking and alcohol dependence. The most important prevention is the early diagnosis and treatment of hypertension. However, the diagnosis and treatment of hypertension and diabetes are costly, both in terms of drugs, medical consultations, laboratory tests and working days lost. Therefore it is unlikely that the majority of those affected in middle-income countries will have access to these preventive measures during the decades to come. What seems a more feasible preventive approach in countries with limited economic resources for health service, is to focus on stopping smoking and promoting physical activity. Like so many other pharmacological treatments, the

208

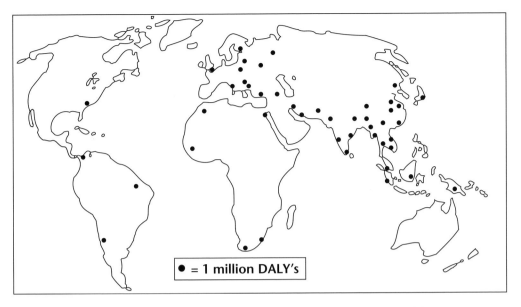

Map 7:3 Cerebrovascular disease causes 45 million disability adjusted life years (DALY) lost per year.
Source: WHO, 2002.

medical prevention of cerebro-vascular disease is too costly where it is most needed.

New treatments for stroke are being developed to decrease brain damage in the acute phase, but these are extremely costly, as they require fast access to well-functioning emergency care. Otherwise treatment is concentrated on controlling complications. Rehabilitation and care of stroke patients is also costly, and in most parts of the world rehabilitation is what the family and community can offer. All of the middle-income countries that are now experiencing a decline in the incidence of infectious diseases and malnutrition are already facing a very costly increase in the burden of cerebrovascular diseases. Cerebrovascular diseases will soon constitute a more prominent part of the disease panorama of middle-income countries than of high-income countries. China and India will experience a higher proportion of heart attacks and stroke, while Europe and North America will experience more dementia and osteoporosis. There is a disease transition going on also among the non-communicable diseases.

7.3 Cancer (5%)

It is estimated that 7 million people in the world die of different types of cancer each year (WHO 2004). More than 50 million have been treated for cancer and about 10 million new cases are discovered each year. Cancer causes about 25% of all deaths in high-income countries and 10% in low and middle-income countries. As cancer mostly affects older people, it only causes 15% of all DALYs lost in high-income countries, and 5% of healthy life years lost in low and middle-income countries (Figure 7.3). With the ageing population in the world and better prevention and treatment of infections, the world incidence of cancer will rise. Another reason for an increase in cancer is that smoking and other cancer inducing factors are spreading in the world.

Cancer is an uncontrolled growth of cells, which may spread from the organ of origin to surrounding tissues and distant organs of the body. The different types of cancer vary according to site and cell type, the growth, pattern of spread and treatment possibilities

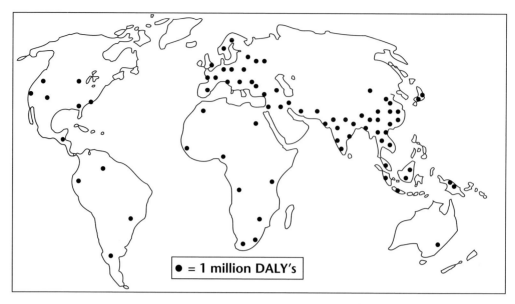

Map 7:4 Cancer causes 78 million disability adjusted life years (DALY) lost per year.
Source: WHO, 2002.

vary greatly, as does the prognosis. The most common types of cancer differ between countries. Men in low and middle-income countries suffer mainly from cancer of the lungs, stomach, liver, and mouth/throat. For men in high-income countries, the most common types of cancer are lung, prostate, colon/rectum and stomach. Women in low and middle-income countries suffer mainly from cancer of the cervix, followed by breast, stomach and lung. In high-income countries, the most common types of cancer for women are breast, colon/rectum, lung and stomach (WHO 1998).

The major risk factors for the most common types of cancer are diet, tobacco, alcohol, occupational hazards, infection and hormones. These risk factors can be modified by prevention. The outcomes of cancers also vary between countries, depending on the ability of the health care sector to detect and treat cancer. Death from cancer of the cervix is largely preventable. In spite of this, most countries in Sub-Saharan Africa do not have the financial resources to offer effective cervical cancer screening programmes. Similarly, the treatment of cancers of the blood,

leukaemia and lymphoma, is now successful in most cases due to new technologies and drugs. However, these new treatments are very costly in terms of drugs, technology and expertise. Although many cancers are curable today, most persons in the world who are affected by these cancers will still die because the investigations and treatments are too costly. Today there is widespread awareness that most people in the world who are infected with HIV do not have access to the new drugs. The same lack of access to life saving treatment is the reality for a number of severe and common diseases in low-income countries, such as cancer, hypertension and diabetes.

The International Agency for Research on Cancer (IARC) is part of the World Health Organization. It is situated in Lyon and leads research and actions to reduce the burden of cancer in the world.[1] IARC holds the best database on cancer in the world and assists countries to develop their cancer registers.

[1]   www.iarc.fr

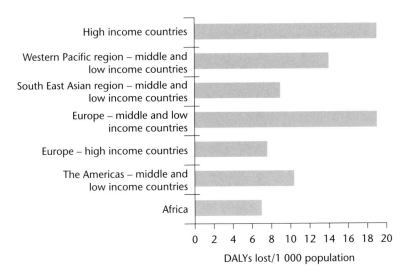

Figure 7.3 DALYs lost per 1 000 population due to cancer by region in 1998.
Source: The World Health Report, WHO, 1999.

7.3.1 Lung cancer (1 %)

Cancer of the lungs and airways is the most common type of cancer in the world. More than 1 million people die of lung cancer each year and tobacco smoking causes most of these cancers. The occurrence of lung cancer in a population reflects the prevalence of tobacco-smoking one to two decades earlier. The heaviest burden of lung cancer is still in high-income countries, but the rapidly increasing number of smokers in middle-income countries in particular is now changing the pattern of lung cancer in the world. Of all cases of lung cancer, 75 % occur in men, but with an increasing use of tobacco by women, there is an increase in lung cancer rates in women, mainly in high-income countries. Screening programmes for lung cancer, using chest x-rays and sputum cytology to detect early forms of cancer, has not proven to be effective. Preventive actions should therefore focus entirely on the reduction of tobacco smoking.

7.3.2 Stomach cancer (0.5 %)

Stomach cancer is the second most common type of cancer in the world. A little less than 1 million people are estimated to die from stomach cancer each year. The highest risk of dying in stomach cancer is in East Asia including Japan and in middle-income countries in Europe. About half of all cases of stomach cancer are estimated to occur in China. This type of cancer is almost twice as common in males as in females. Since the symptoms are sparse apart from unspecific tiredness, weight loss and abdominal discomfort, this cancer is often in an advanced stage before it is diagnosed. The prognosis remains poor even with surgery and chemotherapy.

7.3.3 Liver cancer (0.5 %)

Liver cancer is the third most common form of cancer in the world measured in terms of both DALYs lost and number of deaths. More than half a million persons annually die of liver cancer. This cancer is much more common in low and middle-income countries. The highest incidences are found in China and the Pacific, South-East Asia and Sub-Saharan Africa. Primary liver cancer (hepatocellular cancer) is mainly caused by a chronic infection with the hepatitis B or C

211

viruses. The variation in occurrence of liver cancer is largely explained by the prevalence of chronic infections by these two viruses. Contributing risk factors are a high dietary intake of a mould toxin called aflatoxin. This toxin occurs in badly stored groundnuts. Another risk factor is alcohol use. A vaccine exists against hepatitis B, but not yet against hepatitis C. Early vaccination against hepatitis B is now being included in the vaccination programmes of several Asian countries. In summary liver cancer remains difficult to cure, it may be regarded as an infectious disease, which can be largely prevented by vaccination.

7.3.4 Breast cancer (0.5 %)

Breast cancer represents the most common type of cancer in women in the world. About half a million women are estimated to die of breast cancer each year. In high-income countries, 2 % of women die of breast cancer, but in low and middle-income countries the proportion is only about 0.5 %. A risk factor for breast cancer is not having given birth to children or starting childbearing late. Oral contraceptives, if used from a young age and for prolonged periods, seem to slightly increase the risk of breast cancer in younger women. Breast cancer screening may detect cancer and lead to early treatment, thereby reducing mortality. But breast cancer screening is expensive and not even regarded as cost-effective for women under the age of 50 in high-income countries. Most women in the world have no access to such screening programmes. The results of treatment have improved in the last decades but most women in the world do not have access to these new advances.

7.3.5 Colon and rectum cancer (0.5 %)

Colorectal cancer also causes about half a million deaths per year. This cancer usually appears after 50 years of age in persons who have eaten a high-fat and low-fibre diet. The symptoms may be diffuse before the cancer has become widespread. Since this type of cancer is mainly a lifestyle-determined disease, the promotion of a low-fat, high-fibre diet and exercise may help. While the prevalence of cancer of the stomach declines with socio-economic development, cancer of the colon and rectum increases with the change in diet and population ageing, as we have observed in high-income countries. Today's high rate of stomach cancer in middle-income countries is expected to be replaced by a high rate of colorectal cancer when these countries have gone through socio-economic improvements. The hope is that results from research in today's high-income countries can help to avoid lifestyles that contribute to the development of the same type of diseases, when today's middle-income countries become high-income countries.

7.4 Respiratory Diseases (4%)

The two most important respiratory diseases in the world are asthma and chronic obstructive pulmonary disease (also known as chronic bronchitis and emphysema). Together, they cause almost 3 % of the total DALYs lost, and together with some other respiratory diseases, this group constitutes 4 % of the global burden of disease (WHO 2004).

7.4.1 Chronic obstructive pulmonary disease (2 %)

Chronic obstructive pulmonary disease was ranked number five in causes of death in the world in 2002. This severe disease is characterised by slow but progressive destruction of the smaller airways in the lungs that is mainly caused by tobacco smoking. It results in chronic cough and a decreased breathing capacity. The disease is much exacerbated by acute infections, when the pa-

212

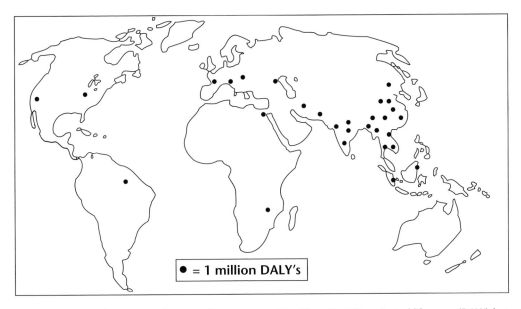

Map 7:5 Chronic obstructive pulmonary disease causes 29 million disability adjusted life years (DALY) lost per year.

Source: WHO, 2002.

tient often requires acute hospital care. Due to increased smoking chronic obstructive pulmonary disease is expected to become the third most common cause of death in the world by the year 2020. Chronic obstructive pulmonary disease caused about 2 million deaths in 2002.

China has by far the greatest burden of chronic obstructive pulmonary disease in the world. To stop the increase of cigarette smoking in China appears to be one of the most important tasks for the improvement of world health. Out of all the healthy years of life lost due to diseases in China, about 8% are estimated to be lost due to chronic obstructive pulmonary disease. The most frightening aspect of the matter is that this number is estimated to rise to 16% by the year 2020 (Murray 1997).

Chronic obstructive pulmonary disease is a disease of middle and old age. Chronic bronchitis and emphysema are the major causes of chronic obstructive pulmonary disease. These chronic diseases cause long-term disability before ultimately leading to

death. Thus, they place a huge burden of care on society.

Chronic bronchitis is defined as: "increased mucus secretion in the airways causing a chronic cough for more than three months of the year during at least two consecutive years, which cannot be explained by any other underlying disease of the lungs." Emphysema may occur alone or in combination with chronic bronchitis or asthma. Emphysema is characterised by rupture and distension of the terminal portions of the airways. Chronic bronchitis leads to an increased susceptibility to pulmonary infection leading progressively to a severe reduction in physical activity due to respiratory insufficiency. Diagnosis is made on the basis of the clinical history, pulmonary x-ray and more advanced laboratory investigations.

Treatment of chronic obstructive pulmonary disease is partly the same as for asthma, although drugs that dilate the airways are usually more effective against asthma. Early antibiotic treatments of respiratory infections and cessation of smoking are the two

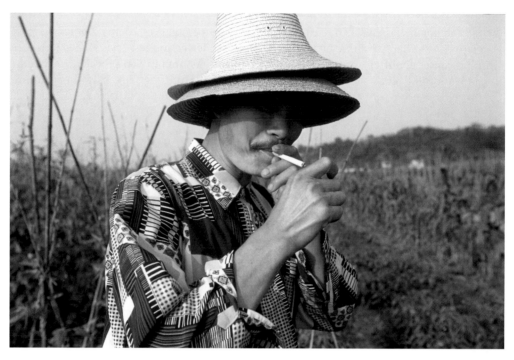

CHINA, Hubei province, Yicheng district, Huang Jiapeng village. Worker in vegetable field taking a cigarette break.

© Trygve Bølstad/PHOENIX.

pillars of treatment. Oxygen therapy at home increases survival and quality of life, but demands great economic and human resources that will not be available for the majority of people with this disease in a foreseeable future.

Smoking is by far the most important risk factor for chronic obstructive pulmonary disease. Other risk factors are chronic respiratory infection, and air pollution. Smoking causes increased mucus secretion in the airways. The mucous membranes of the small airways are damaged and the immunity is decreased, which leads to more respiratory infections. Smokers usually have a bronchial hyper-reactivity and react to tobacco smoke with contraction of the airways.

Chronic obstructive pulmonary disease is more common in men than in women, but the rising trend in smoking among women worldwide will increase the prevalence of the disease among women. The increased

smoking in China explains the increasing burden of respiratory diseases in that country. Smoking is declining in high-income countries and the prevalence of respiratory diseases will be surpassed, and the percentage of DALYs lost exceeded, by the former socialist countries of Europe, Middle Eastern Crescent, India, Latin America and the Caribbean. Smoking and its related diseases are becoming a health problem of middle-income countries in much the same way as traffic accidents today mainly affect middle-income countries.

7.4.2 Asthma (1 %)

Asthma is a common, disabling disease, which affects all ages but causes relatively few deaths. About 240 000 persons are estimated to die each year from asthma (WHO 2004). Most asthma deaths occur in middle-income countries. Worldwide, about 150

214

million people live with asthma (WHO 1998). The burden of disease due to asthma is relatively similar in all regions of the world; it causes about 1% of the DALYs lost in the world. But remember that the DALY measure reflects both incidence of a disease and the success of treatment. The increase in occurrence of asthma in high-income countries in recent decades is not reflected by an increased disease burden. The reason is that most asthma patients in high-income countries are successfully treated with the excellent asthma medicines that are now available to those who can afford them and to those who live in a country where the drugs are subsidised.

Asthma causes periodic, reversible obstruction of the airways. In contrast, chronic bronchitis and emphysema, cause irreversible and progressive obstruction of the airways. The asthmatic obstruction may be triggered by for instance an allergic reaction, by infection, or by exercise. An inflammatory reaction and increased secretions in the airways follow obstruction of the small airways. Pharmacological treatment targets the airway obstruction and the inflammatory and allergic reactions. Inhalation of bronchodilators and steroid hormones as sprays against inflammation has improved the quality of life for many asthmatic patients, but this long-term treatment is expensive. A study of the availability of anti-asthmatic drugs in 24 countries in Africa and Asia showed that the cost of steroid hormone inhalation treatment alone varied between 7 and 100% of an average monthly salary—if it was at all available (Watson 1997).

The prevalence of asthma in children varies between 2 and 12%. There is a worrying trend towards an increased prevalence of asthma all over the world. The reasons for the increase are not yet clearly understood, but studies comparing countries around the Baltic Sea indicate that crowding, lower socio-economic standards and repeated infections in early childhood protect against allergic asthma (Bråbäck 1999). The driving force behind the increased incidence of

asthma in high-income countries may be reduced stimulation of the immune system due to fewer and less severe infections early in life. Asthma is also prevalent in middle-income countries, but in these countries most patients cannot afford modern treatment. This causes the paradoxical pattern of most asthma deaths in middle-income countries, although the incidence is much higher in high-income countries.

7.5 Diabetes mellitus (1%)

An epidemic of type 2 diabetes is spreading across the world. Of the total world population, about 150 million currently suffer from diabetes mellitus, and by the year 2025 this number is expected to double to 300 million. This means that almost 5% of the population of the world will have diabetes. Diabetes is no longer a disease affecting only the high-income countries of Western Europe and North America. Today most people with diabetes live in low- and middle-income countries, and this proportion will increase to 75% by the year 2025 (WHO 1998). Diabetes type 2 will, like lung cancer and traffic accidents, become a disease with its highest occurrence in middle-income countries.

Diabetes mellitus is manifested by high blood glucose levels due to a defect in the production or effect of insulin, the main metabolic hormone. Long-term effects of diabetes include cardiovascular disease, an eye disorder known as retinopathy, kidney failure and disturbed blood circulation and sensory functions in the legs leading to pain and ulcers. The diagnosis is made from elevated blood sugar levels and urine sugar analysis.

Diabetes mellitus occurs as type 1 or type 2. Type 1 usually appears before 30 years of age and requires insulin for treatment. Type 2 starts at an older age and can initially be well managed by either dietary changes or oral medications, or both. Out of all diabetes patients 90% have type 2 diabetes, but

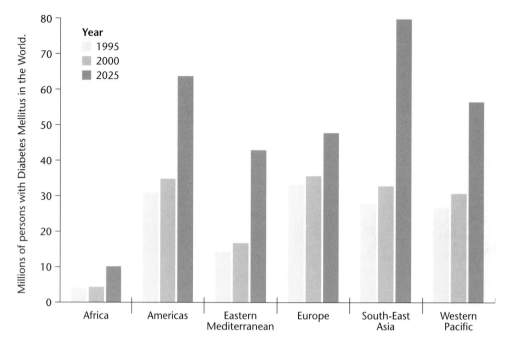

Figure 7.4 Diabetes mellitus, regional estimates from 1995–2025.
Source: The World Health Report, WHO, 1997.

30 % of them eventually need insulin to control their blood sugar levels.

The cause of diabetes mellitus is yet not understood. It is thought that a combination of environmental, genetic and immune system factors jointly cause type 1 diabetes, while immunological factors are unlikely to be involved in type 2 diabetes. Some of the causes of the increase in prevalence of type 2 diabetes are population ageing, obesity, unhealthy diets and physical inactivity. The lifestyle changes that follow with urbanisation and the alleviation of poverty rapidly increase the risk of diabetes. In other words, as soon as people get out of hunger and poverty many tend to 'sit down and eat too much', thereby considerably increasing their risk of developing diabetes. The problem is that a growing proportion of the population in middle-income countries and the better-off low-income countries have enough income to develop diabetes, while they and their countries do not yet have

enough money to treat their disease. No attempted preventive measure for type 1 diabetes has so far proven effective.

The treatment of diabetes is costly and life-long, which places a strain on the finances and delivery of the health care system. Insulin is expensive and difficult to administer correctly in most families in low-income countries. Insulin needs to be kept cold in a refrigerator, something that most families in a low-income country can never afford. If no treatment is available patients will soon die. If insufficient treatment is available, patients will survive but will soon develop severe complications. If they are saved by an amputation, many of the survivors will require kidney dialysis or transplantation. Better treatment of diabetes reduces the risk for complications. Most middle-income countries do not achieve good treatment, which means that they will have to deal with the need for costly treatment of complications. This perspective argues for

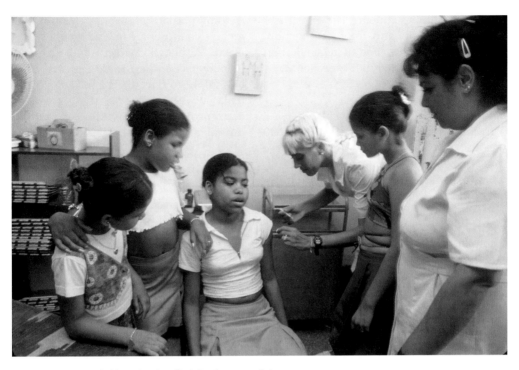

CUBA, Havanna. Child getting insulin injection at a clinic.
© Sean Sprague/PHOENIX.

strong primary preventive actions, especially in middle-income countries. The prevention of type 2 diabetes involves healthy diets and physical activity to maintain normal body weight. It is a great challenge to design and implement prevention campaigns with this message to populations who have emerged out of poverty only ten years earlier. For the first time they can eat as much as they want and do not have to perform physically hard work to survive (compare to the story told in Box 7.1).

7.6 Other non-communicable diseases (13 %)

As much as 13 % of DALYs lost in the world are due to non-communicable diseases that have not already been mentioned in this chapter. In this remaining group we focus

on the following three that are giving rise to the most DALYs lost. The remaining disease conditions each cause less than 0.5 % of the total DALYs lost.

7.6.1 Osteoarthritis (1 %)

The gradual destruction of joints with age, known as osteoarthritis, exists all over the world. Of the DALYs lost in high-income countries about 3 % are due to osteoarthritis. This is not a lethal disease, but it is a very painful and disabling condition. It mainly affects older people. Osteoarthritis affects mainly joints in the hands, feet, knees, hips and spine. The causes of the common type of osteoarthritis that affect older people are unknown. Treatment includes anti-inflammatory drugs in combination with joint rest and weight reduction.

In the last decades surgical replacements of the hip and knee joints have become a very successful treatment. The prostheses decrease the pain and improve function. Following surgery a time of rehabilitation with highly specialised staff is needed.

7.6.2 Cirrhosis of the liver (1 %)

Cirrhosis causes an estimated 800 000 deaths per year around the world. It is three times as common in males as in females. Alcohol explains up to two-thirds of all cirrhosis deaths. Hepatitis B and C are other main causes. The pattern of liver cirrhosis thus closely follows the pattern of alcohol consumption and of the occurrence of chronic life-long hepatitis B and C infections in the world.

Cirrhosis is a progressive destruction of the liver tissue due to fibrosis, i.e. a type of silent scarification. This destruction leads to an impaired blood flow from the gut via the liver to the heart. The liver increases in size, as does the amount of liquid in the abdomen at a later stage. A secondary effect is enlarged blood vessels in the oesophagus, which may result in lethal haemorrhages. Because of impaired liver function, several toxic metabolic substances accumulate in the blood and may cause hepatic coma and death. Treatment involves avoiding further alcohol use and liver transplantation—needless to say, again only available to the few. Preventive measures are concentrated, above all, on reducing alcohol consumption and vaccination against hepatitis B in high-endemic areas.

7.6.3 Cataract (1.5 %)

Cataract is a progressive opacity of the lens of the eye, causing a gradual, painless loss of vision. It causes about 1.5 % of the total burden of disease and is mainly a disease of late middle age and old age. Most of the cataracts in the world occur in low and middle-income countries. The majority of cataract diseases are without known cause, but can be successfully cured by replacing the opaque lens with an artificial lens. An in-creasing proportion of old people in high-income countries are having their lenses replaced. Although cataract is more common in poorer countries, these patients can at best afford to have their lens removed and replaced with thick, expensive glasses. Still, many people turn almost blind because they cannot afford a cataract operation.

A number of common non-communicable diseases that mainly affects old persons have become curable in the last decades. The surgery for cataracts with replacement of the lens with a soft artificial lens is one of the most successful of these new treatments. Hip replacement is another. These two operations mean a lot for the quality of life for old people. It also means that they can take care of themselves to a much higher degree than if they would have suffered from a painful hip or the inability to see clearly. It also means that they will live longer due to the improved life situation. The improved treatment of the diseases of the old makes them healthier and increases their life expectancy and thereby the need for further treatments and operations. This is far from an exclusive medical issue. It is a central part of the economies of the high-income countries where the retirement funds are becoming a major owner in the stock market, where care for the old is becoming a major part of the labour market and where the care for the old is becoming the main issue in the political elections. It is interesting to note that while the public debate in the last decade has given the impression of "cuts" on the health service more and more persons have had their hip, lens and coronary arteries replaced and their life expectance keeps increasing. The expectation for a healthy life in old age is increasing faster than the continuous improvement of the medical and nursing care.

Key references and suggested further reading

Beaglehole R, Yach D. Globalisation and the prevention and control of non-communicable disease: the neglected chronic diseases of adults. Lancet 2003;362:903–8.

Bråback L. Do infections protect against atopic diseases? Acta Paediatr 1999;88: 705–8.

Manson P. Tropical Diseases, 21st edition. London: Saunders; 2002.

Murray C, Lopez A. Global mortality, disability, and the contribution of risk factors: Global burden of disease study. Lancet 1997; 349:1436–42 and 1498–1504.

Reddy KS, Yusuf S. Emerging epidemic of cardiovascular disease in developing countries. Circulation 1998; 97:596–601.

Watson JP, Lewis AL. Is asthma treatment affordable in developing countries? Thorax 1997; 52:605–607.

World Health Report, WHO 1998, 2001, 2002, 2004.

8 Injury (12%)*

I do not know who to trust, the police or the criminals. Our public safety is ourselves…I am afraid that they might kill my son for something as irrelevant as a snack.

From a women's group, Brazil

Injuries have received increasing attention as a global health problem in the last two decades. Injury is defined in Box 8.1. This major health problem was previously remarkably neglected. Injuries were regarded as something the health profession could not do much about, since the preventive measures against injury lay largely in the enforcement of traffic laws and in raising community awareness. The opinion that accidents are inevitable events—strokes of bad luck—is changing, largely due to the increased attention of injury researchers. The systematic collection of data about causes of injuries in registers is still uncommon, particularly in low-income countries. Data quality varies across countries. The Global Burden of Disease study indicates that injury represents about one tenth of the global public health problems (Murray and Lopez, 1996). Its relative importance is projected to increase as that of the communicable diseases diminishes (Plitponkarnpim 1999).

In 2002 injuries caused about 5 million deaths, which correspond to about 9 % of all deaths in the world. Injuries are divided into intentional and unintentional. Intentional injuries, such as homicide, violence, suicide and war, accounted for 1.6 million deaths. Unintentional injuries, such as road traffic accidents, drowning, falls, fires and poisoning, accounted for 3.5 million deaths. Most of the deaths due to injuries (67 %) occurred in males (WHO 2004).

The relative importance on a global basis of each type of injury is shown in figure 8.1. Road traffic accidents are the number one type of injury in the world. Traffic accidents cause about 2.6 % of all healthy life years lost in the world, followed by falls, violence and suicide. The pattern of injuries varies substantially across regions (Table 8.1). High-income countries in the Eastern Mediterranean region, i.e. Gulf countries, have the highest death rates per 100 000 populations from road traffic accidents, but the lowest death rates from self-inflicted injuries. Low- and middle-income countries in the Americas experience the highest death rates from interpersonal violence, but the lowest death rates from poisoning. The middle-income countries of Europe have the

---

Box 8.1

The definition of injury

"a bodily lesion resulting from acute involuntary exposure to energy. The energy can be either a mechanical, thermal, electrical, chemical or radioactive stimulus that interacts with the body in amounts or rates that exceed the threshold of physiological tolerance. In some cases, such as drowning, suffocation or freezing, the injury results from insufficiency of a vital element. An accident is any unexpected event that leads to injury" (Baker et al. 1984).

---

* % in parentheses is estimated share of global burden of disease.

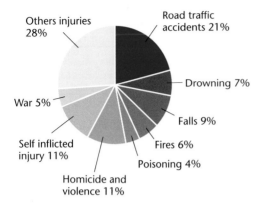

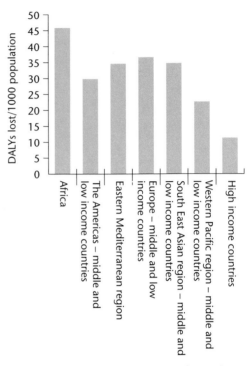

Figure 8.1 DALYs lost by injury causes in 2001 globally.

Source: The World Health Report, WHO, 2002.

highest death rates for poisoning and suicides. Finally, the high-income countries of Europe have the highest death rates for falls that mainly affect the elderly. At the same time these countries have the lowest for fires, drowning, violence and road traffic accidents.

Of all the DALYs lost in 2002, 12% were lost due to injuries. Africa has by far the highest burden of disability and premature deaths due to injury, followed by low and middle income countries in Europe, India and the Eastern Mediterranean region (Fig-

Figure 8.2 DALYs lost per 1 000 population due to injury by region in 1998.

Source: The World Health Report, WHO, 1999.

ure 8.2). A large part of this great burden of injury in Africa is explained by the loss of young persons in road traffic accidents, violence and war. Road traffic accidents are the

Table 8.1 Deaths per 100 000 population by region and cause in 2000.

Region	Road traffic accidents	Falls	Fires	Drowning	Poisoning	Suicide	Interpersonal Violence
Europe high-income	11.2	11.3	1.0	1.0	1.3	12.9	1.0
Europe low and middle-income	16.1	6.6	4.0	9.2	21.5	28.2	15.4
Americas high-income	15.0	6.5	1.3	1.3	3.9	11.6	6.1
Americas low and middle-income	18.1	3.9	1.2	4.3	1.0	5.6	27.3
Western Pacific high-income	15.8	5.3	1.5	4.0	1.1	17.4	1.1
Western Pacific China	18.9	5.7	1.1	12.3	3.8	23.0	2.3
Western Pacific other low+middle-income	14.2	2.8	2.0	4.9	1.2	6.6	13.4
Eastern Mediterranean high-income	34.1	2.7	1.5	1.8	2.0	3.2	4.1
Eastern Mediterranean low+middle-income	18.7	4.3	4.8	4.2	3.8	4.9	6.3
South East Asia India	29.2	2.1	8.3	7.6	7.0	13.6	6.2
South East Asia other low +middle-income	26.6	3.4	8.2	3.8	2.2	5.9	2.9
Africa low and middle-income	26.3	2.7	5.5	13.1	5.6	4.3	18.1

Source: The Injury Chart book: A global overview of the global burden of injuries. WHO 2003.

fifth greatest cause of DALYs lost in the age group 5 to 14 years. War injuries and inter-personal injury are the second and third largest causes of DALYs and deaths lost in the productive age group 15 to 44 years, re-spectively. Because of the wide difference in injury pattern between countries, the pre-ventive measures need to be tailored to the particular problems faced in each country (Murray, Lopez 1996), or rather in each community.

There is evidence from a study of injuries in the age group 15 to 44 years in 54 coun-tries that deaths due to unintentional injury decreased with increasing socio-economic development, as measured by GNP per cap-ita. This relationship becomes even stronger in older age groups. The injury transition starts with a peak in unintentional injuries, when countries have a GNP per capita of 700 to 3000 USD. At higher national in-comes the mortality due to injuries declines rapidly (Ahmed Andersson, 2000). Injuries in children also fall when GNP per capita in-creases. Most middle-income countries are passing through this stage of high mortality

rates due to injury (Plitponkarnpim 1999). Below we describe the types of uninten-tional and intentional injuries that cause the greatest disease burden in the world.

8.1 Road traffic accidents (3%)

Road traffic accidents pose a serious public health problem all over the world. Bicycles are still the most common vehicles of trans-portation. Cyclists, along with the majority of other road users, such as pedestrians, mo-torcyclists, and operators and passengers of rickshaws and carts, lack protection when hit by larger vehicles, such as cars, buses and trucks.

The number of cars used in the world has increased from 50 million in 1950 to more than 400 million in 1998 (Brown 1998). In low and middle-income countries, this in-crease in the number of cars has not always been followed by improvements in road quality. In other words, when countries begin to get richer, more cars are bought,

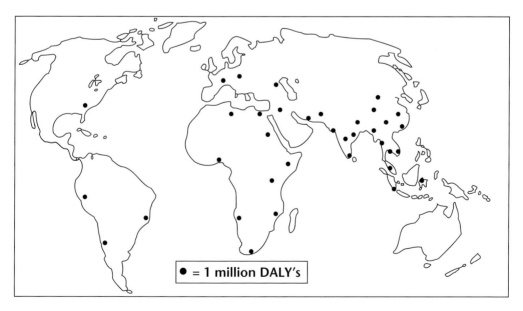

Map 8:1 *Road traffic accidents cause 36 million disability adjusted life years (DALY) lost per year.*
Source: WHO, 2002.

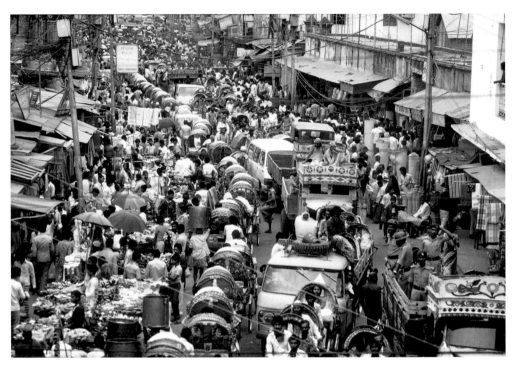

BANGLADESH, Dhaka. Evening traffic in Old Dhaka.
© Heldur Netocny/PHOENIX.

but roads remain bad and traffic regulation weak. In these countries there are no pedestrian safety measures, such as pavements separating people from cars, or marked crossroads with traffic lights and technical inspection of vehicles is missing. The number of accidents due to motor vehicles continues to increase and is projected to rise to become the sixth cause of death in the world by the year 2020.

In 1998 road traffic accidents were the fifth largest cause of DALYs lost in high-income countries, and the tenth largest cause in low and middle-income countries. What is most frightening is that it is estimated that traffic injuries will be the second most prominent cause of DALYs lost in low and middle-income countries by the year 2020. A major reason for this projected increase is the rapid pace of urbanisation and industrialisation. In countries with rapid economic growth, the fall in infectious diseases is largely replaced by injuries, mainly from traffic accidents. For the high-income countries, this evolution took a century, which enabled them to adapt the infrastructure, as well as preventive and curative measures.

Road traffic accidents affect teenagers and young men most severely. For men in the age group 15 to 44 years, road traffic accidents are the most common cause of premature death and disability in the world! The gross national product per capita is positively correlated to the traffic-related mortality per 100 000 population per year, but negatively related to the number of traffic deaths per 1 000 registered vehicles. Traffic-related mortality measured in crude death rates is actually highest in middle-income countries, and in most high-income countries the fatality rate per vehicle has decreased over the last two decades (Söderlund 1995). As noted in Box 2.9 in Chapter 2 the same was the case when Sweden had a na-

224

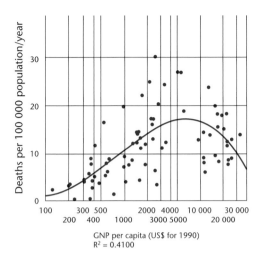 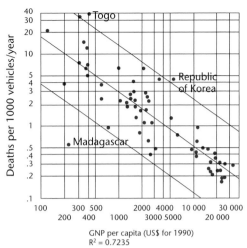

Figure 8.3 Traffic related mortality rates per 100 000 population/year and per capita and traffic related mortality per 1 000 vehicles/year and per capita GNP.

Source: Söderlund, Zwi, 1995.

tional income of contemporary middle-income countries. The traffic deaths peaked around 1950 and it took much creative preventive action to bring the Swedish road traffic death rate down to the low levels found in contemporary Sweden. Low-income countries are expected to move through this same increasing trend of accidents unless preventive measures are taken.

The nature of motor vehicle accidents differs around the world. In low-income countries major causes of accidents are that pedestrians and cyclists are struck by motor vehicles or that passengers fall off the back of open trucks. A larger proportion of children and younger people in low-income countries play on the roads or sell things in the street, and this naturally increases the risk of accidents. In high-income countries accidents affecting drivers of cars, pedestrians struck by cars, farm tractor accidents and young people falling off recreational vehicles are more common (Berger 1996). Motorcycle accidents are common all around the world.

Alcohol intake and road traffic accidents are exponentially linked to each other. The reasons for this increased risk of accidents is

that the alcohol affected driver is slower to react in emergencies and may drive too fast and take more risks. As many as half of all deaths due to traffic accidents in Chile, Zambia and the United States are alcohol related (Berger 1996).

Road traffic accidents can be prevented and case fatality rates improved by a number of measures. These include better design, construction and maintenance of roads and vehicles. The use of helmets for two-wheel vehicles and the use of seat belts in cars have proved effective in reducing mortality and morbidity due to accidents. Other measures include laws about alcohol consumption by drivers, speed limits, improvements in public transport and the use of clothing that is visible in the dark. The importance of preventive measures against traffic accidents is a major priority for the improvement of the global health situation.

8.2 Falls (1 %)

Falls accounted for 1 % of the total loss of healthy years in 2002 (WHO 2004). The death rate due to falls has a positive correlation with economic development. High-income countries have the highest death rates for falls, followed by the former socialist countries of Europe. In high-income countries falls affect mainly elderly women who trip over or fall on ice or stairs. In high-income countries the incidence of falls increases rapidly after the age of 70, and the location of the incident is in most cases the home. The elderly fall either because of internal causes (acute or chronic illness, bad sight, or gait problem) or external causes (tripping over carpets, etc.) (Berger 1996). Hip fractures are the most serious consequence of fall injuries in older individuals. Prevention of osteoporosis in old age has been emphasised to avoid the adverse consequences of falls. Children in high-income countries risk falling from apartment windows or in stairs.

In low-income countries, falls may involve workers falling from coconut trees, children falling from mango trees, roofs or farm animals, and finally home construction accidents (Berger 1996). In low and middle-income countries, falls rank number one in DALYs lost in the age group 5 to 14 years, but they are negligible as a cause of death in these countries. In poorer countries falls causing fractures tend to result in disability because emergency care and rehabilitation are not available to most people.

Preventive measures include modifying the home and working environment, nursing homes, playgrounds, etc. Safety measures include safety equipment in industry, e.g. in construction work, good lighting, and non-slip floors without irregularities. The modification of behaviour, e.g. to induce people to avoid haste and dangerous forms of excitement, is always more difficult to achieve.

8.3   Drowning (1 %)

About 400 000 people were estimated to have drowned in the world in 2002. About 98 % of drowning incidents occurred in low and middle-income countries. Africa has the highest death rate from drowning. Drowning is thus a major poverty-related cause of death. It is related to the inability of parents to spend time guarding their children and to people having to risk their life when fishing (WHO 2004).

In low and middle-income countries, children drown in open wells, rivers and ponds. Preventive measures may involve covering wells with metal or wooden lids, but this costs money.

In high-income countries, drowning accidents typically involve children falling into swimming pools, leisure boat accidents and persons intoxicated with alcohol or other drugs falling into water (Berger 1996). Preventive measures include fencing off pools and teaching swimming skills and using safety vests. Safety promotions to discourage the use of alcohol or drugs in the vicinity of water will also reduce casualty levels.

8.4   Fires (1 %)

In low-income countries, fires occur particularly in slums and poorly built houses. The fast urbanisation in poor countries results in overcrowding. Fires spread quickly between shacks built of inflammable materials in slum areas. Additionally, poorly controlled electricity systems pose a risk of fire. Death rates are highest among the youngest and the oldest, due to difficulty in escaping burning houses. India has the highest death rates per 100 000 population from fires.

Cigarette smoking is a major cause of domestic fires in all countries. In low-income countries, fire accidents occur most often in the home, with clothing catching fire from open cooking fires, kerosene lamps or pressurised stoves, or children falling onto open fires (Berger 1996). Cooking food for the family over an open fire is a major poverty-related health risk for children.

8.5 Poisoning (0.5%)

Poisoning is not as common as other physical causes of injury in the world.

In low-income countries, kerosene, gasoline and pesticides stored at home often cause poisoning. But poisoning also results from naturally occurring toxins from snakes, insects or plants like cassava. In low-income countries, government control of the production, sale and use of highly toxic pesticides is inadequate. It is a tragic paradox that people living in absolute poverty are at risk of diseases induced by natural toxins (Rosling 1995). When they become a little wealthier they can avoid the risk of natural toxin but then they are at risk of commercially acquired toxins. Products that have been banned in high-income countries can easily be found in markets in low-income countries. The protective measure of wearing masks and gloves is too expensive for poor rural populations (Berger 1996). However, pesticides are not only an occupational hazard; easy access to these products makes suicide through the intake of pesticides a major and growing cause of severe poisoning and death, particularly among young women in Asia.

In high-income countries, in contrast, poisoning is rare, with the exception of intentional abuse of alcohol and illegal drugs. Fatal overdoses of illegal drugs like heroin and cocaine have increased in, for instance, the United States since the 1950s (Rivara 1997). The promotion of safe storage of drugs and chemicals in the home, out of reach of children, has been very successful in reducing child mortality in high-income countries. The major poisons are natural toxins, pesticides and illegal drugs in low, middle and high-income countries, respectively.

8.6 Homicide and violence (1%)

Violence may be physical, sexual or mental. Intentional violence leading to death occurs in the form of homicide or suicide. Suicide will be dealt with in section 8.8. WHO has proposed a definition for interpersonal violence (Box 8.2)

According to data from the WHO, violence is strongly associated with the availability of firearms, urbanisation, family disintegration, poverty (or perceived relative deprivation) and social stress. There is a link between inequity and violence. Disadvantaged individuals in a society live under conditions of disempowerment, physical and mental insecurity, fear, frustration and depression. All these factors contribute to violent behaviour. In addition, the use of and trade in illicit drugs is associated with a vicious circle of theft and violence. Alcohol is a very strong contributing factor to both homicide and domestic violence.

The statistics on the occurrence of violence are not very reliable. The reason is that violence is often not reported, because of the victim's powerlessness, stigmatisation or fear. Violence statistics from hospitals, clinics and emergency rooms are a weak instrument to measure the real health impact of violence, because the vast majority of victims of violence do not seek care. Police registers record only reported incidents of vio-

---

Box 8.2

"Violence is the intentional use of physical force or power, threatened or actual, against oneself, another person, or against a group or a community, that either results in or has a high likelihood of resulting in injury, death, psychological harm, mal-development or deprivation." (WHO)

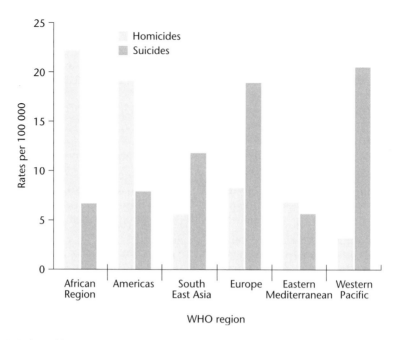

Figure 8.4 Suicide and homicide rate per 100 000 population in different regions of the world, 2000.
Source: World Report on Violence and Health. WHO, 2002.

lence. Mortality data, where it exists, is the most easily accessible indicator of violence, but it must be remembered that this represents only a minor portion of the problem. This is especially true for domestic violence against women and children.

In the United States, death rates due to homicide doubled in the four decades up to 1994. The United States has the highest death rates due to homicide among high-income countries. About 20 000 people are murdered each year in USA. It is those in the 15 to 24-year age group who are most affected, with homicide being the second most frequent cause of death in this group. The risk of homicide in a household is increased by a factor of three if that household possesses a gun, and the risk of suicide is increased by a factor of five. The death rate from murder for men was 12 per 100 000, as against 3.3 per 100 000 for women (Shahpar, 1999). However, since 1993, homicide rates in the United States have steadily declined. A probable explanation for this decline is

that, as the demand for crack cocaine declined and economic conditions improved, many young drug dealers switched to legal employment. Also, weapon searches increased, targeting high-risk individuals, and this deterred the carrying of handguns, so that the incidence of homicide decreased (Cole 1999).

Younger men are the group most profoundly affected by violence. In 1998 interpersonal violence in men was ranked number three among causes of death, and number five among causes of DALYs lost, in the age group 15 to 44 years (WHO 1999). For women interpersonal violence was ranked tenth among causes of death and did not even appear on the list of the fifteen most common causes of DALYs lost. Africa has the second highest death rate due to interpersonal violence, far behind the countries in the low and middle-income Americas. In the low and middle-income countries of the Americas, interpersonal violence ranks first as the cause of death in the age group 15 to 44 years, although the general death rate is lower than in Africa.

Increasing attention is currently being paid to gender-related violence, and it may be fruitful to distinguish four different age groups in which different aspects of violence are significant for women: a) pre-birth; b) childhood; c) reproductive age and d) old age. During foetal life, *pre-birth*, violence is directed towards the pregnant woman in the form of domestic battering. During *childhood*, violence is gender-related, particularly in the form of female infanticide (the killing of newborn baby girls), a phenomenon corresponding to the selective abortion of female foetuses (female foeticide). Beyond the early neonatal period, the threat of female genital mutilation (FGM) is another form of selective violence directed against girls during the first years of their lives. This practice occurs in a belt from north-eastern to mid-western Africa. FGM arises out of old cultural concepts and is currently the subject of much debate and international attention. In the *reproductive age,* gender-related violence concerns above all sexual abuse, prostitution and domestic violence directed against women of childbearing age. According to a population-based survey from countries around the world, 10 to 69 % of women reported physical assault by an intimate male partner at least once in their lives (Heise 1999). Women in *old age* may suffer from physical, sexual, psychological abuse or neglect.

8.7   War (0.5 %)

War is generalised violence. It causes displacement of populations and a general breakdown in law and order, and thus an increase in all kinds of violence. Direct war injuries consist of deaths and war wounds due to the direct conflict or mine injuries. Secondary effects, due to ruptured social and economic structures, splitting of families, destroyed health and social services, and destruction of infrastructure, are usually more prominent than direct war injuries. These secondary effects are not included in official war injury statistics. An estimated total of 170 000 people in the world died due to war injuries in 2002 (WHO 2004).

Sexual violence, including rape, is common in times of war. Reports from the former Yugoslavia, Bangladesh, Uganda, Rwanda, Burma and Somalia describe widespread sexual abuse and systematic rape (Jennings, Swiss 2001). This has long been used as a strategy in warfare. Sexual attacks on women demoralise the cultural roots of a society, leaving strong physical and mental wounds, and one result may be ethnic cleansing. There is a risk of stigmatisation in disclosing wartime rape, and there is vast under-reporting.

The injuries of war seem impossible to prevent, but even in this difficult field there has been progress. As of October 2003 150 countries have signed the 1997 treaty banning the use of antipersonnel landmines. This is a result of a most successful campaign by a non-governmental organisation.[1]

8.8   Suicide (1 %)

Every year about 900 000 persons commit suicide in the world (WHO 2004). This figure probably reflects under-reporting, since many suicides are reported as accidents. The incidence of suicide attempts is 10 to 20 times higher than actual suicide. Attempted suicide is three times more common in females than in males, while completed suicide is three times more common among males than females in most countries. However, in some countries, such as China, suicide is more common in women. In most countries that report suicide data to the World Health Organisation there has been an increase in suicide rates, especially among young men. Japan is one of the few countries where there has been a decrease in suicide rates for both men and women over

[1]   www.icbl.org

the past 35 years. Of those countries that report Hungary, Sri Lanka, Finland and China
have the highest rates of 30 to 40 suicides
per 100 000 population per year. Kuwait and
Egypt have the lowest reported rates, at 0.8
and 0.04 per 100 000 population per year,
respectively (Lester 1997). In general, there
are countries with low, middle and high
rates of suicide in all continents where data
is kept: in the Americas, Asia and Europe.

The method used for suicide varies from
country to country. In low-income countries it is common to ingest liquid pesticides,
while in high-income countries there is a
preference for the ingestion of medications
or the use of firearms (Wasserman 2001).

In most countries suicides are between
two to three times more common in old age
than in youth (Diekstra 1993). This trend is
very prominent in men. In high-income
countries, suicide rates are highest for middle-aged men; in middle-income countries,
it is the elderly who have higher rates; and
in the low-income countries, the younger
age groups have higher suicide rates (Lester
1997). Since overall suicide rates are higher
in old age, the suicide rate is sensitive to the
age structure of a population, which produces a bias in global comparisons if the
rates are not standardised for age. In the age
group 15 to 24 years suicide is not common,
but because the relative mortality is rather
low in this age group, suicide is still among
the five leading causes of death at the age of
20 in many countries (Diekstra 1993).

Mental illness and substance abuse are related to increased levels of suicide. Other su-
icide-associated conditions include easy access to the means of death, such as poison,
and media publicity for suicide. Religious af-
filiation is also clearly correlated to suicide
rates; Islamic countries have lower rates
than the Buddhist countries in Asia, and the
Protestant countries of North America and
Europe have higher rates than the Roman
Catholic countries of Latin America and
Southern Europe. However, there are exceptions. The general improvement in health in
Iran has in recent years unfortunately been
associated with increased suicide rates, especially in young women. Various studies have
shown that suicide rates increase in societies
with higher divorce rates, immigration and
dramatic declines in gross domestic product
(GDP), and decrease with high unemployment rates, where there is a high percentage
of the population aged less than 15 years
and where there are high birth rates. Thus,
studies point to an association between economic development and higher suicide rates
(Lester 97).

References and suggested further readings

Ahmed N, Andersson R. Unintentional
injury, mortality and socio-economic
development among 15 to 44-year olds:
in a health transition perspective. Public
Health 2000;114:416–422.

Baker SP, O'Neill, Karpf RS. The Injury Fact
Book. Lexington Books. 1984.

Barss P, Smith G, Baker S, Mohan D. Injury
prevention: An international perspective.
Oxford University Press 1998.

Berger LR, Mohan D. Injury Control. A Global View. Oxford University Press; 1996.

Brown LR, Flavin C, French H. Worldwatch
Institute. State of the World; 1998.

Cole TB. Ebbing epidemic: Youth homicide
rate at a 14-year low. JAMA 1999;281:25–
26.

Diekstra RFW, Gulbinat W. World Health
Stat. Quart 1993;46:52–68.

Heise LL, Ellsberg M, Gottemoeller M. End-
ing violence against women. Baltimore,
MD: Johns Hopkins University School of
Public Health. Centre for Communica-
tion Programs; 1999. (Population Reports
Series L, No 11).

Jennings PJ, Swiss S. Supporting local efforts
to document human rights violations in
armed conflict. Lancet 2001;357:304.

Lester D. Suicide and life-threatening behaviour 1997;27(1).

Murray C, Lopez A. Global Burden of Disease Study. 1996.

Plitponkarnpim A, Andersson R, Jansson B,
Svanström L. Unintentional mortality in

children: a priority for middle-income countries in the advanced stage of epidemiological transition. Injury Prevention 1999;5:98–103.

Rivara et al. Injury prevention. New Eng J Med 1997;337:613–617.

Rosling H, Tylleskär T. Konzo. In: Tropical neurology. Eds Shakir RA, et al. London: W.B. Saunders 1995; pp 353–64.

Söderlund N. Traffic-related mortality in industrialised and less developed countries. Bull WHO 1995;73: 175–82.

Shahpar Cyrus, Li Guohua. Homicide mortality in the USA, 1935–1994. Am J of Epid 1999;150:1213–122.

Wasserman D edited. Suicide an unnecessary death. London: Martin Dunitz; 2001.

World Health Organization, World Health Report 2004.

World Health Organization. Injury, a leading cause of the Global Burden of Disease. Report:WHO/HSC/PVI/99.11

World Health Organization. World report on violence and health. 2002.

9 Sexual and reproductive health (9%)*

> Lack of public transportation and high costs of private transportation are major constraint to access....Stories are told about pregnant women losing their babies on their way to the health services.
>
> Republic of Yemen 1998

The concept of reproductive health was coined during the mid1980s. It refers to the prevention and treatment of diseases that impair reproduction. The concept has both male and female dimensions. Among males the fertile age extends from puberty to old age. Among females the fertile age is defined by the more limited period between menarche and menopause.

Reproduction denotes the process of producing a new individual. The starting point of reproduction can be said to be the production of sperms and eggs, also known as gametogenesis. It is less clear which point should be designated as the end-point of the process of reproduction. It can be argued that reproduction ends by delivery of the newborn. However, it has been argued that the most vulnerable period in the life of the newborn, infancy or even childhood up to 5 years, should be included in the scope of reproductive health. The dependence of the newborn on the mother for warmth and feeding makes it relevant and reasonable to include health of the mother and her newborn at least up to the end of the perinatal period. This means reproductive health is considered to be up to the end of the seventh day after birth.

Sexuality and reproduction belong to the most private of human spheres. Hence, both issues have been subject to a great number of cultural and religious taboos, making them targets for both praise and condemnation. Down through history, the control of reproduction has been controversial, with a very wide global variation in acceptability. Two global conferences on population in Bucharest 1974 and in Mexico City 1984 were followed by a paradigm shift in the follow-up in Cairo 1994, where the first International Conference on Population and Development (ICPD) was arranged. ICPD constituted in many ways a new era in the global approach to reproductive health. For the first time a human rights perspective was associated with sexual and reproductive health. This has implied a most significant change in attitudes in many countries. (See also chapter 10.)

Many diseases affecting reproductive organs do not necessarily affect reproduction, but have their significance in their sexual transmission (e.g. HIV and other sexually transmitted infections). Therefore, it is now common to refer to sexual and reproductive health (SRH). After the Cairo conference where the human rights perspective became more prominent, the acronym SRHR has come to stand for 'sexual and reproductive health and rights'. It is important to note that sexual and reproductive ill health refers not only to pregnancy-related disorders. In addition to HIV/AIDS and other sexually

---

* % of global disease burden consisting of maternal and perinatal disorders.

transmitted infections (see chapter 5) there are reasons to subdivide this concept into five other aspects of sexual and reproductive ill health:

1 childlessness and reproductive failure: diseases affecting fertility or foetal outcome among females and males, i.e. the capacity of a couple to conceive and to have a successful pregnancy;
2 maternal mortality: deaths during or soon after the end of pregnancy (delivery or abortion);
3 maternal morbidity: diseases affecting women during or soon after the end of pregnancy;
4 perinatal mortality and morbidity: deaths and diseases affecting the foetus or newborn;
5 conditions affecting reproductive organs in both females and males, but not necessarily affecting fertility functions, or occurring outside the fertile age.

9.1 Childlessness and reproductive failure

Infertility is only one part of a greater global health problem, which should more correctly be called childlessness. This problem can be subdivided into at least three principal categories:

1 infertility;
2 pregnancy wastage and
3 child loss.

Infertility is a problem of global proportions, affecting on average 10% percent of couples worldwide. Several highly prevalent diseases have far-reaching influences on female fertility, most of them through an effect on tubal function. While infertility due to lack of egg formation, anovulatory diseases, are fairly common worldwide, unilateral or bilateral tubal occlusion is particularly prevalent in populations where gonorrhoea and Chlamydia infections are common. A distinction is usually made between primary infertility and secondary infertility.

Primary infertility denotes an inability to conceive within two years of unprotected sexual intercourse and without any previous successful conception, while *secondary infertility* refers to such inability after a previous successful conception. Primary infertility in many African settings is reported to be only a few percent, while secondary infertility may reach 20 to 30% of couples in some populations. In Sweden, as in most high-income countries, the proportion of couples not spontaneously capable of conceiving amounts to about 10%. Many of these can be helped with modern technologies such as in-vitro fertilisation, hormonal medication, antibiotic therapy and other measures. The demand for such new reproductive technologies (NRT) is rapidly increasing in many middle-income countries, especially in the Middle East. In Egypt alone nearly 40 in vitro fertilization centres are in operation although these techniques are very costly. Major forces behind the global demand for NRTs are linked to gendered roles and adoption restrictions. This is a prominent example where middle-income countries have to deal with strong demand for new medical technologies at the same time as cheap and cost effective health actions that can prevent a considerable part of the problem have not yet been implemented (Inhorn 2003).

The health of a pregnant woman and the outcome of her pregnancy are threatened by a number of infections and circulatory diseases and adverse environmental conditions. Some infectious agents, e.g. Rubella virus, Syphilis, Herpes simplex virus, Cytomegalovirus, Streptococci bacteria and Chlamydia, are related to adverse pregnancy outcomes. Pregnancy wastage should be understood as any loss of the foetus from conception to delivery, including early and late miscarriage, late foetal death and stillbirth. Several pregnancy-specific circulatory diseases, most of which are related to hypertension, also increase the risk of pregnancy wastage.

The socio-economic determinants influencing reproductive health can be seen most clearly in the global pattern of childlessness. In affluent countries childlessness is almost exclusively an infertility problem. In low-income countries infertility takes a heavy toll, due to tubal obstruction in women and to obstruction of sperm transport in men. In addition to this, however, infections such as syphilis and viral infections are widespread, resulting in much higher figures for pregnancy wastage than in affluent countries. This is particularly true of foetal death and ensuing stillbirth in the second and third trimesters. Because of this, perinatal mortality rates are much higher in poor than in affluent countries.

Male reproductive problems have been somewhat overshadowed by the otherwise very appropriate and adequate focus on female reproductive health. However, it is well known that disorders affecting the male reproductive function are prevalent in most countries. In affluent countries the relative contribution of the male to the aetiology of a couple's infertility problem is considered almost as important as that of the female. The male reproductive function depends on normal production and transport of sperm as well as of the sexual function. Widespread diseases in low-income countries affect both sperm production and transport. Inflammatory changes in testicular tissues and in the epididymis may create obstruction to sperm transport that result in male infertility. Diseases such as mumps and gonorrhoea may affect male fertility by testicular inflammation and epididymitis that block sperm transport. Filariasis may create lymphatic obstruction in the scrotum and the resulting warming of testicular tissue leads to impaired sperm production and infertility.

The global variation in childlessness is insufficiently known. It is dependent on the prevailing norms for sexuality and reproduction, and on existing patterns of genital infections, mainly sexually transmitted diseases.

9.2 Maternal mortality: the tip of the iceberg (2 %)

The crude birth rate in the world is 22 births per 1 000 population. This corresponds to 138 million births per year in the world. In addition there are about 50 million induced abortions and approximately 25 million recognisable spontaneous abortions per year. The total number of pregnancies per year is about 215 million.

The burden of maternal disease and death has gradually become more obvious over the last 15 years. Maternal conditions cause 2 % and perinatal disorders 7 % of all DALYs lost in the world in 2002. The group of maternal disorders account for about the same number of DALYs lost per year in the world as do TB, measles, malaria or chronic obstructive pulmonary disease, namely about 2 to 3 % of the world total (WHO 2004). Several far-reaching international commitments have been proclaimed for the reduction of this burden. Reducing maternal mortality by 50 % by the year 2000 was thus put forth as a principal objective at five world conferences during the 1980s and the 1990s. The problem of setting such a goal for reduction in maternal mortality is that surveys hitherto have only been able to establish grossly and very approximately the worldwide magnitude of maternal mortality.

A maternal death is the death of a woman from any cause while pregnant or within 42 days of termination of the pregnancy by abortion or delivery. Earlier 'incidental' and 'accidental' causes were not counted, and suicides, for instance, were not included. With the increasingly evident problem of deaths caused by domestic violence, the concept of 'pregnancy-related death' is now in use, regardless of the cause of death.

The global variation in maternal mortality is extreme. Historically, data from both middle and low-income countries are scarce. Sweden has one of the world's oldest and most reliable registers of maternal deaths, dating back to around 1750. At that time,

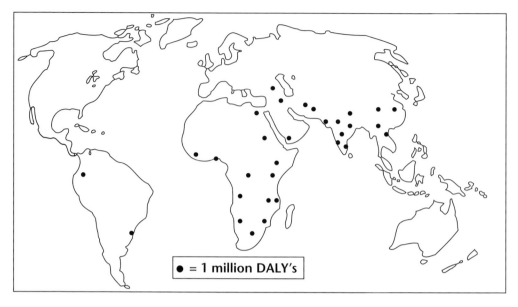

Map 9:1 Maternal disorders cause 31 million disability adjusted life years (DALY) lost oer year.
Source: WHO, 2002.

Sweden had a maternal mortality ratio, as defined below, of around 1 000 per 100 000 live births. This is the same figure as is estimated for Mozambique today. Most high-income countries in northern Europe today have maternal mortality ratios below 10 per 100 000 live births.

Globally, most recent estimates indicate that there is an annual toll of maternal deaths amounting to around 500 000, about 1% of the total number of deaths in the world in a year. An estimated 99% of these deaths occur in low and middle-income countries, implying that a maternal death is an extremely rare event in high-income countries. It is a cause of death that can be brought to almost zero.

An illustrative example of the decline in maternal mortality in Sweden is presented in figure 9.1. It is noteworthy that the decline in maternal mortality ratio was from around 1 000 in 1750 to about 5 today. The decline from about 1 000 in the year 1750 to a maternal mortality ratio of about 150 per 100 000 live births around 1900 constitutes a decline of 85%. This occurred well before

the advent of modern technology such as blood transfusion, antibiotics, modern hospital care, safe abortion, contraceptives and antenatal care. During this period of industrialisation, the most important single cause of maternal mortality decline was the creation of the Swedish midwifery system. One example of the association between maternal mortality decline and percentage of midwifery assistance at birth is shown in figure 9.2 (Högberg 1986).

The historical example of medium-level health care providers in Sweden in the form of midwives is important when considering the unmet need of 'safe motherhood' where there are no doctors.

9.2.1 Measures of maternal mortality

Maternal mortality ratio represents the number of maternal deaths per 100 000 live births. This ratio (MMR) measures the risk of death among pregnant and recently pregnant women after delivery or abortion. The strength of this measure is that it expresses the quality of pregnancy care and delivery

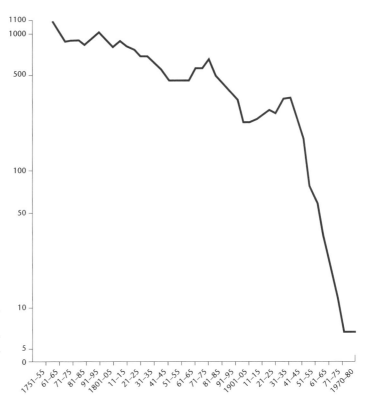

Figure 9.1 Maternal mortality in Sweden between 1751 and 1980, deaths per 100 000 live births, five year mean, logscale.

Source: Högberg 1986.

care, 'safe motherhood'. MMR is not sensitive to fluctuations in fertility.

Maternal mortality rate represents the number of maternal deaths per year per 100 000 women aged 15–49. This expression is rarely used since it reflects both the risk of death among pregnant and recently pregnant women after delivery or abortion and the proportion of all women that become pregnant in a given year. It can consequently be reduced either by making a wanted pregnancy safer (as for MMR) or by lowering fertility. It measures the contribution of maternal mortality to the overall mortality among women of reproductive age.

Lifetime risk of maternal death measures the risk over a woman's entire reproductive life span and is also related to the total number of pregnancies. The total fertility rate tends to be high in association with a high infant and child mortality for two principal reasons. Firstly, there is a psychological replace-

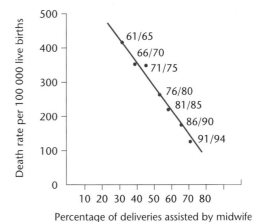

Figure 9.2 Maternal mortality (septic deaths excluded) as a function of the presence of a midwife at home delivery in an area in nothern Sweden 1861–1894 (the dots along the line indicate five-year intervals).

Source: Högberg 1986.

ment effect, whereby compensation is made for the loss of a child through a new pregnancy. Secondly, there is an endocrine effect: when a breastfed infant dies, the sucking stimulus on the nipple ends, with an ensuing reduction of circulating prolactin hormone. Such a reduction facilitates the return of ovulation, enhanced fertility and a probable new pregnancy. The final result is that the lifetime number of pregnancies tends to increase in societies with high infant and child mortality. The lifetime risk of maternal death is then increased, and the individual risk of each pregnancy should be multiplied by the lifetime number of pregnancies. In the least developed countries, the lifetime risk may be as great as one in ten, while in Northern Europe it is in the order of one in 10 000.

There are several hurdles in measuring changes in maternal mortality. *Firstly*, the MMR is most often below 2 % (2 000 per 100 000 live births), even in the poorest countries. Large samples are therefore needed to make reliable estimates, and the costs of large sampling are high. *Secondly*, where maternal mortality is high, the majority of mothers die at home or at least outside the health care system. These women's deaths are known to be under-reported and in most low-income countries there is no regular reporting of any deaths outside hospitals. Underestimates in the range of 30 to 50 % are also found in high-income countries and in middle-income countries the under reporting is even higher. In many cases we have to multiply publicly available figures by a factor of 2 or 3 to estimate the mortality. *Thirdly*, it is difficult to know whether a death is maternal or non-maternal, and misclassification is a problem in all types of countries. The fact that the woman was pregnant may be simply overlooked, forgotten or not recognised. This is particularly probable when crime is involved, as in cases of clandestine abortion or homicide in the context of domestic violence.

There are several ways to overcome the problems mentioned. Very often, national es-

timates of maternal mortality are based upon available but deficient and non-representative hospital data, which has little to do with the maternal mortality at the community level. In low and middle-income countries three specific survey methods are used for measurements of maternal mortality, each with specific advantages and disadvantages.

To assess the magnitude of maternal mortality in countries where it is not reported, *the sisterhood method* is a cost-effective way. Persons are interviewed regarding maternal deaths among their adult sisters. It can be carried out as one part of a household survey, which makes it a comparatively cheap way of measuring maternal mortality. The disadvantage, however, is that it is fairly imprecise, giving a range of uncertainty of up to ± 20 %. Furthermore, it reflects a reality that may be a decade or more out of date. The most important disadvantage is, however, that it does not give any clue to operational activities or interventions to reduce maternal mortality, since it provides numbers but not circumstances.

Another method is *the household survey*, which is costly and time-consuming. A few household surveys on maternal mortality have been published. One of the best-known examples is the Addis Ababa study, which resulted in an estimated maternal mortality ratio of 566 maternal deaths per 100 000 live births. This study was based on 45 maternal deaths identified in a survey of 32 000 households. Even such a huge undertaking has a wide 95 % confidence interval, which in this study was calculated to range from 374 to 758 deaths per 100 000 live births (Kwast 1986).

A more effective way of reaching valid conclusions for interventions is the *reproductive age mortality survey* (RAMOS). Such studies imply the identification—from village surveys, from demographic sites, from vital registration or from cemetery surveys—of all deaths among women of reproductive age, often defined as 15 to 49 or 12 to 55 years, depending on prevailing patterns of reproduction. After identifying such deaths, trained interviewers are sent to each identi-fied household of a female death and the cir-cumstances of death are clarified, with an emphasis on the distinction between mater-nal and non-maternal deaths ('verbal au-topsy'). In demographic sites such verbal au-topsies are often done routinely for each identified death. Empirically, this approach is the best method for subsequent interven-tion, since such 'autopsies' often give infor-mation about aspects of avoidability and other practical circumstances, which can be applied to interventions. When using pro-spective registration of maternal death among 77 000 women during six years in the largest demographic site in Tanzania the confidence interval for MMR was 600 to 1 100 per 100 000 live births (Mswia 2003). This clearly shows that maternal mortality is 'too rare' to be affordable to monitor year by year in low-income countries. It is probably only meaningful to make national estimates for ten-year periods.

9.2.2 The principal maternal 'killers'?

Knowledge of the global proportions of the causes of maternal death is extremely lim-ited, but the main causes are well known (Box 9.1). Haemorrhage following delivery and uterine rupture during delivery are com-mon in remote areas, where life-saving hos-pital services are beyond reach. Hygiene at delivery, even when birth takes place under primitive conditions, may reduce the inci-dence of life threatening infections ('child-bed fever'). Life threatening infections fol-lowing abortion and delivery have been shown to be on the increase in areas with a high prevalence of HIV infection. Brain malaria during pregnancy and immediately following the delivery is also a growing prob-lem, especially in Africa. The regional varia-tion of the life threatening type of hyperten-sion, eclampsia, is striking. There are a much greater number of maternal deaths due to eclampsia in lowland coastal areas, while eclampsia is rare or even non-existent in most highland areas investigated.

9.3 Maternal morbidity: the base of the iceberg

Maternal morbidity refers to all complica-tions of pregnancy, delivery and abortion. It is noteworthy that the major portion of ma-ternal ill health is found *after* pregnancy, be it concluded by delivery or by abortion.

The global variation in maternal morbid-ity is virtually unknown. This is particularly true for low-income countries, while statis-tics from high and middle-income countries are better. Morbidity-specific figures are pre-sented below.

An overview from low-income countries has shown that around 40 % of women had acute health problems during pregnancy, of which 10 to 15 % developed chronic health problems, including specific conditions such as fistulae, prolapse, or incontinence directly resulting from the pregnancy. These

---

Box 9.1

The six prominent causes of maternal death

1 postpartal haemorrhage (bleeding due to the failure of the uterus to contract following delivery)
2 post-abortion septicaemia (infection due to an unsafe abortion)
3 postpartal septicaemia (infection due to childbed fever)
4 eclampsia (circulatory death due to pregnancy-induced hypertension)
5 uterine rupture (bleeding due to obstructed labour)
6 brain malaria (infection due to pregnancy-related deterioration of immunity)

---

seemingly high figures can best be understood if recognised that they include common but still serious conditions like pregnancy anaemia, malaria, malnutrition, pregnancy-induced hypertension, pregnancy induced diabetes, syphilis and a number of other infectious diseases. The figures also constitute a reminder that severe maternal morbidity is a much more prevalent problem than maternal mortality.

In various projects aimed at improving maternal and perinatal outcome of pregnancy, maternal morbidity has been suggested as a tool to measure the impact of programmes. Maternal morbidity is, however, difficult to define and to interpret. There is a significant degree of inter-observer variation in diagnosing various maternal diseases, and technologies are not always available to establish a correct diagnosis (e.g. measurement of haemoglobin concentration for the diagnosis of anaemia). Maternal morbidity can be divided into four categories: pregnancy-related, unsafe abortion-related, delivery-related and puerperium-related diseases.

9.3.1 Pregnancy-related diseases

Studies in the USA and in Canada show that about 25 % of women with low-risk pregnancies suffer from disease during pregnancy, mostly anaemia, hypertension or urinary tract infection. The latter is known to be associated with adverse pregnancy outcomes such as early delivery, low birth weight at delivery and various infectious complications involving the genital tract.

The prevalence of hypertension varies considerarbly between different studies. Diastolic pressures greater than or equal to 90mm/Hg have been found in about 25 % in high-income, 15 to 20 % in middle-come and 5 to 10 % in low-income countries.

Anaemia is defined by the WHO as a haemoglobin level in the blood of less than 110 gram/litre. WHO estimates that up to 60 % of pregnant women in several studied low-income countries are anaemic. It seems that this prevalence has not changed over the last decades. If more serious pregnancy anaemia is considered (<70 gram/litre), the prevalence is below 5 %.

9.3.2 Unsafe abortion-related diseases

At least 50 million induced abortions are performed in the world each year, and half of them constitute unsafe interventions. This implies an unmet need for fertility regulation. It is a huge challenge to the world to counteract dangerous abortions carried out by untrained persons and to prevent the mortality and morbidity resulting from them. Preventive measures include health education and fertility regulation as well as provision of safe abortion.

The diseases associated with unsafe abortion consist above all of ascending genital infections. These can be expected to occur in at least 30 % of cases, which would correspond to close to 10 million women per year. There is evidence that such post-abortion infections frequently result in occlusion of the fallopian tubes, with resulting secondary infertility. As a rough estimate, this much-feared complication results in at least 2 million women each year becoming infertile as a direct consequence of an unsafe abortion.

The global variation in the occurrence of unsafe abortion is unknown. The criminal nature of the intervention makes under-reporting a significant factor both in routine statistics as well as in special surveys. Maternal deaths related to unsafe abortion are presumably most prevalent in Africa and in Asia, each of which is estimated to account for 40 to 45 % of all abortion-related maternal deaths, amounting to around 90 000 per year globally. It is almost impossible to find estimates of trends in numbers of unsafe abortions. The advent of cheap medical abortion technologies such as the use of the drug misoprostol will presumably contributes to a reduction in the occurrence of unsafe abortion. The increasing prevalence of HIV infection would tend to make lay abortions more dangerous, with more post-abortion infectious complications.

9.3.3 Delivery-associated diseases

The most typical morbidity occurring during labour and delivery results from abnormally prolonged labour due to constitutional or functional disturbances. Depending on the exact definition, 10 to 15 % of pregnant women suffer prolonged or obstructed labour. Underlying factors may include youth, short stature, or diseases. Eclampsia may deteriorate into convulsions and severe anaemia may lead to acute cardiac failure.

9.3.4 Puerperium-related diseases

Two problems predominate the period after the delivery known as puerperium. These problems are bleedings and infections. Failure of the uterus to contract adequately, due to uterine atony, may result in abnormal haemorrhage. This typically occurs shortly after delivery and in approximately 10 % of all deliveries. Abnormal bleeding is defined as a loss of more than half a litre of blood. If drugs promoting uterine contraction are routinely used to prevent atony, the bleeding prevalence can be brought down to approximately 5 %. On average, about the same prevalence is found for retained placenta, often associated with excess haemorrhage.

Postpartal bacterial infection of the uterus may lead to puerperal fever ('childbed fever') and deteriorate into genital sepsis, a life threatening general infection. It may occur several days after delivery and even beyond the first week after delivery, and is frequently under-reported. In low-income countries it is estimated to affect approximately 5 % of women after delivery, while it is rarer in middle-income countries and almost non-existent in high-income countries.

One particularly significant puerperal disorder is *uterine prolapse*. Its prevalence is generally unknown, but studies in some countries (e.g. Egypt) have revealed that it is clinically significant in more than 50 % of women with previous childbirth. Another tragedy is damage of the soft tissues of the birth canal due to prolonged labour. This can lead to a permanent hole between the bladder and the vagina, a so-called vesico-vaginal fistula, or between the rectum and the vagina, a recto-vaginal fistula. These complications affect particularly young short women during their first delivery, as there is a risk that the not fully-grown pelvis leads to prolonged delivery.

If an estimated 40 % of the 138 million annual births involve complicated pregnancies (around 55 million) and this figure is added to the estimated number of spontaneous abortions (25 million), then a total of at least 80 million pregnancies with acute problems occur each year in the world.

9.4 Perinatal morbidity and mortality (7 %)

Reference is often only made to before or after birth. It should be noted that the concept 'perinatal' alludes to the foetus/infant and the mother. Current use of 'perinatal' often excludes maternal aspects by focusing on foetal/infant events. Maternal morbidity or mortality is often not included in perinatal medicine; although more than 50 % of all maternal deaths occur in the perinatal period. One reason is that two types of med-

---

Box 9.2

Definition of the perinatal period

"The perinatal period is the period extending from the gestational age at which the average foetus attains the weight of approximately 500gram (equivalent to 22 completed weeks of gestation) to the end of the seventh completed day of life."

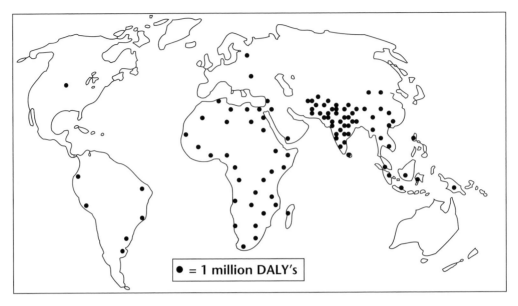

Map 9:2 *Perinatal conditions cause 97 million disability adkjusted life years (DALY) lost per year.*
Source: WHO, 2002.

ical specialists divide the responsibility for the care of the mother and the child.

It is obvious that the road to health in the perinatal period is dependent upon the health of the mother. Her health during pregnancy depends on her living conditions before becoming pregnant. The young girl that suffers from malnutrition during childhood will be at risk of skeletal stunting, deficiency diseases such as rickets (Vitamin D deficiency) and infections resulting in pelvic asymmetry. Such a girl will often run a high risk in later pregnancies. The road to perinatal health for the young mother is threatened by a number of complications potentially affecting both the mother and the foetus. Either of the two may die from complications originating in the woman's early years.

The enormous global burden of perinatal ill health is well illustrated by the fact that perinatal disorders top the list of conditions that cause most DALYs lost in the world (WHO 2004). The burden of 'perinatal disorders' is estimated to be more than three times as big as the burden of maternal disorders. If compared only among females the relation-

ship is approximately the same. In general, stillbirths and neonatal deaths during the first week of extra-uterine life tend to be approximately equal. The total number of perinatal deaths annually in the world is estimated to be about 2.5 million, with the bulk of the problem occurring in Southern Asia, followed by Sub-Saharan Africa (WHO 2004).

9.4.1 Low birth weight

The health problems of the foetus/neonate occurring in the perinatal period are almost always associated with maternal disease. This is especially so for low birth weight (LBW), which is defined as a newborn weight of up to 2499 gram. The proportion of newborns with a birth weight below 2500 gram varies considerably from country to country. It is often used as an indicator of the general health situation and living standard in a given country. It has been calculated that about 95 % of all LBW births, or 20 out of 21 million per year, occur in low and middle-income countries. This problem is particularly important in southern Asia, where 20 to 30 % of newborns have a birth weight below 2500 gram. Any population with an LBW incidence above 7 % is at risk of having a high perinatal mortality, which could be counteracted by analysing the roots of the LBW problem. In low-income countries a significant share of this problem is thought to be associated with the problem of smallness for gestational age (SGA), due to a combination of maternal malnutrition, anaemia, malaria, placental insufficiency, pre-eclampsia and also unknown factors. Babies who are small for age (SGA) are those who have a birth weight below the 10th percentile at any gestational age. Very limited data exist, however, regarding the aetiological role of various maternal diseases for the development of SGA. Only a proportion of SGA newborns suffer from intrauterine growth retardation (IUGR), which is a condition associated with disturbance of placental function. Some normally growing foetuses may still be in the SGA category for genetic reasons and may be considered small but healthy.

Among LBW newborns, there is a variety of causes of perinatal infant death. Vulnerability to infection, particularly maternal genital infections, seems to play a predominant role in some deprived populations. Such maternal infections may lead to uterine contractions and finally to expulsion of the baby, sometimes with intrauterine growth retardation. Asphyxia, hypothermia and infections, especially neonatal tetanus, are other causes of neonatal death.

There are few tools available to predict LBW. Anthropometry is one useful approach in this regard ('tape-measure obstetrics'), by which the growing abdomen of the mother can be measured at regular intervals. In this way the distance between the symphysis bone and the upper part of the uterus can be monitored to recognise early deviations in foetal growth.

9.4.2 The small baby

Newborns with a birth weight below the 10th percentile consist of various groups of infants, among whom the long-term prognosis may vary from severe persistent growth retardation and psychomotor retardation to completely normal growth and development. In many cases, it is not possible to predict the outcome before the child has reached the age of 6 months or more. With a high prevalence of LBW, a high prevalence of developmental disorders may be expected.

Asymmetrical growth retardation. The baby's weight is abnormally low in relation to its length. Where severe maternal malnutrition is prevalent, e.g. in parts of India and Africa, these infants constitute a significant proportion of the LBW category. Their length and head circumference are in most cases normal for full-term infants. These newborns have for some reason suffered intrauterine malnutrition, frequently without any obvious maternal disease. This pattern is also encountered in multiple pregnancies, in pre-eclampsia and in other conditions featuring an inadequate placental nutritional supply to the foetus. These newborns may be born at term or pre-term. They may also suffer from deficient access to oxygen from the umbilical cord during delivery and the first minutes of breathing following birth. This is known as neonatal asphyxia and it may be the reason for late neurological complications contributing to long-term disability. The prognosis in cases with late growth retardation is, however, good. With adequate care, the child will grow fast and regain most of the initial weight loss. However, if prenatal malnutrition is followed by severe postnatal starvation, the situation rapidly become precarious and the risk of permanent brain damage is high.

Genetically small newborns. Short mothers and fathers often have small children. These infants will remain small and their prognosis is generally good. However, in this group, there is also a subgroup of infants with very early intrauterine growth retardation, due to either diseases or parental genetic aberration, the true causes of which cannot be determined.

9.4.3 Pre-term birth—being born too early

The word pre-term refers to any gestational age earlier than 37 completed weeks of pregnancy. The word 'premature' is not synonymous with 'pre-term'. In actual practice, 'premature' is often (poor) jargon for 'less than 2,500 gram', which is correctly designated 'LBW'. The word 'premature' should therefore never be used, since it is obsolete, unclear and misleading. Reference should instead be made specifically to weight (e.g. LBW) or gestational age (e.g. pre-term).

It may be of clinical interest to know whether a LBW baby is born pre-term or at term. The estimation of gestational age is thus important, and if the maternal menstrual data is reliable there is no problem in calculating it. If the data is absent or inaccurate, it may be of some help to use a maturation-scoring system. At present there is, unfortunately, no maturity-scoring system tested in both developed and developing countries. No system gives a better estimate of gestational age than ± 2 weeks.

The global variation in the prevalence of pre-term birth is substantial. In settings where ascending genital infections prevail, up to 20 % of births may be pre-term. In settings where such ascending genital infections are less common, the prevalence may be less than half of that.

In current practice in most settings where resources are scarce, efforts to save pre-term babies start when they have reached approximately 28 weeks of gestation, corresponding to a birth weight of around 1 000 gram. The mortality among newborns with a birth weight of less than 1 000 gram is close to 100 % in the general health service in low-income countries. But even with very scarce resources the survival can be improved by simple and cost-effective methods such as the skin-to-skin (mother-newborn) method, known as the 'kangaroo' method (Christensson 1998).

9.4.4 Hypothermia

Over the last decade, hypothermia has been recognised as a problem in new-borns even in tropical countries. It is usually defined as a temperature below 36.5°C. Insufficient attention has previously been paid to the problem of low temperature, since room temperature in these countries is usually high, at least during the day. Body temperature has usually been measured with conventional rectal thermometers, which do not record temperatures below 35°C. Thus, the temperature of a baby admitted to a neonatal ward may be reported to be 35°C, although the actual temperature may be much lower. Perinatal death is clearly associated with hypothermia. It has been shown that pre-term babies with a rectal temperature of less than 36°C had a mortality rate of more than 75 %. If they were kept warm, the mortality rate dropped to less than 20 %. Avoiding hypothermia is probably the most important and most feasible single factor in reducing neonatal mortality among LBW newborns in resource poor settings. It has been estimated that during the last decades, the prevention of hypothermia has contributed to a 25 % increase in survival rate in high-income countries. The 'kangaroo' method (see above) has meant a most significant improvement in the maintenance of thermal control, particularly for the smallest newborns.

9.4.5 Perinatal infections

Worldwide, infections are one of the main causes of maternal death and perinatal infant death. The availability of antibiotics was a major advance in reducing perinatal deaths. The anti-tetanus vaccine was another major technical advance. Recently, there has been some progress in research into fairly low-cost medications aimed at reducing the risk of vertical transmission of HIV infection from HIV-infected mothers to the newborn. However, huge logistical and motivational problems still remain for the wide utilisation of these drugs. Puerperal endometritis with sepsis is a largely preventa-

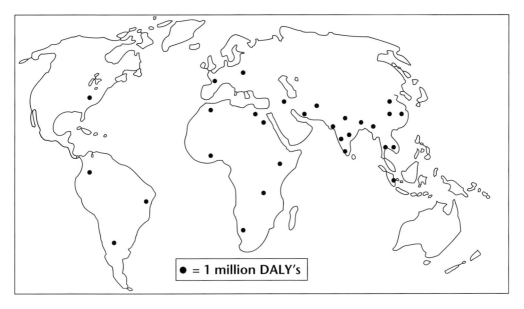

Map 9:3 Congenital abnormalities cause 29 million disability adkjusted life years (DALY) lost per year.
Source: WHO, 2002.

ble complication, which kills many mothers. Unhygienic handling at birth is also an infection risk that may be fatal in combination with other negative circumstances, such as LBW.

Both transplacental and transcervical infections are common during pregnancy in low-income countries. Many viruses that infect the mother may cross the placenta, while only few bacterial or parasitic infections, such as syphilis and malaria, can pass this route. Ascending infections make the birth canal an important route of entry for any bacterial or occasionally even viral infection the mother may have in her vagina or cervix. At birth, a baby may thus carry an infection acquired during pregnancy or while passing through the birth canal.

The healthy, well-nourished, breast-fed, term newborn that is kept warm enjoys good protection against infections during the first few months of life. This is due in part to the antibodies transferred to the infant through the placenta or via breastmilk. The colonisation of the skin and intestinal tract of the infant by the bacterial flora of

the family is essential for the protective mechanisms of the infant. On the other hand, the defence mechanisms of LBW and/ or malnourished newborns are poor. The threat of a serious infection is increased by the high risk of acquiring hypothermia and poor suckling ability, leading to starvation. All this contributes to impaired defence mechanisms in the newborn. In such cases, overcrowded neonatal units are particularly dangerous places, since cross-contamination from one infant to another or from staff members to the child is common.

At birth, there is an increased risk of infection for the mother and for the infant. Infections are commonly transmitted from patient to patient in hospitals. It is important that the newborn be colonised with maternal bacteria that are less harmful than the hospital ('nosocomial') bacteria. Some measures, such as separation of the child from the mother, care in closed neonatal units and the use of protective clothing, have proven to be ineffective. Such routines have seriously impaired opportunities to establish close contact between the mother and newborn and thereby optimal conditions for breastfeeding.

The global variation in perinatal infections is substantial. Syphilis may reach only 1 to 2% prevalence in India, while corresponding figures in many communities in Sub-Saharan Africa may reach ten times that prevalence level. The implications of multiple infections in the mother during the perinatal period consist of both maternal (post-partal) and congenital infections—acquired in utero—of the newborn, delivered alive or stillborn.

9.4.6 Congenital disorders (2%)

Depending on the nature of the disorder, the proportion of congenitally acquired abnormalities in the foetus varies between 5 and 15%, the most common being malformation of the heart. The aetiology is genetic, environmental and in many cases unclear. Traditional customs of marriage between close relatives are known to increase the risk of genetically induced perinatal mortality, and presumably also of congenital abnormalities. The number of congenital disorders leading to death is estimated at half a million, equal to the number of estimated maternal deaths per year.

9.5 Other conditions associated with reproductive ill health

9.5.1 Sexually transmitted diseases

The two categories of sexually transmitted infections (STIs) are fatal and non-fatal. Three potentially fatal STIs are HIV infection, cancer of the cervix and syphilis, the last of which is also potentially fatal to the unborn foetus. The remaining STIs are non-fatal and include gonorrhoea, chlamydial infection and bacterial vaginosis. The STIs are described in Chapter 5.

9.5.2 Sexual and reproductive ill health among adolescent women

It is important to distinguish this age group (up to 19 years), since young women have a disproportionate share of the reproductive mortality and morbidity. Unwanted pregnancy, sexual abuse and violence, genital mutilation, social marginalisation due to unwanted pregnancy and complications of pregnancy, septic abortion and fistula complications at delivery are pertinent examples. It is rewarding to note that in some countries (e.g. Mozambique, Uganda, Kenya, and Tanzania) efforts are currently being made to establish 'youth clinics' or 'adolescent centres' to cater to teenage reproductive ill health.

9.5.3 Genital malignancies (0.5%)

This category of diseases represents a significant threat to female reproductive health unrelated to fertility and pregnancy as such. About 400 000 new cases of cancer of the uterine cervix are estimated to occur annually in the world. In practice, screening aimed at early diagnosis and cure is too costly for low-income countries. Even if the bulk of these women die outside the fertile age, cervical cancer has serious consequences for female reproductive health. This is particularly pertinent in the light of recent evidence that this disease is due to human papilloma virus (HPV) infection, presumably transmitted sexually. In this perspective, it is noteworthy that long before AIDS the world had this potentially fatal, sexually transmitted disease selectively killing women. Progress has recently been made towards the development of a vaccine against HPV.

9.5.4 Female genital mutilation

'Mutilation' is defined as the removal of a part of the human body that is not diseased. Female genital mutilation has previously been known as 'female circumcision'.

Female genital mutilation (FGM) is a traditional surgical procedure that involves the

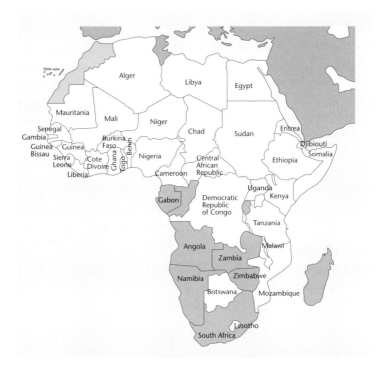

Figure 9.3 African countries in which female genital cutting has been reported since 1979. White areas have reported cases, green areas no cases reported.

Source: Shell-Duncan 2001.

partial or total removal of clitoris and vulva (Box 9.3). It has emerged as a serious challenge in the area of reproductive health and rights. FGM has currently achieved great prominence in the sphere of human rights worldwide. The precise origin of the practice is unknown, but appears to date back to ancient Egypt earlier than 2000 BC. FGM is deeply rooted in the local traditions and culture of the people practising it. It is part and parcel of their cultural heritage.

There are immediate and long-term complications to FGM, due to bleeding, infection and pain provoked by the intervention, often performed under primitive, unclean conditions.

The geographical variation in genital mutilation is significant. As can be seen from the map in figure 9.3, genital mutilation in different forms is concentrated in a belt across Africa from Somalia in the northeast

to Nigeria and other West African countries. It does not coincide with the distribution of any specific religion, though it has been argued that it is by and large an Islamic tradition. This is not true, since for instance, it is not practised in Saudi Arabia or in other major Muslim countries. It is also encountered in areas of other religious faiths. Female genital mutilation is practised on 98 to 100 % of women in countries like Somalia and parts of Sudan, while its occurrence is very variable in countries like Tanzania and Kenya. The variation in severity of mutilation is also significant, even within countries.

FGM has been classified as a violation of children's rights and as a violation of human rights. There is no doubt that FGM is a harmful traditional practice. It is well documented that FGM has both short-term and long-term health complications. In the short-term perspective, bleeding and acute

---

Box 9.3

Classification of Female Genital Mutilation according to the WHO

Type I—The clitoral prepuce is removed, sometimes along with part or the entire clitoris.

Type II—Both the clitoris and part or all of the labia minora are removed.

Type III—The clitoris is removed and the labia minora are amputated and incisions are made on the labia majora to create a raw surface. These raw surfaces are either stitched (with silk or thorns) or kept in contact until they seal (infibulation).

Type IV—Unclassified FGM, e.g. pricking, piercing or incision of the clitoris and or labia, cauterisation, scraping and/or cutting of the vaginal entrance, or introduction of corrosive substances and herbs into the vagina.

---

infections are known to take place in a significant proportion of cases. In a long-term perspective, pain on sexual intercourse (dyspareunia) and complications of delivery are among the more significant problems.

A specific problem is the issue of *re-infibulation*. This involves the repetition of infibulation after giving birth, i.e. the re-suturing of the vulva after cutting up the closed, infibulated vulva. The law in several European countries prohibits the performance of re-infibulation. The justification for this restrictive attitude is that re-infibulation after each birth implies a gradual worsening of the long-term complications of FGM.

Recent research in Sudan indicates that there has been a significant change in attitudes and practice regarding FGM. New generations, and particularly males, have been found to be negative to the continuation of FGM, and many African women's organisations are now active in abolishing FGM.

9.5.5 Male circumcision

Male circumcision is one of the most common surgical interventions in the world. In contrast to female genital mutilation there is evidence that it may have advantages in some contexts and the side effects are limited. In spite of this there are controversies around this procedure. The Canadian and the American Association of Paediatricians, have come to the conclusion that it has no

benefit for the child—unless, of course, there is some specific indication, and that it is a violation of the UN Convention of the Rights of the Child.

In sharp contrast to these views from pediatricians in high-income countries there is an increasing amount of epidemiological evidence for a positive effect on HIV prevention. The most recent major review from infectious disease specialists from London School of Hygiene and tropical medicine conclude *"There is compelling biological and epidemiological evidence of the protective effect of circumcision on the acquisition of HIV infection and ulcerative STDs. It is unlikely that any single control measure will reduce HIV transmission sufficiently and therefore circumcision needs to be investigated as part of a package that includes education, condom promotion, and STD control. The potential adverse effects of promoting male circumcision need to be carefully monitored. In spite of the difficulties associated with promoting male circumcision as a measure to control HIV and STDs, this promising strategy should not be ignored."* (Quigley 2001).

A more recent Cochren review concludes *"The results from existing observational studies show a strong epidemiological association between male circumcision and prevention of HIV, especially among high-risk groups. However, observational studies are inherently limited by confounding which is unlikely to be fully adjusted for"* (Siegfried 2003). As three randomised controlled trials of the effect of male circumcision are ongoing they recommend that active promotion of male circumcision should wait until a positive effect has been confirmed by these studies with a scientifically much stronger design. This seems to be a wise conclusion at the present state of knowledge.

9.6 Sexual and reproductive health: the human rights issue

During the Cairo International Conference on Population and Development (ICPD) in 1994, the issue of 'reproductive rights' was brought forward with success. Issues previously not discussed, such as unsafe abortion and domestic violence, gained ground as important examples of violations of rights. The Cairo conference was followed by a women's conference in Beijing, at which these issues were further promoted. A number of challenges in reproductive health and rights began to be discussed in a light that had previously been impossible at international meetings.

With the exception of maternal and perinatal health, the human rights challenges in reproductive health care consist of the availability of safe abortion, prevention of childlessness, prevention of transmission of HIV, early detection and cure of STIs, and screening for pre-cancerous lesions of the cervix.

There are many obstacles to enhanced sexual and reproductive rights. One such obstacle may be a lack of co-operation between obstetricians and paediatricians, and between doctors and other staff. All experience shows that a continuing dialogue involving all categories of staff, as well as clients, patients and their families is a prerequisite for good reproductive health care.

In several low-income countries, the low status of midwives and nurses constitutes a serious problem. Underpayment and irregular wages often lead to absence from work in order to earn a living in other ways. Perina-

tal care needs staff, and in hospitals there must be staff around the clock. Inexperienced staff in inadequate numbers has little chance of solving the problems of overcrowding and lack of drugs and equipment. Provision of reproductive health care is thus a question of both rights and economic resources.

The improved status of women, women's education and a focus on access to life-saving skills and emergency care can significantly reduce maternal mortality during the coming decades in middle income countries with adequate health policy. A 50 % reduction in neonatal mortality and the eradication of neonatal tetanus within 5 years are examples of goals formulated by WHO. These can be attained even in low-income countries, provided affluent countries offer substantial increases in support to the health care budgets of these countries. However, without economic development, sustainable fulfilment of human rights pertaining to sexual and reproductive health will remain unattainable.

References and suggested further reading

Bergström S. Reproductive failure as a health priority in the Third World. East African Medical Journal 1992;69:174–180.

Bergström S, Höjer B, Liljestrand J, Tunell R. (Eds.) Perinatal health care with limited resources. London: MacMillan; 1994.

Christensson K, Bhat GJ, Amadi BC, Eriksson B, Hojer B. Randomised study of skin-to-skin versus incubator care for rewarming low-risk hypothermic neonates. Lancet 1998;352:1115.

De Brouwere V, Van Lerberghe W (Eds.). Safe Motherhood Strategies: A Review of the Evidence. Antwerpen: Itgp Press; 2001.

Egerö B, Hammarskjöld M, Munck L. AIDS: the challenge of this century. Prevention, care and impact mitigation. Department for Democracy and Social Development, Sida, Stockholm: 2001.

Högberg U, Wall S, Broström G. The impact of early medical technology on maternal mortality in late 19th century Sweden. Int J Gyn Obst 1986;24:251–61.

Inhorn MC. Global infertility and the globalisation of new reproductive technologies: illustrations from Egypt. Soc Sci Med 2003;56:1837–51.

Kahlid SK et al. WHO analysis of causes of maternal death: a systematic review. Lancet 2006;367:1066–74.

Kwast BE, Rochat RW, Kidan-Mariam W. Maternal morbidity in Addis Ababa, Ethiopia. Stud Fam Plan 1986;17(6 Pt 1):288–301.

Lawson JB, Harrison KA, Bergström S. (eds.) Maternity care in developing countries. London: Royal College of Obstetricians and Gynaecologists (RCOG); 2001.

Mswia R, Lewanga M, Moshiro C, Whiting D, Wolfson L, Hemed Y, Alberti KG, Kitange H, Mtasiwa D, Setel P. Community-based monitoring of safe motherhood in the United Republic of Tanzania. Bull World Health Organ 2003;81:87–94.

Mundigo A, Indriso C (Eds.) Abortion in the developing world. New Delhi and London: Zed Books; 1999.

Quigley MA, Weiss HA, Hayes RJ. Male circumcision as a measure to control HIV infection and other sexually transmitted diseases. Curr Opin Infect Dis 2001;14: 71–5.

Shell-Duncan B, Hernlund Y. Female Circumcision in Africa—Culture, Controversy and Change, edited by Shell Duncan and Hernlund. London: Lynne Riener Publisher; 2001.

Siegfried N, Muller M, Volmink J, Deeks J, Egger M, Low N, Weiss H, Walker S, Williamson P. Male circumcision for prevention of heterosexual acquisition of HIV in men. Cochrane Database Syst Rev 2003; (3):CD003362.

WHO. Female genital mutilation: report of a WHO technical working group meeting: Geneva: 17–19 July 1995. Geneva: World Health Organisation; 1996.

WHO. Interpreting Reproductive Health. WHO/CHS/RHR/99.7, Geneva; 1999.

WHO. Maternal Mortality in 1995. WHO/RHR/01.9, Geneva; 2001.

WHO. Reproductive Health Indicators for Global Monitoring. WHO/RHR/01.19, Geneva; 2001.

WHO. World Health Report 2004.

10 Global population change

> *Having 10 daughters but no son is the same as having no children.*
>
> Poor woman, Vietnam 1999

The new interest in the size of the human population on our planet emanates from the early 1950s. The reason was the rapid population growth, particularly in southern Asia and Africa. India was the first low-income country in the world to have a national family planning association in 1952. Incidentally, the International Planned Parenthood Federation (IPPF) was founded the same year, and the Rockefeller Foundation in the United States established the Population Council. Many big international organisations, such as the World Bank, WHO and UNICEF, initiated support activities in the area of birth control in the 1960s. The United Nations Fund for Population Activities (UNFPA) was formed in 1969.

Today the fertility rate has decreased considerably in most countries in Asia as well as in the Middle East and Latin America. The total fertility rate (TFR) in India has fallen from more than six children per woman in 1960 to about 3 per woman today. On the way from the unsustainable 6 children per woman to the sustainable fertility rate of 2 India has already achieved 75 % of the necessary change over a 40 year period. The drop in fertility in Bangladesh from 6.5 to 3.5 during the last two decades came unexpectedly and was surprisingly fast in spite of the prevailing high child mortality, illiteracy and poverty. Major middle-income countries like Brazil and Indonesia today have less than 2.5 children born per woman. A large part of the economic success of a number of Asian countries, the so-called tiger economies, has been attributed to "the demographic gift". The African island country of Mauritius is a prominent example of demographic gift following investments in female education. Fertility declined, between 1963 and 1972, from 6.2 to 3.2 children per woman. This unprecedented fertility decline was followed, in the 1980s, by dramatic economic growth. Mauritius history challenges the belief that economic growth is an essential precondition for fertility decline (Lutz 1994).

The fast drop in fertility rates, combined with falls in mortality rates, has had a distinctive effect on age structures in the populations of these Asian countries. There is a substantial lowering of child-dependency ratios, in other words there are more adults in relation to children. At the same time there are not so many old people in the population. Later, there is a rapid aging of populations. This ageing is now rapidly underway in many Asian countries with fast socio-economic development. Between the lowering of the proportion of children and the increase in the proportion of old, the countries benefit from several decades with a highly favourable age distribution. This period is known as the "demographic gift". The high proportion of workers in the productive ages makes the economy grow faster and makes it affordable to provide good schools for all children (Chu 2000).

Four to five decades ago many regarded the population growth as the main problem in the world. Today when the UN set the Millennium Development Goals (table 1.5) fertility is not even included among the 8 goals, 15 targets and 44 indicators that are selected for the monitoring of world development. This constitutes a tremendous change in perspective. The change is mainly due to the fast decline of fertility that has taken place. But the change is also due to a deeper understanding of the driving forces behind development where the negative and positive effects of population composition are given less importance today than 40 years ago. How did the view on population policy change?

It is a characteristic of the early 1950s that the public debate in the rich countries saw a rapidly increased commitment to 'population issues'. The understanding of *fertility determinants* was limited. Rather, the population growth was seen as a supply-demand problem, and governments and non-governmental organisations (NGO's) launched vigorous campaigns to achieve the widest possible contraceptive coverage. Along with improved contraceptive technology, several Western countries embarked upon extensive birth control projects, Sweden for many years being the biggest donor per capita in this field.

The global interest in 'population issues' culminated in 1974 with the World Population Conference in Bucharest, when the controversy between affluent and poor countries came to the surface. The majority of impoverished countries counterbalanced the population control-oriented approach of some experts and politicians. They called for recognition of the problems of widespread poverty and injustice in global distribution. The Indian minister of health, Dr Karan Singh, stated: "The best pill is development." In the years to come, influential circles gradually modified their positions and powerful Western debaters admitted profound changes of opinion.

In retrospect, it is instructive to note that while Karan Singh expressed the above slogan, the architects of the Indian emergency—implemented in the mid 1970s—were already well organised in several states in northern India. This 'emergency' implied essentially an abolition of several laws protecting human rights, so as to permit compulsory sterilisation by law. In other words the Indian government did consider population growth so alarming that a war-like state of emergency was declared to permit the vi-

olation of basic reproductive rights. In the wake of the Bucharest conference, there was also a growing alertness among leaders of low-income countries regarding the nature of the population growth. India and China followed their own paths, opting for control in the name of national interests, while other countries opted for recognition of family planning as a human right to be integrated into maternal and child health care (MCH). Still others continued their pronatalist stand and did not adhere to the idea of birth control as a component of socio-economic improvement.

Ten years later, in 1984, the next World Population Conference was held in Mexico City. Now there was more agreement among low-income countries and affluent countries about the need to limit population growth and to achieve development. A decade later, in 1994, the next population conference took place in Cairo, the International Conference on Population and Development (ICPD). This was the first 'population' conference to acknowledge the need to broaden the scope of the debate from merely demographic issues to women's and men's reproductive health and rights. The Cairo conference was, in theory, a true paradigm shift away from birth control targets to a women's rights perspective, encompassing controversial issues like abortion, sexual violence and women's empowerment. Far-reaching commitments were pronounced by the rich countries. These commitments were further enhanced by two following world conferences in 1995, the Social Summit in Copenhagen and the Women's World Conference in Beijing.

The Cairo conference was also innovative in that commitments were made to follow up the plan of action of the conference with activities entitled 'Cairo Plus Five', which took place in 1999. The idea was to investigate whether or not financial and legislative commitments had been implemented, and to review activities programmed as a consequence of the plan of action adopted in Cairo. So far there have been more rhetorical statements than discernible concrete actions taken by the high-income countries. A concern is the lack of international funding for commitments, while many middle-income countries make domestic priorities that change the fertility determinants and provide family planning to the couples that request it.

10.1 Global population growth

A population growing at a constant percentage growth rate will double in size at regular intervals. The mathematical representation of this process on a graph is an exponential curve, theoretically ending in an almost infinite population in a comparatively short period of time (Figure 10.1).

In the last thousands of years the world population increased at a rather slow rate, presumably amounting to an average of 0.1% per year. This rate is assumed to have prevailed until the late 17th century (table 1.1). The improvements in general living conditions following the industrial revolution have resulted in a slowly declining mortality and a rising global population growth rate. This trend was accentuated during the 20th century. The world popula-

tion increased by about one billion from the early 1970s to 1987, and by another billion by the year 2000. The projections foresee the addition of another billion by 2010. This is foreseen to occur in spite of the dramatic decline of the growth rate of the planet's population from 1960 to 2000. A good way to clarify the implications of population growth rates is to state the doubling period, i.e. the number of years over which a population will double in size at a specific growth rate (as mentioned in chapter 3.10). The formula used for estimating of the doubling period in years is simple:

$$\text{Doubling time of a population} =$$

$$= \frac{69 \text{ years}}{\% \text{ annual growth}}$$

A growth rate of 1% will result in a doubling in 69 years, while a 3% growth rate will double the population in about 23 years. A growth rate of 3.8%, which was the case in Kenya in the early 1990s, meants a doubling in 18 years. The latest estimate for Kenya indicates that the growth rate is 2.3%, corresponding to a doubling time of about 30 years.

Using merely currently available data may be misleading. A simplistic application of

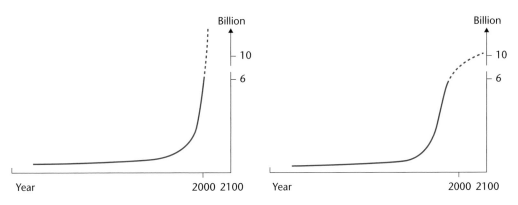

Figure 10.1 The exponential graphs of the 1960s and 1970s depicted the global population growth as an "explosion" (graph on the left). The currently valid graph takes into consideration the decline in global population growth (graph to the right), which by all probability implies the achievement of a stable world population by the year 2100.

Source: Adapted from Lutz, Sanderson and Scherbov, 2001.

the 'doubling time mathematics' earlier led to a frightening scenario and constituted the basis of a doomsday perspective launched by Paul Ehrlich (1970). This theoretical litany has turned into a major success in global development, the decreased rate of global population growth. It is obvious that the exponential graph had to be corrected to correspond to a forthcoming steady state. A comparison of these two graphic models can be seen in Figure 10.1.

It is obvious that the exponential graph was almost correct in predicting the estimate of around 6 billion inhabitants in the world by the year 2000 and in making the prognosis that the world will reach approximately 8 billion inhabitants by the year 2020. These figures may appear threatening, but they conceal the fact that fertility has fallen in recent decades in all countries except in Sub-Saharan Africa. Globally, the population growth rate has declined from 2.0% in the 1960s to 1.5% in the early 2000s. The total fertility rate (TFR) in the world was 6 children per woman in 1960, reached 4 per woman in 1985 and has fallen to 2.8 in 2002. In the most probable UN projection, the TFR will reach 2.3 children per woman by the year 2025. This demonstrates that the doubling time mathematic does not make sense for the world any longer, since it assume the growth rate to be constant. As we have seen it is not. The 'replacement level of fertility' when a population remains stable in size over time is about 2.1 children per woman. This is the level it is assumed that the world will have reached by between 2025 and 2050. The leading independent demographer Wolfgang Lutz's (2001) best forecast is that the world population will stop growing in the second half of this century and that the world at 2100 will have 8 billion people but the uncertainty range will be from 6 to 12 billion. More interesting than the exact number is that one third of the world population in 2100 will be older than 60 years.

The rapid change in population growth globally implies that the population pyra-

Table 10.1 Global population change 1950–2050 in percent.

Age group (years)	1950	2000	2050
0–14	34	30	21
15–59	57	59	54
60–79	8	10	21
≥80	1	1	4
Population in billions	2.5	6.0	9.3

Source: UN Department of Economic and Social Affairs Population Division. World Population Prospects: The 2000 Revision. New York: UN 2001. See also: Diczfalusy 2002.

Table 10.2 Population change in high-income countries 1950–2050 in percent.

Age group (years)	1950	2000	2050
0–14	27.3	18.3	15.6
15–59	60.0	59.2	41.3
60–79	11.7	19.4	33.5
≥80	1.0	3.1	9.6
Population (millions)	814	1.191	1.181

Source: UN Department of Economic and Social Affairs Population Division. World Population Prospects: The 2000 Revision. New York: UN 2001. See also: Diczfalusy 2002.

mids will change significantly over the decades to come. As can be seen from Tables 10.1 and 10.2, the world will witness quite a significant change, which is more pronounced in high-income countries than in low-income countries. These examples indicate a powerful trend towards world population ageing, most clearly demonstrated in the case of Japan. From Table 10.3 we can see that in the year 2050 the number of children in Japan aged 0 to 14 years will have declined over one century to only one-third of what it was in 1950. During the same time interval, the proportion of people above 60 years of age is estimated to increase from 8% to 58%, a *seven-fold increase*. The corresponding global increase in people above 60 years of age is three-fold, from 8.7% in 1950 to an estimated 25.2% in

254

Table 10.3 Population change in Japan 1950–2050 in percent.

Age group (years)	1950	2000	2050
0–14	35.5	14.7	12.5
15–59	56.3	58.3	29.8
60–79	7.7	23.2	42.3
≥ 80	0.5	3.8	15.4
Population (millions)	84	127	109

Source: UN Department of Economic and Social Affairs Population Division. World Population Prospects: The 2000 Revision. New York: UN 2001. See also: Diczfalusy (2002).

2050. The world will change tremendously in the next 60 years. Remember that in contrast to many other scientific disciplines demography is good at predicting the future many decades ahead. What was predicted 30 years ago has largely come true.

10.2 Poverty and the demographic trap

More than ten years ago, at the time of UN's meetings on the Convention on the Rights of the Child and the Rio Conference on environment, the concept of the 'demographic trap' was launched by the British specialist in international health, Maurice King. His trap analogy implied a priority setting among prevailing global threats in strong favour of population control.

It is known that fertility decisions depend on a number of determinants and it would therefore be more adequate to address any alleged trap as constituted by the constellation of the most important fertility determinants. Considering such determinants, there is general agreement that poverty, high child mortality, female illiteracy and the low status of women are directly related to high fertility. The arguments by King 10 years ago may have been the last time someone seriously suggested isolated focus on population control in low-income countries. The theories on poverty by Amartya Sen have put high fertility and population growth in a more complex perspective (See chapter 1.1). High fertility does constitute a part of the vicious circle that keep the poor in poverty but it must be realised that in the short perspective it is rational for poor families to give birth to several children (Caldwell 1999).

In poor countries, rapid population growth lowers and keeps earnings at survival level. The reason is that the poor have to compete with each other for the scarce work opportunities. Population growth forces small-scale farmers to compete for the scarce land. Poverty and population growth will overtax natural resources, leading to soil erosion that diminishes long-term productivity. In such a setting poor couples prefer having large families due to a complex set of circumstances. In the constant struggle for survival, impoverished populations tend to see children not only as the meaning of life but also as an economic asset. Poor families see each additional child as an opportunity to broaden, diversify and thereby strengthen their means of support. More children mean better capacity to watch the goats, to keep the birds away from the rice field, to catch extra fish for the evening meal and to sell the tomatoes at the local market. When times are bad for some of the children, they may be better for others in the family. This 'strength in numbers' strategy may reduce the chances of pulling the whole family out of poverty, but that is a small price to pay if it reduces the risk of falling into starvation. High fertility is thus a rational strategy for the survival of the family. Thus poor families do not want many children in order to be taken care of at old age. They want many children in order to live to old age.

10.3 Population growth and natural resources

Population projections by the UN for the year 2050 range from 7 to 11 billion. The fertility rate in the world has over the last 40 years fallen from 6 to 3. Young people increasingly want to wait to have children, and want to have smaller families even in low-income countries. Still, more people and higher incomes worldwide are multiplying humanity's impacts on the environment and on the natural resources that are essential to life. In some parts of the world, fresh water, fisheries, forests and the atmosphere are already strained. Based on these observations, it is obvious that in the era of the 21st century we shall witness even greater pressures on natural resources. Let us take a closer look at some of these resources: water, cropland, fisheries, forests and climate.

– *Water:* an estimated 500 million people face relative water scarcity. It has been calculated that, by the year 2025, between 2 and 3 billion people may be living in areas where potable water is scarce. For some millions of people in the Middle East and in parts of Africa today, the lack of available fresh water is a concern that is going to become more acute and more widespread. Much of the fresh water now used in water-scarce regions comes from deep-water sources, which are not being refreshed by the natural water cycle. In some countries, where the water shortage is severe, high rates of population growth may exacerbate the declining availability of fresh water.

– *Cropland:* in countries where arable land is scarce, the number of people is projected to increase between 0.5 and 1.0 billion by the year 2025. The soil on today's cropland must remain fertile to keep food production secure. The minimum amount of land needed to supply a vegetarian diet for one person without the use of any artificial chemical inputs or loss of soil and soil nutrients is estimated to be 0.07 hectare or slightly less than a quarter of an acre. An estimated 420 million people today already live in countries that have less than that per person. Increased food production must come from increased yield per hectare.

– *Fisheries:* in 1997, global fish production climbed only modestly, almost entirely because the farming of fish expanded in the world, notably in China. Most fisheries worldwide are considered to be fully exploited or in decline. More food will not be extracted from the sea, unless the fishes are fed artificially.

– *Forests:* based on the current number of people living in countries with forest scarcity, and on a medium population growth projection, this population could triple from about 1.7 billion people to around 4.5 billion in 40 countries with less than 0.1 hectare of forested land per capita. This figure is an indicator of a critically low level of forest cover.

– *Climate:* the world has seen a continued upward trend of carbon dioxide emissions. The increased per capita emission accelerated the accumulation of greenhouse gases in the global atmosphere. With 4.6% of the world's population, the United States accounted for about 22% of all emissions from fossil fuel combustion and cement manufacture, by far the largest CO_2 contributor among nations. Emissions remained grossly inequitable, with one-fifth of the world's population accounting for more than 60% of all emissions in 1996, while another, much poorer fifth accounted for less than 2%.

One of the main arguments for poverty alleviation in the world is that this is the only way to stabilise the world population because "birth control" without poverty alleviation is doomed to fail. At the same time contraceptives should be made available for all, so that men and woman can make rational choices to keep their families small as soon as their life conditions so allow.

10.4 Migration: the 'push' and the 'pull' factors

The main human solution to population growth has been migration (see chapter 1.5–6). Today people may migrate from one area to another area for various reasons. A distinction has been made between 'push' factors and 'pull' factors. The former term refers to factors forcing people away from an area of origin, and a further subdivision has been made between 'hard' and 'soft' push factors (Box 10.1).

The 'hard' push factors are well known as such, though their migratory consequences may not be well known, as regards magnitude and direction. War and starvation belong to tragic events which force people to flee. Environmental disasters occur mostly in middle and low-income countries. Floods, drought, soil erosion and desertification are widespread and recurrent problems. A report from the International Organisation for Migration has disclosed that 'environmental migration' will be caused by several serious disruptions affecting the living conditions of millions of people: elemental, biological, slow-onset accidents; disruptions caused by 'development', and environmental warfare.

Among the 'soft' push factors, increasing hardship due to economic recession may act in combination with persecution to increase migration in many parts of the world. Sudan, Burma, the former Yugoslavia and El Salvador are examples of areas where this factor has contributed to migration. Along with the 'push' factors, some authors have also distinguished 'pull' factors. Obviously, pull factors tend to reflect push factors. For instance, differences in salary/wealth may constitute both push and pull factors. Relaxed immigrant regulations in some attractive countries may represent an important pull factor. Such factors may change in the future, due to a potentially significant future demand for labour in richer countries. Today people migrate from collapsed countries to low-income countries, from low-income to middle income and from middle income to high income countries. There is also migration from high-income to higher income countries such as medical doctors moving from Sweden to the richer neighbour Norway. Such a stipulated demand of labour where there is money, should be seen against the background of the quickly ageing population in many countries, to which reference has previously been made (see section 10.1).

In high-income countries, attitudes towards immigration are generally in favour of strong regulations and increasing limitations on the numbers that are allowed to enter. The same attitude can be found in Costa Rica against immigration from Nicaragua and in South Africa against immigration from Mozambique. The complex pattern of interacting 'push' and 'pull' factors will in all probability increase international migration in the foreseeable future.

10.5 Fertility determinants

The concept of 'fertility determinant' is complex. A number of different, interacting phenomena, sometimes mutually reinforcing, sometimes not, constitute the reality of

---

Box 10.1

Push factors for migration

Hard factors	*Soft factors*
War	Persecution
Starvation	Poverty
Environmental catastrophes	Social loneliness

---

which the level of fertility is a consequence. For instance, if the prevalence of secondary infertility (see chapter 9) is high, as in several central African countries, the average total number of children a woman will have over a lifetime may be low. In such settings, however, widespread sexually transmitted infections (STIs), leading to secondary infertility, may run parallel with other diseases of poverty tending to increase perinatal mortality and thus infant mortality. High infant mortality figures are empirically related to high fertility rates (Caldwell 1999).

One recent study from India, based on National Family Health Survey (NFHS) data, demonstrates that fertility levels in India can be explained by four major direct determinants: the proportion of females who are married; the incidence of induced abortion; the fertility-inhibiting effect of breastfeeding; and the prevalence of contraceptive use. The NFHS data suggest that without these listed determinants, fertility levels would have risen to higher levels than at present. It was concluded that if the effect of delayed marriage had been removed, without any other change in 'fertility behaviour', the fertility level would have increased.

In Sub-Saharan Africa, a panorama similar to the Indian one has been demonstrated in recent overviews of fertility determinants. Data from the Demographic and Health Surveys (DHS) during 1986 to 1995 indicate a distinctly decreasing trend to lower fertility in Southern Africa, transitional fertility decline in East Africa, and a less dramatic decline in West Africa. In the analyses, it was noted that Central Africa has surprisingly low fertility, a finding that should be seen in the light of the high figures found for secondary infertility in these countries. For Sub-Sahara Africa, it was concluded that major fertility determinants were: age at marriage, postpartum factors such as breastfeeding and sexual abstinence, postpartum amenorrhoea, education, child survival and contraceptive use.

Recent research has also focused on one specific fertility determinant, to which in-

sufficient attention has hitherto been paid: induced abortion. In one study comparing the development of fertility in Egypt and Zimbabwe, it was found that the observed declines in fertility over the years 1988 to 1994 are most probably due to increases in abortion rates. As the availability of safe induced abortion is limited in both countries, the conclusion is that abortions induced under unsafe circumstances are on the increase. Several studies involving in depth interviews with women admitted to hospitals for allegedly 'spontaneous' abortions have shown that more than 50 % of them had undergone induced abortion.

Country-specific analyses of fertility determinants indicate that dramatic changes have occurred. It is noted in one study that fertility in Bangladesh has declined by 44 %. This decline is brought about by increased age at marriage, delayed childbearing, breastfeeding with lactation amenorrhoea, and increased contraceptive use.

It is not possible to single out any specific fertility determinant as being crucial for fertility decline over time and across all countries. It is obvious, for example, that over the period 1900 to 1960 Europe saw a very steep fertility decline in the absence of modern contraceptives. A critical review of achievements in the area of population control in the last decades, indicates that the initial focus on contraceptive technology has been criticised as an obsession with a technique that implies that fertility is regarded as a disease, requiring particular remedies. This has conveyed a research orientation towards technical solutions to essentially motivational problems. In contrast to this technical focus it has been found that when the motivation exists, couples find ways to control their fertility whether a strong family planning programme exists in the country or not. It is interesting that the fertility rates have fallen from more than 6 children per woman in 1970 to less than three in 2000 in countries as different as Indonesia, Vietnam, Iran, Morocco, and Peru.

It has been further argued that the one-sided approach did not recognise one particularly perceived need in the impoverished populations targeted: reproductive failure and childlessness. Childlessness in low-income countries is a three-pronged problem comprising infertility, pregnancy wastage and child loss. Infections killing children under five years significantly contribute to child loss, thereby making such diseases important in the area of reproductive failure and childlessness. The latter concepts thus cover much more than gynaecological problems.

Another experience gained is that the motivational aspect has been given insufficient attention. It remains a fact that, for the poorest families in low-income countries, children may be the only tangible capital available, not only as child labour and as an economic guarantee, but also as security in old age. It has often been overlooked that children—however malnourished and deprived of decent living conditions—may still imply a net advantage in poor families. However deplorably they are cared for, they may still produce a net surplus of income and social status. The problem of child labour has gradually come into focus, and it has been demonstrated that having many children in employment, seen from a mere capital-generating point of view, can be a rational decision.

The so-called Caldwell hypothesis has gained widespread recognition. It postulates that human reproduction (number of children born) is associated with capital flow from children to parents and vice versa. If the net capital flow from children to parents is positive, children may constitute an economic advantage resulting in more obvious unwillingness to limit fertility. On the other hand, when children cost (e.g. in school fees and clothes, child labour being illegal), parents may tend to limit their number.

It has been learnt that a key concept in the freedom of fertility decisions is perceived need. In campaigns to force couples to accept contraception, it has been noted

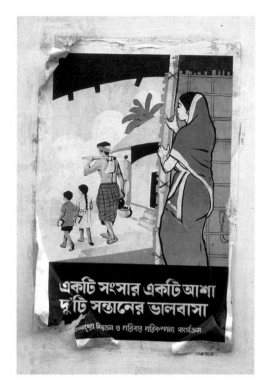

BANGLADESH, Chittagong province. Poster propagating the small nuclear family.
© Heldur Netocny / PHOENIX.

that insufficient motivation results in low acceptance of fertility regulation. In order to overcome this hurdle, campaigns have been launched to generate demand. This shows clearly the conflict between perceived and alleged needs. The conflict allows us to raise a number of critical questions:

1 Does family planning/birth control in a given setting enhance the self-determination and well being of women, or does it remove control of fertility from women, placing it in the hands of birth control providers?
2 Is there a difference between birth control needs as perceived by potential recipients and by birth control providers?
3 Can alleged needs (not perceived by potential recipients) be discerned in programme documents?

4 Does family planning/birth control exist as a means of reducing social pressures resulting from economic and political inequities that family planning programmes are unwilling to confront?
5 Is family planning/birth control a substitute for economic and political reforms responsive to the self-perceived needs of the poor?

10.6 Will AIDS stop population growth?

In countries characterised by rapid population growth, both fertility and mortality trends will be decisive for changes in population growth. In settings with a high prevalence of HIV/AIDS, mortality rates among sexually active, mostly young people, has increased considerably, and because of maternal-foetal transmission, the numbers of infected new-borns have also increased. The combined risk of intrauterine, intrapartal and postpartal transmission of HIV for an African newborn is in the range of 40%, while the risk for a newborn in an affluent country may be only half. The explanation is unclear, but it seems that the coexistence of genital wounds and concomitant sexually transmitted infections enhance the transmission from maternal tissues to foetal tissues during passage through the birth canal. With anti-retroviral medication, now widely available in high-income countries, vertical transmission can be reduced. In other words, the vast majority of newborns of infected parturient women can avoid infection. However most of these children will be or become orphans and run a considerable risk of dying from other causes. They are also likely to remain completely or partly illiterate, as there are no parents that can pay for their education

Even if the consequences of a high HIV prevalence may seem far reaching, it is still obvious that prevalence rates around 20% will not stop population growth in the presence of fertility rates around 5 children per woman. With a population growth rate of 2.5 to 3%, which is a common figure in Sub-Saharan Africa, a prevalence of 50% will be required in order to reduce population growth to zero. Only a few locations in Africa currently exceed 50% HIV prevalence, and only in such areas can one foresee a decline in population. It is, however, clear that prevalence rates around 20 to 25% may have a quite clear demographic impact and may half the population growth, for instance from 3% to 1.5%. It is important, however, to recognise that such calculations may be misleading. Except for purely AIDS-related deaths, there is a parallel phenomenon related to deteriorating socio-economic conditions among the surviving older generation and among non-infected children left as orphans (about 12 million in Africa alone) or migrating for survival. Social networking and support from various non-governmental organisations may reduce this parallel mortality risk. The demographic impact of HIV will thus depend not only of the direct effect of the virus but perhaps as much on the indirect effects.

In summary, it is clear that AIDS-affected communities will experience deaths directly due to AIDS and indirectly due to other diseases among groups made vulnerable by malnutrition, poverty and abandonment. The deterioration may be aggravated by the non-availability of drugs and health care in units already overburdened by a large number of AIDS cases. Even more important is whether the highly affected countries will be able to maintain a general progress in economic and social terms in the presence of such a strong impact from HIV.

10.7 Fertility control: a human right or a human obligation?

The concept of 'control' is that it has an implication of setting limits to or checking and intervening at a defined stage of development. In one sense, the word is positive: to keep an eye on the undesirable. There are few who would question the inherent good in pollution control, pesticide control, nuclear arms control, etc. But when it comes to birth control or population control, the issue becomes more controversial. In whose interest is the control to be executed? To whom is it desirable to control numbers of impoverished individuals rather than to control impoverishment? It may be argued that potential threats should be controlled and limits should be set to avoid undesirable events. Such a threatening event would be over-population or too many births. In this sense control implies intervention in one of the most private of spheres. Much of the controversy surrounding population control undoubtedly stems from control measures taken without due attention to the integrity and the privacy of fertility decisions, particularly among the poorest in the world, for whom children often represent security, hope and an asset for the future.

Few, except those who are opposed for religious reasons, would deny the great value of fertility regulation technology, if used appropriately. There are, however, reasons for concern. The resistance among impoverished populations to comply with population policies formulated at the national level and executed in a manner unrelated to health priorities at the local level has led to severe conflicts. India provides an illustrative example of this renaming process. After the compulsory sterilisations of the mid-1970s, the concept of family planning became so strongly associated with coercion that it could hardly be used at all. The prevalence of contraception sank to extremely low levels in the population and a process took place in which the word 'planning' was substituted by the word 'welfare'. Consequently, books on the subject of 'family welfare methods' mention condoms, pills, IUDs, sterilisation, and so on, while saying nothing about other aspects of family welfare in the more common sense of the word. Likewise, 'family welfare centres' pro-

vide welfare only in the limited sense of female contraceptive surgery, which in actual fact consists of two—and only two—activities: abortion and sterilisation. It is important to note that when the coercion stopped in India fertility continued to decline. During many decades the Chinese government has put a continuous pressure on couples to reduce the number of children. It seems as if coercion was more successful in China either because it was combined with a stronger reduction of child mortality or just because there was no freedom of speech to protest against the political force put upon families' reproductive decisions.

Family planning is undoubtedly a valuable asset, particularly in the process of women's emancipation. It is laudable that it is considered a human right. However, there is historical evidence that the provision of this human right has implied the deprivation of freedom. A look into the process of freedom in fertility decisions may raise some doubts.

In the early era of 'birth control' campaigns in South-East Asia, much attention was given to *information, education and communication* (IEC) campaigns in order to spread the message of the advantages of family planning. Due to unresponsiveness among the poor and the unsatisfactory outcome of these campaigns, they were intensified to also include *persuasion* and more aggressive interventions to convince resistant individuals in the target population to accept family planning. With selective payments to those who accepted family planning but not to maternal and child health care (MCH) attendees, to family planning workers but not to MCH care providers, some improvement in the birth control campaigns were achieved. When persuasion through incentives (and subsequently disincentives) did not produce the desired results, the next logical step was to increase the pressure on families with many children to include compulsory sterilisation by law. The human right to family planning was provided to the population by coercion in more countries than China and India.

The resistance that was met by these birth control campaigns entailed extensive manipulative measures, which were all geared towards the creation of demand where this was insufficient. Through this approach, the governments and even foreign donors did not pay due attention to the perceived (versus alleged) needs of poor people:

1 intensive mass communication aimed at target audiences;
2 persuasion efforts with incentives (such as the distribution of food to a starving population in order to achieve sterilisation targets); and
3 coercion in the form of legalised violence.

The three levels were related to each other, even if the degree of violation of the needy poor populations became progressively more brutal. The isolation of *perceived* needs (recipients' opinion) from *alleged* needs (donors' opinion) runs parallel with a clearly visible tendency to the status quo, giving most family planning programmes the character of no-change programmes.

The concept of an 'incentive' would presumably seem like a positive word to most people, implying an encouragement of efforts, e.g. made in the assumed societal interest for the common good. In impoverished societies with extremely small margins for survival, incentives may have much more controversial implications. In such societies, there are areas of widespread poverty and starvation, where incentives undoubtedly can be coercive. If incentives really were an attempt to enhance interest in maternal and child health (including family planning) in the population, incentives should naturally be paid to support the broad concept of MCH/FP. Instead selective fertility regulation incentives (and disincentives) have been introduced in several poor countries, questioning the only tangible capital the poor may be able to generate: their children. In the escalated form that incentives/disincentives issues took in India in the mid-

1970s, the *de facto* coercion did not result in a fall in birth rate but rather a fall of government. The political implications of deprivation of freedom in fertility decisions can hardly be illustrated more succinctly.

Today, India has changed its population policy completely, at least on paper. The overriding principle is now the 'target-free approach', implying a focus on reproductive health in general and on maternal and perinatal health in particular. The previous demographic target-oriented approach has been abandoned and incentives have been virtually abolished. The future will show whether this new orientation will be sustained.

In today's Asia, China remains a prominent example of a country in which strong pressure is exerted on the population to comply with the 'one child' ideal. This coercion is also associated with a system of incentives and disincentives in order to achieve demographic goals. Other countries in the Far East where far-reaching demographic targets have influenced reproductive health care are Vietnam and Thailand. There are more abortions per capita in Vietnam than in any other country in the world, and pregnancy interruption has in reality come to play an important role as a fertility regulation method. In Bangladesh, a country in which abortion legislation is extremely restrictive, the application of the concept of 'menstrual regulation' is widespread. Without knowing whether a woman whose menstruation has ceased is pregnant or not, a suction device can be inserted into the uterine cavity to 'induce' menstruation. In most of these women an early pregnancy has already been established, and in these cases menstrual regulation is in reality an induced abortion.

10.8 Birth control versus motherhood control

While it is self-evident that zero fertility will automatically mean zero maternal mortality, it is less clear what impact family planning will have on the maternal mortality ratio. This ratio is defined as the number of maternal deaths per 100 000 live births. In a study from Bangladesh in the early 1980s, it was shown that the impact of family planning was unexpectedly limited. Two villages were compared; one was subjected to intense family planning promotion over several years, while in the other no family planning propaganda was distributed. In the village where family planning was promoted, fertility was reduced by 26 % in relation to the reference village. Unexpectedly, the maternal mortality ratio was identical in the two villages.

The explanation was that the intensive family planning drive had not conveyed any increase in safety at birth. The findings imply that wanted pregnancies did not enjoy any better protection in the family planning village than in the reference village. Family planning could even have been counterproductive to safer motherhood, because the few resources (doctors and nurse-midwives) available may have been co-opted to family planning activities. In fact, in the area studied, 75 % of women dying in childbirth did not see a doctor before their death and almost 90 % had no access to modern health facilities.

It is a well-known fact that most maternal deaths occur at medium parity (one to four births) and at medium age (20 to 35 years). This is derived from various findings, of which one, from a study in Bangladesh 1968 to 1970, is particularly revealing. It was calculated that if *all* births had been averted in women below the age of 20 or above the age of 39, and beyond a parity of 6, the maternal mortality ratio would only have declined from 570 to 430 per 100 000 live births. Even with this extremely non-realistic achievement of virtually cutting off all births in these groups of women, a very limited gain in maternal mortality would have resulted.

Even if we assume an impoverished country with a high maternal mortality in the high parity range, we can still conclude, as

shown in various data-simulation studies, that elimination of all women with more than 5 children may mean a less than 5 % reduction in maternal deaths. This and similar findings indicate the limited value of targeting grand multiparous women for sterilisation in order to reduce the overall maternal mortality. However, it must be emphasised that, beyond all doubt, a significant number of women with many children want fertility control. It can be concluded that it is not the age/parity distribution of births that explains the low maternal mortality in the developed world. It is a well-documented fact that grand multiparity is associated with high maternal mortality figures in impoverished countries, but not in more affluent countries. An illustration is the very low maternal mortality in the high parity range in Sweden and other developed countries. It has been shown in Nigeria that high parity is associated with high maternal mortality, but only if child mortality is high. This has been confirmed in historical epidemiological studies in Sweden 1800–1900: what kills the mother is not parity but poverty.

In Sweden, the maternal mortality ratio has dropped from levels of around 1 000 to about 5 maternal deaths per 100 000 live births over a period of 250 years. The bulk of this decline (more than 90 %) occurred before any kind of modern contraception was available. It is true, however, that the combined effect of increased availability of contraceptives and access to safe, legal abortion services meant a very important contribution to the final reduction in maternal mortality over the last 50 to 60 years in Sweden. A similar pattern has been found in several other industrialised countries.

The need for health-oriented empowerment of women and men to plan for optimal reproductive health and voluntary spacing of births is uncontroversial. The controversial point lies in the priority given to birth control relative to more comprehensive maternal health care. In a review as early as 1987, Winikoff and Sullivan concluded, "efficient health care is more effective than family planning in preventing maternal deaths."

References and suggested further reading

Caldwell J. Paths to lower fertility. BMJ 1999;319:985–7.

Chu CY, Lee R (eds). Population and Economic Change in East Asia. New York: Population Council, 2000. Supplement to Population and Development Review, vol. 26, 2000.

Diczfalusy E. Population growth: too much, too little or both? IPPF Medical Bull 2002; 36:1–2.

Egerö B, Hammarskjöld M (eds). Understanding Reproductive Change: Kenya, Tamil Nadu, Punjab, Costa Rica. Lund: Lund University Press; 1994.

Helig G. DemoGraphics software 1998. (www.magnet.at/heilig)

Lutz W. Mauritius finds the magic mix. People Planet 1994;3:10–2.

Lutz W (ed.). The Future Population of the World: What Can We Assume Today? International Institute for Applied Systems Analyses. London: Earthscan Publications Ltd.; 1994.

Lutz W, Sanderson W, Scherbov S. The end of world population growth. Nature 2001; 412:543–545.

Lutz W, Qiang R. Determinants of population growth. Philos Trans Royal Soc Lond B Biol Sci 2002;357:1197–1210.

Sen G, Germain A, Chen LC (eds). Population Policies Reconsidered: Health, Empowerment and Rights. Harvard University Press; 1994.

Sen G, George A, Östlin P. Engendering International Health—the Challenge of Equity. MIT Press; 2002.

UNFPA The State of World Population. (www.unfpa.org)

UN Department of Economic and Social Affairs Population Division. World Population Prospects: The 2000 Revision. New York: UN; 2001.

UN population division. (www.un.org/ popin)—Information on current publications in the UN system on population development.

11 Health policy and health systems

> *We do not go to the hospital because it is necessary to bring our own linen, dishes and sometimes even a bed.*
>
> A young woman, Mauynak, Uzbekistan

Since time immemorial, humans have made joint efforts to control diseases. A review of health policy might therefore start in any ancient civilisation. For example the Greek goddesses Hygeia and Panacea represent the two major health policy options: to prevent diseases or to treat the diseases that appear. By challenging magical explanations, Hippocrates directed interest to the environmental causes of diseases. He argued that regulations and public actions by communities could reduce the occurrence of diseases. He also claimed that the practice of curative medicine requires codes of conduct. In other words, he suggested health policies for his society. Health policy concerns the ways societies organise preventive actions, sets codes for curative practice, and how health considerations are integrated into all types of political decisions. The corresponding professional and scientific field is known as public health.

11.1 The birth of modern public health

In the 19th century the new understanding of the causes of infectious diseases led to new options to prevent these diseases. In 1801 Jenner published his classical work on vaccination against smallpox, and publicly organised vaccination programmes followed. In most of Europe public provision of safe drinking water in urban areas followed soon after John Snow's elucidation of the mode of transmission of cholera in London in 1855. By 1900 sanitary legislation had become part of all modern societies. The elucidation of modes of transmission of parasitic diseases like malaria and bacteriological diseases such as tuberculosis also facilitated new forms of disease control. The reduction of malaria occurrence was achieved by actions against mosquito breeding sites and tuberculosis could partly be prevented by the pasteurisation of milk.

The first attempts to build the Panama Canal were stopped by severe outbreaks of yellow fever in the labour camps. Before anyone knew that a virus caused the disease, the Cuban researcher Carlos Finley discovered in 1881 that mosquitoes transmit yellow fever and that public measures against mosquito breeding could reduce the transmission of the disease. The application of vector control enabled the construction of the canal. A memorial of Finley's discovery stands at the Pacific end of the canal as a permanent reminder of the importance of evidence-based health policy for human progress and economic growth.

The advances in understanding infectious disease that occurred in the last century gradually increased the separation of the curative and preventive approaches of medicine. Different public organisations emerged for hospital service and disease control in the industrialised countries of Europe and North America, as well as in the countries under colonial administration. In the last 50 years, there has been a further organisational split in high-income countries between control of infectious diseases and the prevention of non-communicable diseases. Most high-income countries, including Sweden, have a national institute for the control of infectious diseases and a separate national institute for public health with a focus on non-communicable diseases. The institutes for infectious diseases are generally laboratory-oriented and focused on correct diagnosis, whereas the public health institutes are dominated by behavioural sciences and attempts to change behaviour associated with disease risks. Therefore the prevention of HIV is, in a country like Sweden, largely taken care of by the National Institute of Public Health.

The explosive developments in curative medicine in the 20th century led to a rapid increase in curative health services, especially hospitals. The curative services gradually consumed a larger and larger share of the gross national product of the richer nations and employed a growing proportion of the labour force. In the second part of the 20th century, the health sector had become an important part of the economies of the richest nations, and the pharmaceutical industry an important part of the industrial sector. While the impact of health policy rapidly improved the health status in the industrialised countries, the improvements in health in the poorer countries under colonial dominance were modest before the Second World War. Following the formation of the World Health Organization and the independence of most former colonies health dramatically improved in most parts of the world. The main changes in international health policy in the last half century are chronologically reviewed in the following sections.

11.2 Vertical approaches to disease control (1946 to 1977)

The policy and organisational structure of the World Health Organization was initially disease-oriented. In the WHO headquarters in Geneva, there was one department for each major disease, e.g. smallpox, tuberculosis and malaria. Each group of disease spe-

cialists at WHO guided similar national groups of disease experts in the Ministries of Health of the member states. Each of these groups organised separate national control or eradication programmes for each disease. Each disease programme had separate offices in different parts of each country, with their own mobile teams visiting every community in their part of the country. This type of organisation is known as 'vertical disease control'.

The vertical control strategy became a complete success for the viral disease smallpox that had been causing repeated epidemics in the world for thousands of years. Following systematic vaccinations against smallpox in all countries and a final intensive search for the last cases in Somalia, smallpox could be declared eradicated from the world in 1978. In contrast to the success with smallpox, and in spite of initially promising results, WHO failed to eradicate the parasitic disease malaria and the bacterial disease tuberculosis. Most of the failures regarding these two diseases were later attributed to the vertical organisation of the programmes. So why was the vertical strategy a successful policy for smallpox but not for malaria and tuberculosis? And why is the same vertical control strategy now being successful in eradication of the poliovirus.

The fight against smallpox and polio relied entirely on an effective vaccine. The fight against malaria relied on both an effective drug, chloroquine, which was given after blood tests had identified malaria parasites, and an effective insecticide (DDT) against the vector, i.e. the mosquito that transmitted the disease from human to human. Tuberculosis was to be controlled by detecting cases early using x-rays taken in mobile laboratories that could bring the new technology to the villages, and by prescribing new effective drugs that could cure the disease: isoniazid, which was taken as tablets, and streptomycin, which had to be injected.

Let us consider what these campaigns looked like from the perspective of a family

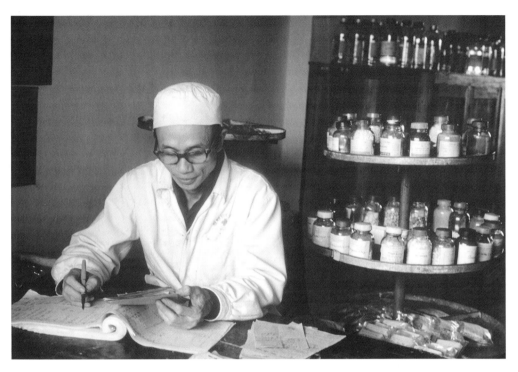

VIETNAM, My Van, on the road to Haiphong. Pharmacist at the regional hospital. Here principally traditional medicines are being used, some produced locally.
© Heldur Netocny/PHOENIX.

in an Indian village in the 1960s. One day, the smallpox team would arrive in the village. After a brief explanation, they asked everyone to line up for vaccination. Those who could prove that they had previously been vaccinated against smallpox, by presenting the typical scars on their arms, were exempted. The others were vaccinated by scratching the vaccine into the skin. The newly developed freeze-dried smallpox vaccine was cheap and did not have to be kept in continuous refrigeration. The simple bifurcated needle made it possible to get exactly the right amount of vaccine for each inoculation, and one inoculation was enough to provide long-term immunity, and the successful vaccination left a scar. The absence of a scar later helped to identify anyone who had not been vaccinated. The only thing required of the persons was to lift a shirtsleeve and tolerate minimal pain for

half a minute. Side effects were rare and limited. People knew about smallpox and noted with satisfaction that those vaccinated were completely protected against the disease.

A few days later the malaria team would arrive. Following a brief explanation, a health officer with a mobile DDT spraying apparatus on his back would enter the first home and all the walls would be sprayed with a gluey film containing DDT. The rationale was that the Anopheles mosquitoes, after feeding on the blood of a family member, would die from the DDT when resting on the wall to digest the blood after the meal. Other malaria team members would ask the village population to line up for capillary blood sampling. The blood slides were examined for malaria parasites and the bitter tasting chloroquine tablets would be given to treat those found to have malaria parasites in their blood, even if they had no symptoms. Although malaria was a severe problem, the population often perceived that the attempt to eradicate malaria caused more problems than the disease itself.

Some weeks later, the TB team would come to the village for a one-day visit in their bus. They asked people to queue for an x-ray of their chests taken with a mobile x-ray machine. Those with TB-suspected lesions on the X-ray film would be prescribed injections with streptomycin for two months and tablets against TB for a full year. When the team had left, there was no one to consult about side effects of the drugs. The fact that many improved within a month, and thereafter were not motivated to continue taking the long course of tablets, meant that many initially cured TB patients relapsed within months. Relapses of the disease were common, and resistance to the drugs developed fairly fast.

It was frustrating for the families in most villages around the world that these 'vertical visits' would only treat one disease at a time. Resources for handling most of their diseases and for the promotion of health by improving hygiene and nutrition were not made available to them. However, the reason for the failure to eradicate malaria and control tuberculosis was not only that the populations tried to avoid the actions or stopped treatment too early. The unexpected problem was the development of resistance among mosquitoes to DDT, among malaria parasites to chloroquine, and among tubercle bacteria to the first generation of drugs against tuberculosis. Strains of the Anopheles mosquito that flew out the window without resting on the DDT sprayed walls took over the role of transmitting malaria from the strains that were killed by DDT while resting on the wall. Medical science, as well as science in general, had yet to learn about ecology.

Smallpox, which for many years had been looked upon as the good example of how diseases should be eradicated, soon became the exception. The amazingly efficient vaccine developed by Jenner 180 years earlier proved easy to administer to the entire population of the world. The fact that refrigeration was not needed and that the scar made monitoring of vaccination coverage easy, were immensely important for the success. The simplicity of the preventive action and the low degree of community participation required, explain why smallpox eradication succeeded. The other programmes failed because they consisted of more complicated actions that required much more participation by the population.

At the same time as the eradication of malaria and TB failed, the wealthiest countries of the world were facing similar difficulties in controlling their new health problems. These were the problems induced by increased tobacco smoking and intensified traffic. In spite of intensive attempts to screen for pulmonary cancer, operate early and combine surgery with chemotherapy, the pulmonary cancers continued to kill more and more people. Attempts to prevent the carcinogenic effect of cigarette smoking by putting filters on cigarettes also proved futile. The only remaining policy option was widespread health education aiming at reduced smoking. This behaviour change became even more important when the role of smoking in cardiovascular diseases was gradually revealed through epidemiological studies. Advances in trauma surgery could only cure a part of all the injuries resulting from increased automobile traffic. The only policy option left was prevention: to regulate the traffic through speed limits, promotion of safety belts and actions against drunk driving.

Disease-oriented curative care was not available for many of the new diseases in the rich countries. Curative treatment existed but could not be afforded for most of the infectious diseases in the poorer countries. Technical prevention without behavioural change failed in the rich countries and could often not even be tried in the poorer countries, as their meagre health budgets were consumed by a few rapidly growing hospitals in the major cities. At the end of the 1970s, the time had come to change the vertical disease oriented approach as it, for different reasons, was failing across the world.

11.3 Primary health care strategy (1978 to 1982)

In 1978 it was possible for the Director General of WHO, Dr Halfdan Mahler from Denmark, to gather an international consensus for the need to change health policy. He did so by arranging an international meeting in the Asian part of the Soviet Union. In this 1978 conference, held in Alma-Ata in present Kazakhstan, the ministers of health of the world agreed that WHO should launch a primary health care strategy. The strategy was presented with the bold slogan: "Health for all by the year 2000".

The primary health care strategy was conceptualised in some basic principles. Health care should be made accessible to all and be designed in a way that the communities could afford. It should be based on community participation, i.e. the population should be made active in promoting health rather than acting as receivers of services. The policy emphasised that 'intersectoral actions' for health, involving other sectors of society such as education and agriculture, were as important as the actions performed by the health sector itself. The strategy also emphasised the need for equity, i.e. a fair possibility for everyone to access health services and achieve a healthy life. Seen in hindsight it is interesting that no emphasis was placed on gender issues and almost nothing was said about how the health care activities should be financed. Governments were assumed to take the full responsibility for providing health care. The content of primary health care was defined in eight elements that are listed in Box 11.1.

In many rich countries the primary health care strategy led to a new focus on general practitioners as the backbone of health services. Family medicine developed as a speciality of its own for physicians in many countries, which increased public investments to achieve better coverage by family doctors. A focus on preventive aspects could also be found in the richer countries. The actions that increased traffic safety in the richer countries can be seen as one of the most successful applications of the new primary health care policy. The decrease in the proportion of the population that smoke cigarettes and the successful promotion of breastfeeding are other examples of successful implementation of the intersectoral aspect of the primary health care strategy.

In the less affluent countries, the main effect of the primary health care strategy was to inspire governments to reorganise health services in order to make it accessible to the whole population. This effort was partly supported by development aid from the

---

Box 11.1

The eight elements of primary health care

E – ducation
L – ocal disease control
E – xpanded Programme of Immunisation against childhood diseases
M – aternal and child health care, including family planning
E – ssential drugs
N – utrition and food supply
T – reatment of common diseases and injuries
S – anitation and safe water supply

---

richer countries. In the first years following the Alma-Ata conference, many of the new efforts focused on training village health workers, also known as 'barefoot doctors' in the Chinese version of the Primary Health care strategy (Anonymous 1977). This included attempts to achieve safe deliveries through collaboration between the modern health service and traditional birth attendants. Although some positive effects came out of these efforts, it soon became obvious that there are only a few low-cost 'shortcuts' available for the improvement of health. Barefoot doctors did not function without strong political organisation of the local community as in China, or with financing from the government budget as in Iran. Local communities in the least developed countries, failed to provide economic support to their newly trained community health workers. For economic reasons many of these health workers eventually worked mainly with curative care for which their training was insufficient. The most successful implementation of the primary health care strategy occurred in middle-income countries like Costa Rica and Iran. In most low-income countries, the public budget for health failed to provide trained health staff in peripheral health centres and health posts with acceptable salaries. Many began to sell the drugs that should have been distributed free of charge to patients, and many governments failed to purchase sufficient drugs for free distribution. These failures of community-based health services in the poorest countries yielded an urge among donor organisations in the richer countries to focus support on a few essential aspects of primary health care that could make an impact on global health within a matter of years. UNICEF became the organisation that took the lead in this policy of 'selective primary health care'. The leader of UNICEF, Jim Grant (Jolly 2003) focused on a few 'golden bullets', as the concept was coined in the donor jargon of that period.

11.4 Selective primary health care (1983 to 1992)

The wishful thinking in the primary health care strategy soon became obvious in the least developed countries. In fact it was not until the study of macroeconomics and health was published in 2001 that WHO really calculated what basic primary health care would cost (Sachs 2001). When assessing available interventions that could achieve measurable results, UNICEF launched its GOBI-FFF policy in 1982. This was in a way a return to a more vertical approach, but no longer with a focus on single diseases. The strategy met with criticism from those liking the ideology of primary health care, but the focused policy of UNICEF proved to be very useful for actions. The GOBI-FFF components listed in Box 11.2 affected a number of diseases through each of a few specific actions.

UNICEF organised effective promotion campaigns for this policy at global, national and local levels. Jim Grant mobilised extensive external funding for all the components of the policy, and most developing countries implemented all the actions. Following the first intensive debate about ideological aspects, a productive discussion followed about evaluation of the coverage and impact achieved by the different components. While the coverage became relatively high, the impact differed, due to different inherent effects of each 'bullet'.

Growth monitoring of children at regular visits to child health clinics was widely implemented but proved largely to be a failure. Although it achieved high coverage, it had limited impact on the health and nutrition of the children of the poor. The weighing was done, but it was recorded and interpreted with poor quality. The emerging advice was difficult or impossible for poor mothers to follow. Studies in poor communities showed that health education alone, without growth monitoring, was just as successful in promoting good health and nutrition among children.

Box 11.2

The 'golden bullets' of the selective primary health care policy

Growth chart,	for monthly monitoring of the weight increase of infants and young children.
Oral rehydration,	against the dehydration caused by watery diarrhoea.
Breastfeeding,	to improve nutrition and protect against infectious diseases.
Immunisation,	against tuberculosis, tetanus, diphtheria, whooping cough, polio and measles
Female education,	mainly to increase primary school enrolment for girls
Feeding programmes,	especially dietary supplements to vulnerable groups
Family planning,	provision of both education and anti-conception methods

---

Oral rehydration therapy to combat acute diarrhoea seems to have contributed to a reduction of child mortality worldwide. However, not as much as expected, because most of the diarrhoeal deaths were found to be due to chronic diarrhoea linked to malnutrition rather than to acute dehydration. The process of diarrhoea management in middle and low-income countries has been a dynamic process, where evaluations and research have resulted in changes in policy, and above all in an ability to apply policy according to local circumstances. Therefore the focus on oral dehydration eventually became a successful action.

Breastfeeding was successfully promoted and protected throughout the world. This may be considered as the most successful application of the primary health care policy at a global level, in both its comprehensive and selective forms. The reason may be that most mothers like breastfeeding and the vigorous promotion in all countries met with a positive response at the grass roots' level. In addition there was strong scientific support for the benefits of breastfeeding that could counteract opposition from commercial forces. However, the emergence of the HIV epidemic and the contributing role of breastfeeding in its transmission from mother to child (so called 'vertical' transmission) has now created great difficulties in the protection of breastfeeding.

Immunisation, mainly against polio and measles, became a major success. Following the joint efforts by WHO, UNICEF and national governments the proportion of vaccinated children increased from 5% to about 70% in a 15-year period. Once more, this was done by a dynamic policy process in which health system research played a very important role. Through regular evaluations and applied research, small but decisive adjustments were made concerning when children should be vaccinated against different diseases, and how vaccination should be organised in each country. The development of new ways of delivering vaccination in different social settings also helped to improve the coverage. UNICEF also facilitated a number of technical improvements such as kerosene refrigerators, high quality cold boxes and other materials required for reaching remote rural populations in poor countries. Finally the UN organisations helped to implement a cost reducing purchasing system, where the annual need of vaccines for several countries was purchased at the same time. The resulting reduced price for vaccines constituted an important part of the success.

The World Health Assembly decided to eradicate polio in 1988, following the success of the vaccination programme for most of the world's children. This focus on one disease at a time brought global health policy back to the aspirations it had before the primary health care strategy was launched. Now, 15 years later, WHO has come very close to the eradication of polio. This shows that global disease eradication is possible when a cheap, effective and easily administered vaccine is available (WHO 2003).

The three F's were gradually added to UNICEF's policy. They have enjoyed different levels of success. The enthusiasm for feeding programmes for children based on screening for malnutrition by growth monitoring has faded due to lack of measurable effects. Female education remains a major priority but it is slow to implement, as it requires major changes to occur at both national and local level. Recent years have seen a much deeper understanding of the determinants of the health situation of women. The right of girls to education remains a top priority, although it is difficult to measure the health impact of this core dimension of social development in isolation. The last F, Family planning, has been adopted rapidly in most middle-income countries, and fertility rates in the world are falling everywhere, except in some countries in Sub-Saharan Africa. The reduction of the number of children born per woman stands as one of the major successes in human development during recent decades.

The economic constraints of the least developed countries were, however, found to be so severe that the achievements of the selective primary health care strategy could only be sustained by continued external financing of recurrent costs. UNICEF and other donor organisations paid not only for vaccines and refrigerators but also for transport. In many low-income countries the primary health care staff were given 'allowances', i.e. supplements to salaries for administering the vaccines.

By the beginning of the 1990s, it had become obvious that the main obstacles to access to health care in low-income countries were financial and managerial. Centralised public health systems could not effectively provide these services. Most evaluations showed that coverage had been achieved at the cost of quality, and that quality could not be restored without more money. The World Bank was, surprisingly, the international organisation that took the initiative in promoting policies to meet these new challenges.

11.5 Health system reforms (1993 to 2000)

In the last decades of the past century the international health policy discussions were focused on health system reforms. This term summarises all forms of change in organisation, delivery and financing of health services with the aim to improve the quality of and access to health care. Such health system reforms are still ongoing in many, if not most low- middle- and high-income countries. The reforms include a number of measures, the main ones summarised in Box 11.3.

Box 11.3

Four major components of health system reforms

1 A decentralisation of management and financial responsibility in the public system from national to local level.
2 An increase and diversification of fees in the public system
3 A shift of the public-private mix of services to more privately financed and privately provided services.
4 An improved cost awareness and use of cost-benefit analysis

---

Concerns about the rising costs of health care and the aim of structural adjustment programmes to reduce public spending have largely driven these health system reforms. In most countries they formed part of the general political process of this period. Health reforms have focused on a reduction in bureaucratic planning. Budgeting and financing systems were changed in favour of introducing competition and more need-based methods of allocating resources. Changes in financing, decentralisation and increased competition appear to be three functions most commonly associated with health system reforms.

For the poorest countries, in particular those in Africa, different international organisations have tried to diagnose the ailments of the health systems and they have imposed a variety of prescriptions. Over the last 20 years, UNICEF and WHO have proposed priority programmes such as GOBI-FFF and the integrated management of childhood illness (IMCI), respectively. The World Bank prescribed a different list of the most cost-effective public health and clinical interventions in the book 'Better health in Africa' (World Bank 1994). The effectiveness of the different interventions were discussed in more general terms by the World Bank in the World Development Report of 1993, which has to be considered as a landmark in global health policy analysis. Other comprehensive interventions recently proposed by WHO are the 'Roll back malaria initiative' and 'Stop TB programme'. All of these programmes have broad objectives but are vertical interventions with both curative and preventive components. Such externally funded projects and programmes require a functioning health system in order to achieve the effect of all the evidence-based interventions suggested by WHO and other international organisations. Functioning health systems mean well educated and reasonably paid staff that are wisely deployed in relation to where the population lives. It also means good management, i.e. regular provision of drugs and other consumables as well as maintenance and acquisition of the necessary buildings and equipment.

But it is obviously difficult to put all the proposed technical interventions into practice, if the health system is malfunctioning, even if the vertical interventions provide targeted financial support to low-income countries. It has also been noted that external funding of many special projects tend to disrupt the activities that function in weak health systems. The staff got very little salary for doing their regular job such as attending deliveries, treating the sick and running the health education. Therefore they would attend any short course whether relevant or not just to get the 'sitting allowances' offered by the external donor agency that financed each of these courses as a 'development project'. In many weak health systems in low-income countries staff earned more money from participating in short externally funded project activities than they did by doing their job during the rest of the year.

Faced with these effects on failing health systems with too many vertical projects, new ways of international co-operation were planned. This was made possible in low-income countries that decentralised the economic management from national to district level. They have adopted a new way to use donor funding that is known as 'sector-wide approaches' (SWAps). Instead of donor agencies putting funds into a number of specific projects the SWAp concept entails putting donor funds together into one 'basket' for each district, to be used during the year according to local needs. This gives the responsibility and possibility for district health authorities to prioritise health interventions using resources provided by the government and/or the 'basket' provided by a group of donor agencies. First impressions of these SWAp programmes are positive. It has also become clear how limited the international financial support is to the health services in the poorest countries. Most of the money for health services is paid by national governments and the patients themselves.

The health reforms have often been accompanied by attempts to introduce varying levels of user fees to relieve the government budgets of some of the costs for the health care system. However, poor communities have often reacted negatively, sometimes even violently, when governments have introduced charges for services that were previously offered free of charge. In many low-income countries unofficial fees were already being charged and the introduction of official fees often caused a confusing situation where the patients had to pay both unofficial and official fees.

The main conclusion from the ongoing health system reforms in low-income countries is that the general effectiveness of governance in the country is the limiting factor. Important aspects of this are the degree to which authorities in districts can handle public funds effectively and correctly. This largely depends on having competent administrative staff available. It also partly depends on how well the public audit system functions and how free the mass media are. Good governance depends largely on the transparency of how decisions are made and implemented regarding health at local and national level, and to what extent the quality and coverage of services are reported and debated in the mass media. This means that improvements in a country's public health service are very difficult to achieve without improvements in the general management of public services and, perhaps, changes in the political system.

In many of the poorest countries non-governmental organisations such as religious organisations and charity foundations operate hospitals and peripheral health service in a more effective way than do the public institutions. However, these former missionary hospitals and clinics charge increasing fees to finance their services. These non-governmental institutions tend to increase the quality of services rather than the number of hospitals and clinics. Hence the former missionary health service is gradually providing service mainly to the middle and upper class in low-income countries. In contrast privately operated outpatient clinics are rapidly increasing in number in these countries and relatively low trained staff work in these institutions. Paradoxically these private-for-profit facilities often have a higher proportion of poor patients than do the former missionary health clinics. Many of the poorest patients do not consult any trained staff before buying their medicines from unofficial drug sellers at the local market. The services provided by traditional healers are also changing in character in many countries and are partly becoming very commercialised. In many low-income countries the different forms of health services are difficult to categorise into conventional private, public or modern-traditional categories. Most governments therefore, have great difficulties in predicting how their reforms will affect the whole health system, which is composed of a dynamic mix of services by government, non-government, private-for-profit and traditional providers. Both policy analysis and operational research runs the risk of dealing with minor parts of the health system since the poor majority of the population mainly use informal or illegal provision of drugs and services, which are the only means that are affordable to them.

In conclusion, we find that while WHO has set global targets for health, it is only after 50 years that the organisation has prepared systematic numeric estimates of how much it will cost to achieve these goals (Sachs 2001). WHO's commission on macroeconomics and health (WHO 2002) concluded that a sum corresponding to 30 USD per capita is needed to provide basic health services. At present most low-income countries only manage to invest 5 USD per capita of public money per year and the population pay on average another 5 USD out of their own pocket when they are sick. The contribution from international development aid is only a few additional dollars.

Table 11.1 Estimates for domestic public and private spending on health service compared to funding from international organisations.

Country group	Public spending (per person, 1997, USD)	Private spending (per person, 1997, USD)	Donor spending (per person, 1997, USD)	Total spending (per person, 1997, USD)
Least developed countries	6	3	2	11
Other low income countries	13	9	1	23
Lower-middle income countries	51	41	1	93
Upper-middle income countries	125	115	1	241
High income countries	1 356	551	0	1 907

Source: Sachs 2001.

The present contribution of development co-operation financing from high-income countries is almost negligible as shown in Table 11.1.

Two questions arise when it becomes clear that the funding needed to enable basic health care to effectively reduce avoidable mortality requires an increase in donor funding that is several times larger than the current level.

• Will the rich countries be willing to contribute the money?
• If the money is made available in an optimal form and given the organisational difficulties, how many low-income countries will be able to absorb the new money appropriately, without increased waste and corruption?

11.6 Health status and health care

High expenditure on medical and health care does not necessarily lead to good population health. Japan spends 6.5 % of GDP on health care, while the United States spends more than twice as much. Still the US population has a shorter life expectancy than Japan's (Evans 1994). The effect of health care upon health status has been a hotly debated issue. It has been shown that improved diet, better housing and sanitation, and general socio-economic progress in the latter part of

the 19th and early part of the 20th century had a much greater impact on life expectancy than modern medical care. In fact, a steep reduction in morbidity and mortality from a variety of infectious diseases was shown by McKeown (1979) to have taken place even before the identification of the relevant pathogens and the introduction of any effective treatment or preventive measures. The identification of determinants of health and general socio-economic progress were found to have had a greater significance for health than many of the technical medical interventions, such as antibiotics.

Today poverty is regarded as the main cause of ill health or, as sometimes stated, poverty is the most dangerous pathogen in the world. About 20 percent of the world's population live in absolute poverty with an income of less than USD 1 per day. The first of the UN Millennium Development Goals is to reduce poverty. More specifically the goal for 2015 is to have reduced by half the proportion of people that in 1990 lived on less than the purchasing power of one US dollar a day. Poverty reduction is now taking place in different parts of the world, but there has been very little positive development in Sub-Saharan Africa. Undoubtedly poverty causes diseases and diseases cause poverty but the role of the health sector in alleviating poverty is by no means clear. To provide health services for the poor, to legislate for better health, to provide information

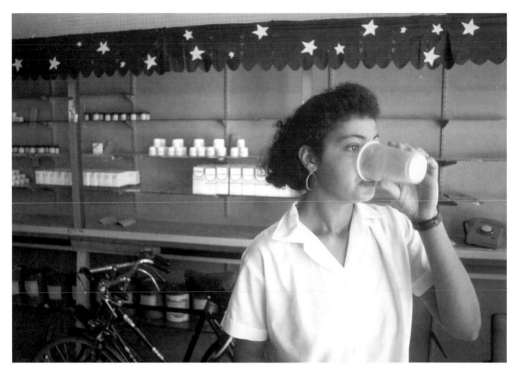

CUBA, San Salvador de Los Banios. Pharmacy with nearly empty shelves.
© Eric Miller/PHOENIX.

and to target diseases that specifically affect the poor are actions that have been, and are being, tried: results so far are largely disappointing. It is much easier to improve health for those with a better economic situation (Gwatkin 1999, Victora 2003).

With a more traditional disease oriented analysis, and studying diseases for which there are effective treatments, it has been consistently found that preventable deaths have fallen at a faster rate than other deaths. In a large sample of low and middle-income countries, scientific and technical progress have been shown to explain almost half of the reduction in mortality between 1960 and 1990. To analyse the impact of a health system focusing on the health sector alone would therefore provide a different result from that of a health system that includes public health interventions such as improved water and sanitation, and the promotion of healthy lifestyles. Yet this is not

enough. The analyses also have to include all socio-economic factors that have other main objectives but that have strong indirect effects on health such as education, economic growth, human rights and gender equity.

Thus, the definition of a health system becomes all-important when it comes to assessing its impact on health. It seems that more evidence is available on how to best spend money and resources in the health sector than on how to optimally allocate money between health, education, and other social sectors.

11.7 Health economics

The health sector constitutes almost 10 % of the world economy. Economics is obviously a central discipline for the analysis of what is effective in improving health. Health eco-

276

nomics covers many aspects of health, from defining the meaning and value of health, to studies of how well resource utilisation within health services function. Like other health sciences research, health economics has mainly focused on the situation in high-income countries. Studies have focused on large-scale insurance markets, on the differences between private for-profit and non-profit hospitals, and on mechanisms for regulating highly complex health systems. However, important advances have also been made in the analysis of how resources are best used in middle and low-income countries (Culyer 1999).

Health economics is especially demanding to apply in low-income countries, as substantial parts of the economic transactions in the health sector are informal. It requires a thorough understanding of the complex context to do an economic analysis in poor countries, however when this is carried out it can contribute immensely to rational policy. Health economics is potentially most useful where the resources are most scarce. The discovery that the provision of impregnated bed nets could reduce the malaria deaths in children in low-income African countries at first gave an impression that the malaria problem in Africa could easily be reduced by this preventive method. A simplistic saying is that "prevention is better than cure", but the question for the poor is of course "is prevention cheaper than cure?". Health economic analysis (Goodman 1999) unfortunately revealed that the cost for saving one healthy year of life by provision of insecticide treated bed nets was 19 to 85 USD. However, the cost for saving one DALY by improvement of curative services was estimated to be only 1 to 8 USD. The treatment of the sick child therefore remains a ten times more cost-effective approach, even if the prevention of malaria by using bed nets intuitively appears more cost-effective. Sadly the health economic analysis showed that the necessary package of interventions to decrease the bulk of the malaria burden is not affordable

in very low-income countries. This finding that the prevention of child deaths from malaria in Africa requires substantial assistance from external donors was a major reason for the recent focus on increasing international funding for health by creation of the Global Fund for the fight against Aids, TB and malaria (see chapter 12).

Health economics has had an important influence on approaches to health service provision and national governments as well as health service managers have adopted the methods and tools of health economics. The international comparisons of health systems, which highlight the impact of different institutional arrangements on health outcomes as well as methods of assessing the health impact, are of great importance for global health policy. The same could be said about the economic analysis of public health interventions to control infectious and nutritional diseases in different socio-economic contexts.

The best advice we can give to a young health professional wanting to make a career in international health is to study some economics. Yet the development of health services and health systems also requires methods and concepts from other academic disciplines outside the conventional health sciences. These are political sciences, sociology, anthropology, economics and system and managerial analysis of different kinds. The combined application of a range of methods to understand the functioning of the health sector is called health system research and health economics is a central component of this area of research.

11.8 Health system research

Earlier analyses of health systems focused on how a health system was organised and how resources were allocated to and within that system. The objectives of the health system were generally taken to be cost-effectiveness, including both technical and operational efficiency as well as in most in-

Table 11.2 Matrix of health systems.

Economic level	Health systems policies (degree of market intervention)			
	Entrepreneurial and permissive	Welfare-oriented	Universal and comprehensive	Socialist and centrally planned
High-income	United States	Germany Japan	Great Britain New Zealand	
Middle-income or transitional	Thailand Philippines	Brazil Egypt	Israel	Cuba
Low-income	Nepal, Vietnam	India	Sri Lanka Tanzania	

Source: Roemer 1993.

stances equity. Roemer (1991, 1993) defines a health system as "the combination of resources, organisation, financing and management that culminates in the delivery of health services to the population". WHO defines a health system as "all actions in a society that are primarily intended to improve health" (WHO 2000). Consequently, the main functions of the health system are resource production, organisation of programmes, economic support, management and delivery of services.

Resource production comprises the different groups of manpower, the health facilities, drugs and medical equipment and knowledge. The basis for organisation is the ministry of health, around which are grouped other government ministries and agencies, voluntary agencies, professional associations and enterprises. The economic support to the health system comes in varying proportions from (1) taxation, (2) compulsory social insurance, (3) voluntary insurance, (4) fees and (5) charitable donations. Within the management function falls health planning, administration, regulation and legislation. The delivery of services, i.e. running hospitals and other health facilities, is mostly subdivided into three levels: primary, secondary and tertiary health care. The levels may also be called primary health care, local hospitals and specialised hospitals.

Roemer distinguished four major types of health systems:

- the entrepreneurial and permissive;
- the welfare-oriented;
- the universal and comprehensive;
- the socialist and centrally planned.

With a classification based on economic resources, a matrix could be constructed (Table 11.2) with countries at different levels of economic development fitted into the different categories of health systems. With the recognition that the informal and traditional medicine sectors are excluded, this analysis led to the conclusion that public systems dominate in Asia and Africa, as well as in the formerly socialist countries and a few high-income countries. The poorer countries are often characterised by government provision of medical care in generally under-financed and overcrowded facilities.

Health insurance systems dominate in the high-income countries of Western Europe and North America, Australia and parts of Latin America. Most of these have a combination of private and public insurance system. Various systems of user fees are applied. The United Kingdom and Sweden are sometimes seen as intermediate forms with their combination of national health services and a national health insurance systems. The British National Health Service covers the entire population, but general practitioners have a contractual relationship with the government, and consultant doctors may have private patients in special pay beds in government hospitals. Sweden had a similar system until the 1990s, although for most practical purposes private practice played an insignificant role. But from the 1990s onwards, the Swedish system is being gradually changed. Health system reforms that change the provision and financing of health care are being carried out in many countries in order to contain costs and/or improve quality and access to health services. The carry home message is that health systems vary in many respects even between countries that are relatively similar in other aspects and the systems also continuously change over time in each country.

11.9 New approach to health systems

The World Health Organization in its World Health Report 2000 launched a new approach to the measurement of the performance of a health system. The name of the report was 'Health Systems: Improving Performance'. In this report, the health system was for the first time defined as comprising all the organisations, institutions and resources that produce health actions. A health action is defined as any effort whose primary purpose is to improve health, whether hospital service, primary health care, public health services or intersectoral initiatives. The methodology used and the concepts introduced have been well described by Christopher Murray (2003).

This means in effect, that a given action can be counted as part of the health system or not, depending on the motivation behind it. If a set of traffic lights at a dangerous road junction is set up in order to reduce accidents that cause injuries and possibly deaths, that action becomes part of the health system. On the other hand, if the lights are set up primarily to achieve a more even pattern of traffic flow, then it does not become part of the health system, even if it may save lives. This definition is theoretically attractive but it remains difficult to use when analysing resource allocations in most

countries. In fact even with this new definition of a health system many major health determinants, such as education, housing and human rights, are not even theoretically included because even if they have strong positive effects on health their main purpose is not to improve health. The WHO year 2000 definition of a health system does not merge health services and public health; it includes all of the health services but not all aspects of public health. Bearing that in mind the new definition still has advanced the analysis of the health sector and its role in development. The new definition of health system has been criticised for drawing the focus away from public health towards the financing of curative services that are the economically dominant part of all health systems. In response to this Christopher Murray, the leading researcher behind the definition, says "well the health system as now defined constitutes 10 % of the economic activity of the world and we need systematic ways to assess if the spending of all those resources delivers what we want". In this view (WHO 2000), the three fundamental objectives of a health system are:

- To improve the health of the population (health attainment);
- To respond to people's expectations (responsiveness);
- To provide financial protection against the costs of ill health (fairness of financing).

A health system must not only achieve the best possible level of health. The system should also achieve the smallest feasible difference between individuals and groups regarding attained health. It is thus not only a question of the average life expectancy in a country but also how life expectancy varies between different groups in the country. To achieve the three objectives the health system needs four basic functions, delivery of services, resource generation, financing and stewardship. These four concepts are reviewed below in section 11.9.1–4.

11.9.1 Delivery of health services

The delivery of health services requires cost effective organisation with the optimal content. Cost-effectiveness means choosing the interventions that give most value for money, and giving lower priority to those that contribute little to improving people's health. Cost-effectiveness analysis is but one tool in the improvement of the health system, but it is a tool that is more under than overutilised. In the health service, the cost per healthy life-year saved in a rich country could vary between USD 250 for screening and treating newborns with sickle-cell anaemia, and USD 5 million for control of radioactivity emission. In a poor country in Africa, the cost for a life-year saved through short-course drug therapy for malaria can be as low as USD 3 (Goodman 1999), while other interventions like anti-retroviral treatment may cost many hundreds of dollars per healthy year saved (Creese 2002), i.e. to get the same result. Combining calculations of cost with measures of effectiveness of interventions and using them to guide policy decisions is a very recent development.

11.9.2 Resource generation

This entails the training of staff and their deployment, the production of drugs and medical equipment, and the provision of facilities for health care. In the end, it is the combination of human and physical capital and consumables within the public and private sectors that is important. The combination of these different types of resources, known as the 'health care resource profile', varies widely between countries. For example, the US spends more than any other country on any resource input, with a particularly large amount for medical technology. Sweden has a large stock of human resources and beds, and together with Denmark, high spending on drugs. Mexico has a high ratio of physicians, while in contrast Thailand and South Africa have a low ratio of physicians. In South Africa, nurses greatly outnumber physicians. In Egypt and Mex-

ico, for example, the proportions are reversed.

Another resource is pharmaceuticals that represent up to 40% of government and private out-of-pocket expenditures in low-income countries (World Bank 1993, Govindaraj 1997). If expenditures on salaries are excluded, then pharmaceutical expenditure often dominates the public health budgets even in middle-income countries. In high-income countries drugs usually represent less than 10% of the costs of health services. The most efficient resource mix will vary over time and across countries, depending on relative prices among inputs, country-specific health needs and national priorities. But it is clear that there is considerable waste and inefficiency in most national health systems. A study of pharmaceuticals in Africa (Shaw and Elmendorf 1993) concluded that waste and inefficiency were so great in the procurement, storage, prescription and use of drugs that only about 12% of the total amount spent by governments actually resulted in the right type of treatment for a patient.

11.9.3 Financing

The third major function is financing. Global health care expenditures are estimated to have risen from 3% of total world income (GDP) in 1948 to 8% in 1997. The present cost of health service in the world corresponds to a total of around USD 2.5 trillion ($2 500 000 000 000). This makes health care one of the major economic sectors in the world.

The main purpose of financing is, of course, to pay for health care and to ensure access to health care for all individuals. The system of financing should ensure equitable access to health care for all citizens in a country. In order to do this, the financing system has to take care of three distinct financing functions: revenue collection, pooling of resources and purchasing health interventions. The five main sources of funds for revenue collection are (1) general taxation,

(2) compulsory health insurance, (3) voluntary health insurance, (4) out-of-pocket payment (user fees) and (5) donations. Most high-income countries rely heavily on either general taxation or compulsory social health insurance contributions. General taxation in the OECD countries on average accounts for more than 40 % of GDP. However, the corresponding figure in the low-income countries is on average less than 20 %. Therefore, tax revenues in low-income countries are usually not sufficient to finance necessary health care expenditures.

By necessity, the health systems in low-income countries rely to a high degree on out-of-pocket financing. This means that patients have to pay cash when they are sick, whether they need antibiotics or a caesarean section. For countries relying mainly on general taxation the ministry of finance manages the collection of money and the allocation to the ministry of health is performed through the government budgetary process. During the health care expansion phase of the 1970s and 1980s, many countries built up health care systems that required heavy government financing.

'Free' health care was declared the aim even in the poorest countries. This was the time when the belief in the state capability to finance and provide health care was at its peak. But in hindsight, we can now see that these countries, especially those in Africa, never acquired the capacity to finance the health care systems they had started to develop. Salaries fell to levels that were much less than the value of the drugs the staff was supposed to administer for free. A large proportion of the staff sold the drugs that should have been distributed for free or started to demand 'envelope money' as unofficial fees. In this way many public health services were unofficially privatised to a very high degree.

Pooling of resources is an insurance function, whereby the risk of having to pay for health care is borne by all the members of the pool and not by each contributor individually. In other words the healthy have to pay for the treatment of the sick. Pooling is essential to avoid catastrophic health expenditures in cases of serious illness. When people pay out-of-pocket, there is no pooling. When a poor woman needs a caesarean section, it becomes a catastrophe for the family economy. It should be noted that insurance systems do not imply that the rich will pay for the poor.

Purchasing involves the choice of method to pay the providers of health care. It has been shown, for example, that a fee-for-service system, in which patients pay the provider for each visit and service rendered, encourages the provision of unnecessary services. A major division can be made between systems that rely on prepayment and those that do not. Out-of-pocket payment is usually the most socially destructive way to finance for health service. Such systems are making the poor pay more in relation to their income than the rich. Health service fees expose people to the greatest financial risk and health service may save lives at the cost of pushing a family into poverty. Children may no longer go to school because their mother needed a caesarean section during the last delivery. Thus, the way revenues are collected largely determines the degree of equity of any health system. Here, WHO is unequivocal in its advocacy of prepayment as a means of protecting the poor, who otherwise might not be able to purchase health care when needed.

11.9.4 Stewardship

Stewardship means leadership through policy, regulation and co-ordination. It is a new notion in health policy. The concept itself has religious roots. In the Old Testament of the Bible, Joseph became Potiphar's and then Pharaoh's steward: the self-less servant who manages assets in the best interest of the master without owning them. In WHO's language, stewardship as 'the effective trusteeship of national health' is a major role of governments. Stewardship requires a long-term vision and influence, primarily by ministries of health. This role implies setting rules and ensuring their compliance by the public as well as the private sectors. Stewardship is both about providing the essential drugs free for the poor in the public sector and assuring that no fake drugs are sold in the private sector. Few countries have developed effective strategies to deal with the private sector in health care, making this area a priority in most countries.

With these factors included in the analysis, WHO also compares countries according to what they achieve as measured in health status, in their responsiveness to people's expectations and in their fairness of financing. A complex system for numeric measurement was developed and the first calculations in the World Health Report 2000 relied partly on very weak data. Yet, two main rankings were developed, the first one being for overall attainment or what WHO terms 'goodness' and 'fairness' combined. This was intended to reflect how well a health system achieves a long, disability-adjusted life expectancy, or a high level of responsiveness (or a high degree of equality in either or both) or a fair distribution of the financing burden. These factors were weighted after a survey of 1 000 respondents, so that health (disability-adjusted life expectancy) received half the weight, and responsiveness and fair financial contribution 25 % each.

The ranking of health attainment resulted in a list with the high-income countries all coming high up on the list, while the poorest countries are found at the bottom. What WHO terms performance, i.e. achievement relative to resources, is the ultimate measure of the analysis. In colloquial terms: 'who gets most bang for their buck'.

The ranking of performance thus gives a different ranking from that of attainment as described above, although the two measures tend to be quite closely associated. The rich countries still figure in the upper part of the table, and the poorest countries still end up far down the list.

In this ranking, France was number one, followed by Italy. Surprisingly, the Nordic countries were ranked relatively poorly: 11 (Iceland), 15 (Norway), 23 (Sweden), 31 (Finland) and 34 (Denmark). The United States ranked only number 37, despite spending far more per person for health care than any other country. Not surprisingly, Sierra Leone came last. But the uncertainty intervals were considerable.

This serious attempt to analyse the performance of health systems is a clear step forward. With its more inclusive definition of health systems, it comes closer to the actual determinants of health. But in the absence of sufficient quality data, efforts to rank countries were premature. The study (WHO 2000) was based on complex statistical analyses of hundreds of assumptions and values, interviews with thousands of people, including many WHO staff, and on assigning weights to the different parameters, which in the end were compressed into a few simple indices. The statistical basis for these complex calculations was obviously deficient, in particular for the poorest countries.

Some critics have referred to the high French and Italian rankings as the 'olive oil effect', the possible result of the renowned and presumably healthy Mediterranean diet, rather than as a function of the health system as such. Even with this broader definition, curative health services are given a heavy weight. For example, fairness in financing and responsiveness apply only to the curative part of the health system. It is likely that the emergence of new data will result in changes, possibly great changes, in the country rankings.

It is interesting to note that WHO in the yearbook of 2003 is returning to the primary health care concept from 1978 (WHO 2003). This is a more political than technical framework for health policy. It may take several years to generate the data that is needed to make the more evidence based assessments of health system performance that were suggested in the 2000 report. Annual publishing by WHO of national health accounts, that means the basic economic data about the health systems of all countries, will create a basis for such assessments.

11.10 Public and private health care

Today, the balance between public and private health care provision and financing is a major health policy issue in almost all countries. It is generally referred to as the issue of public/private mix. But in global health policy this is a debate of fairly recent origin. The Primary Health care Strategy from 1978 did not even mention private provision of health care. It was taken for granted that governments were the sole or main providers of health care. If two types of health care were discussed it was mostly regarding the concepts of traditional and modern medicine. However, this changed radically during the 1980s and 1990s. The World Bank and others pointed to 'government failures' such as bureaucratisation and inefficiencies in the public provision of health service. The suggested alternative was to introduce more market mechanisms in health care. Those arguing for health systems based on government provision and financing of services, such as those found in Sweden and the United Kingdom emphasised the 'market failures' associated with health markets. They claimed that market solutions that function in other sectors would result in market failures if applied in the health sector.

In essence, the three causes of market failure presented in Box 11.4 speak against viewing most parts of health care as a commodity to be bought and sold in the marketplace.

Box 11.4

Market failure

Market failure is a concept in economic theory. The background is the theory that a totally free market, in which suppliers and customers meet at the marketplace, is the most effective mechanism to make products and services available at prices customers are willing and able to pay. Economists recognise three situations where the free market is not the most effective mechanism to allocate resources and to decide what and how much to produce.

1 *Externalities* are effects, positive or negative, which occur outside the actual transaction. Immunisation against measles is a typical example of a health action with strong positive externalities. If I vaccinate my child, I protect not only my child but also my neighbours child and visitors children from contracting this potentially lethal disease. Society as a whole benefits from parents who choose to immunise their children against measles. In a pure free-market situation, this would lead to under-provision of this particular service. Consequently, measles vaccination presents a good case for government involvement.

2 *Public goods* are those products or services that cannot be divided and sold, and where the consumption by one individual does not prevent other individuals from enjoying the benefits. Clean air and defence are typical examples of public goods, and the eradication of a disease such as smallpox is another. Polio will never be eradicated if individuals are asked to buy immunisations for polio at market prices; the global community has to step in to ensure the benefits that will ensue for all of mankind to achieve the goal.

3 *Information asymmetry* occurs if the medical professional knows more about the need for and probable benefits from a certain treatment than the patient; the latter will then not be in the best position to assess whether the price for the service is what is worth paying.

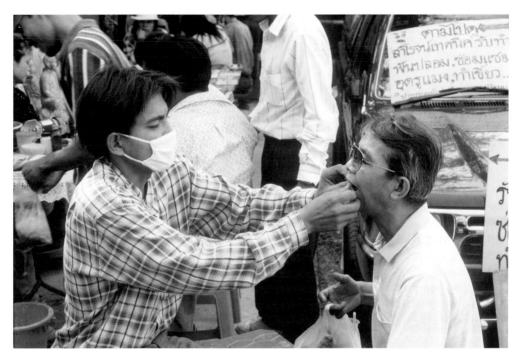

THAILAND, Bangkok. Street dentist.
© Jean-Léo Dugast/PHOENIX.

Even for the most hard-nosed neo-liberal economist, there is a clear case for government involvement in health care, in particular with regard to the financing and regulatory aspects. The public/private issue is often confusing, unless the differences between health services provision or health services financing is made clear. Examples are given in Table 11.3 (Newbrander 1992).

All kinds of public and private combinations are possible, and there are developments in each country in different directions. In many countries public provision of financing-dominated health care formerly tended to be sanctified, and it was seen as inappropriate to do business in this connection. Costs were seen as unimportant, and it was even considered unethical to introduce economic considerations in the choice of treatment and in the organisation of health services. The best possible care was supposed to be provided to all citizens. This attitude

contributed to several of the government failures.

In theory, the definitions of public and private should be clear. 'Public' refers to government ownership, and 'private' to everything else. In reality, the picture is more obscure. Government may involve public entities at different levels, from the national level down to the districts or municipalities. Shared ownership between public bodies and private interests is also possible. Former government staff may take over and collectively run former government clinics.

The private sector in itself has many faces. For-profit bodies, i.e. companies, own and run facilities in some countries for the purpose of making a profit. In other countries, religious societies or foundations may dominate private ownership of health facilities. Large not-for-profit organisations tend to act more like government bodies. Individual profit motives in the formally not-for-profit

Table 11.3 The components of public/private mix.

Financing	Provision		
	Public	Private	
		Not-for-profit	For-profit
Public	Free health care in a government facility	Government subsidy to a church hospital	Contracted private providers of free care
Private	User fees in a government hospital	Private insurance	Paying for surgery in a private hospital

Source: Adapted from Newbrander 1992.

sector may influence policies through what is known as 'rent-seeking'.

The international health debate has hitherto been dominated by discussions about governments role in the provision of health care. These discussions have often not reflected reality. The private sector tends to be more important in both the provision and financing of health services in low-income countries than in the high-income countries. In a country like China, 80 % of health financing is private. In most countries, between 30 and 90 % of total pharmaceutical spending comes from private sources. Traditional medicine is mostly a private activity and in some countries informal provision of services and sale of drugs dominates the government and officially registered private services.

Today, efforts are being made to find new and more effective relationships between the public and private sectors, e.g. in the form of contractual relationships or managed markets, with services of various kinds being contracted out to the private sector.

No one has been able or willing to provide a prescription for the role of the private sector that could be applied in different countries. Apart from historical political influences, the differences in culture, social and economic factors make for different solutions in different countries. But there appears to be one common conclusion: that although the private sector can complement public health provision and provide some types of service better, it cannot lead the health sector in a direction that will maxim-

ise its contribution to the health of the population.

The stewardship role of the government, including its regulatory institutions, becomes all-important in guiding the health system to maximum efficiency within each given context.

11.11 Is it possible to construct an effective health system?

There is no simple and clear guide of how to organise health systems. It is difficult, probably even impossible, to assess a health system in a scientific way and arrive at clear conclusions as to where it is better or worse. What is clear is that, with a public health budget of less than USD 10 per person per year, it is impossible to provide decent basic health service for all of the citizens in a country. And, indeed, today many low-income countries are to be found in this situation. A Minister of Health in one of Africa's poorest countries used to tell the allegory about a man that was trying to sleep during a cold night with a very small blanket (Box 11.5).

For countries spending a hundred times or more on their health care, it seems clear that they should be able to organise their health systems in such a way that all of their people have access to reasonable health care. But even in such cases, it is hard to come to any definite conclusions. And cer-

---

Box 11.5

Trying to sleep under a small blanket

It was a cold night. The man first covered his legs and feet with his small blanket, but he could not fall asleep because his head was too cold. He moved the blanket to cover his head but then his whole body started to shiver. He decided that it was wiser to place the blanket over his body, but in vain, his feet and head remained too cold to enable him to sleep.

In panic he then decided to stretch the blanket so that it covered his whole body. But the blanket was not elastic and his stretching resulted in him tearing the blanket into useless small pieces. With a number of useless minute pieces of blanket he suffered sleepless throughout the cold night.

An allegory about the available choices for a Minister of Health in an African low-income country.

---

tainly cultural and socio-economic variables have great significance for the appreciation of the services by the population. Nevertheless, the evidence seems to point to the following conclusions, as a preliminary guideline for policy-makers.

1 There is no set optimal ratio between public and private provision of health services; it varies depending on circumstances.
2 Governments have an important role to play as stewards of the health care system, including responsibility for regulation of private providers.
3 Equitable access to health care can only be achieved when the government takes a major responsibility for the financing of health care, raising revenue through taxation or through compulsory health insurance schemes.
4 Out-of-pocket payment for health care should be limited to a minimum. Prepayment is preferable to out of pocket payment. Pooling of resources is essential in order to distribute risks and avoid catastrophic health care costs.
5 Fee-for-service payment encourages overtreatment and unnecessary interventions.
6 Fragmented purchasing functions create inefficiency.

References and suggested further reading

Anonymous. A barefoot doctor's manual (Translation into English) Philadelphia: Running Press; 1977.

Berman P (ed). Health Sector Reform in Developing Countries. Making Health Development Sustainable. Boston: Harvard School of Public Health; 1995.

Creese A, Floyd K, Alban A, Guinness L. Cost-effectiveness of HIV/AIDS interventions in Africa: a systematic review of the evidence. Lancet 2002;359:1635–43.

Culyer AJ, Newhouse JP (eds). Handbook of Health Economics. Elesvier; 1999.

Dubos R. Mirage of Health. Utopias, Progress and Biological Change. New York: Harper Colophon Books; 1979.

Evans RG, Barer ML, Marmor TR (eds). Why are some people healthy and others not? The determinants of health of populations. New York: Aldine de Gruyter; 1994, p. 201.

Goodman CA, Coleman PG, Mills AJ. Cost-effectiveness of malaria control in sub-Saharan Africa. Lancet 1999;354:378–85.

Govindaraj R, Chellaraj G, Murray CJL. Health expenditures in Latin America and the Caribbean. Soc Sci Med 1997; 44:157–169.

Gwatkin DR, Guillot M, Heuveline P. The burden of disease among the global poor. Lancet 1999;354:586–9.

Jolly R (ed). Jim Grant – UNICEF visionary. Jim Grant foundation; 2001.

Koop CE, Pearson CE, Schwarz MR (eds.). Critical Issues in Global Health. San Francisco: Jossey-Bass, A Wiley Company; 2001.

Lee K, Buse K, Fustukian S (eds). Health Policy in a Globalising World. Cambridge: Cambridge University Press; 2002.

McKeown T. The Role of Medicine, Basil Blackwell; 1979.

Nitayarumphong S (ed). Health care Reform. At the frontier of research and policy decisions. Bangkok: Office of Health care Reform, Ministry of Public Health; 1997.

Newbrander W, Parker D. The public and private sectors in health: economic issues. International Journal of Health Planning and Management 1992;1:37–49.

Powell F, Wesser AF. Health care Systems in Transition. SAGE Publications; 1999.

Lees DS. Health through choice. Institute of Economic Affairs, Hobart Paper no. 14, London; 1961.

Sachs JD. Report of the Commission on Macroeconomics and Health. 2001. www.cmhealth.org

McPake B, Mills A. What can we learn from international comparisons of health systems and health system reforms? Bulletin of the World Health Organisation 2000; 78:811–820.

Murray CJL, Evans DB. Health System Performance Assessment – debates, methods and empiricism. WHO; 2003.

Roemer MI. National Health Systems of the World, Volume I. The countries. Oxford University Press; 1991.

Roemer, MI. National Health Systems of the World, Volume II. The issues. Oxford University Press; 1993.

Saltman RB, Ferroussier-Davis O. The concept of stewardship in health policy. Bulletin of the World Health Organisation, 2000;78:732–39.

Sachs J. Report of the commission on macroeconomics and health. WHO; 2001.

Shaw RP, Elmendorf AE. Better health in Africa. Experiences and lessons learned. World Bank; 1994.

Townsend P, Davidson N. Inequalities in Health (The Black Report). Harmondsworth: Penguin Books; 1982.

Victora CG, Wagstaff A, Schellenberg JA, Gwatkin D, Claeson M, Habicht JP. Applying an equity lens to child health and mortality: more of the same is not enough. Lancet 2003;362:233–41.

Walt G. Health Policy: an introduction to process and power, London: Zed Books; 1994.

Wildavsky, A. The art and craft of policy analysis. MacMillan Press; 1979.

World Bank. World Development Report. Investing in health. Oxford University Press; 1993.

World Bank. Better Health in Africa: Experience and Lessons Learned. The International Bank for Reconstruction and Development, Washington, DC: 1994.

WHO. Primary Health care. Report of the International Conference on Primary health care, Alma-Ata, USSR, 6–12 September 1978.

WHO. World Health Report 2000. Health Systems: Improving Performance.

WHO World Health Report 2003.

12 Global health collaboration

For older readers the yellow vaccination certificate that not very long ago had to accompany any intercontinental travel was the most visible example of international health collaboration. The certificate with the logo of the World Health Organization, stands for one very obvious justification for co-operation in health. Preventing the spread of infectious diseases was one of the original reasons and remains a major reason for countries around the world to work together in the field of health.

To some the eradication of smallpox in 1977 under the leadership of WHO, the successful work of UNICEF to reduce children's deaths and suffering through cost-effective interventions and protection of breastfeeding, and the enormous power of the World Bank, to guide countries' expenditure on health care stand as visible examples of multinational health collaboration over the last decades. For others membership in organisations such as the Red Cross or one of the many faith-based organisations that are heavily involved in health service all over the world, may provide the framework for a personal involvement in global health collaboration.

Sometimes these efforts appear important or even vital—such as the teams that are sent out to deal with outbreaks of Ebola or the Severe Atypical Respiratory Syndrome (SARS). In other cases the bureaucratic processes in international organisations or doubtful policies merit criticism. What merits most critique is that the world has not managed to do more to reduce the sufferings from diseases.

This chapter provides an overview of the need for global health collaboration and reviews the main current players. An empha-sis is put on what previously was called aid relationships, nowadays termed international development co-operation. But it should be remembered that much of these collaborations originate from self-interest such as the need to combat infections in other countries. This may however not be a bad motivation. Other forms of collaboration may also be motivated by reasons other than altruism, such as a quest for profit or political influence.

12.1 The role of global health collaboration

The health sector today represents one of the largest sectors in the world economy, having a total turnover that is today around two and a half trillion US dollars and it employs some 35 million people worldwide (table 12.1). The health sector constitutes almost 10 % of the world economy.

Out of the 6 billion people in the world 5 million live in low and middle income countries. These 5 billions suffer from 93 % of the global burden of disease but have only access to 11 % of the total resources for health care. More than 40 % of the world's health care resources are spent in the United States. In 2001 the health care spending in the US accounted for an unprecedented 14.1 % of the total US economy. This means an average of over USD 5 000 per person, which is some 500 times more than the amount spent on health care per person in the poorest countries in the world. The most important message in this chapter is that the entire international health collaboration only accounts for 6 billion USD. Even in the low-income countries the interna-

Table 12.1 Summary of the economic size of the health sector in world economy.

	Total sum in current USD	Percent of the above
Total global income	30 000 000 000 000	
Global health care costs	2 400 000 000 000	8 %
Health care in low & middle-income countries	106 000 000 000	4 %
Global development aid health care	6 000 000 000	6 %

Source. Commission for Macro Economics and Health, WHO 2001.

tional contribution to the health sector is only 10 % of the total health spending. The relative insignificance of this contribution in relation to total health spending in the poorest countries, tells us that by far the greatest share of the costs of health care is borne by the individuals and countries themselves. This is true for practically all countries, and particularly the large ones, such as China and India, where external support accounts for only a minute share of their total health care costs. In China the international health collaboration only accounts for less than 1 % of the expenditure in the health sector. (Pouiller 2002).

For all of Sub-Saharan Africa, excluding South Africa, 20 % of health expenditure comes from external sources. There are a few countries in Africa where the contributions from external agencies and organisations account for a greater share of total health care costs. An extreme example is Mozambique, where foreign aid accounts for 70 % of the health budget.

However, the flow of money between countries is likely to have a greater significance than one might think. The aid funds are not obligated beforehand for salaries or other fixed costs, and can therefore be used more flexibly and for strategic purposes. They can also help to propagate new ideas, to finance pilot projects and to disseminate and try out ideas and solutions across national borders. These aspects enhance the value of the international flow of funds in relation to ordinary health budgets. It has been suggested that their role in influencing priorities and policies is greater than the figures may lead us to believe.

The overall official development assistance (ODA) in the world has continued to fall, by almost 20 % in real terms, from USD 62 billion to USD 53 billion since 1992. Today, it has reached an unprecedented low of 0.22 % of the combined national product of the high-income countries that contribute money to international development assistance. This statistics is compiled by Organisation for Economic Co-operation and Development (OECD) that has a Development Assistance Committee (DAC) providing statistics on international development assistance.[1] The share of the health and population sectors has risen from 7 % in 1990 to 11 % in 1997 (Musgrove 2001, DAC 2002).

When it comes to the health services as such, certain areas have traditionally been popular for donors, such as programmes against leprosy or blindness as well as hospital constructions. Today external assistance tends to prioritise preventive rather than curative programmes, rural areas rather than cities, and specific interventions rather than general reinforcement of systems. Highly visible actions, for example the initiative to eradicate polio, have been particularly attractive areas for donor financing, while it has been more difficult to get support for general health systems infrastructure, except from the development banks. At present support for HIV drugs is getting considerable funding in spite of a lower cost effectiveness compared to many other possible health interventions.

[1]   www.oecd.org/dac

12.1.1 History

Modern efforts to deal with epidemics can be traced back to the City of Venice in 1423. In that year the city established a permanent quarantine station for infected crews and goods on naval vessels. Ships arriving in Venice from infected ports were required to sit at anchor for forty days before landing. This practice, called quarantine, was derived from the Latin word *quadraginta*, meaning forty. The station was placed on an island with a monastery called "San Lazaretto Nuovo" outside Venice. The quarantine station became known as in "lazaretto" and this word developed a wider meaning. "Lassarett" is the word for public hospital in Swedish and in many other languages. More far-reaching measures, in the form of pest houses, mass house quarantines and *cordons sanitaires* around metropolitan areas, were taken to prevent the spread of bubonic plague in Europe in the 1630s.

Modern health collaboration between countries is a consequence of the first European outbreaks of cholera starting in London 1832.[1] Cholera constituted the immediate reason for the convocation of the first international sanitary conference in Paris in 1851. But it took almost 40 years and a number of international health conferences to produce the first agreement: the International Sanitary Convention, in 1892.

Another international convention dealing with plague was adopted five years later, but then it took only a few more years for the first structures for a continuous international co-operation in health to be established. It was the International Sanitary Bureau for the Americas, the forerunner of today's Pan American Health Organization (PAHO), which was founded in 1902 in Washington DC, and the Office International d'Hygiène Publique (OIHP), which was established by eight countries in Paris in 1907. The latter remained even when the League of Nations was created and set up its Health Section in Geneva, which was active

in the period between the two world wars. The international sanitary convention was revised in 1926 to include provisions against smallpox and typhus, and in the 1930s a new sanitary convention for aerial navigation came into force.

During the Second World War the international health work was neglected. However, in 1945 the United Nations Conference on International Organisation in San Francisco unanimously approved a proposal by Brazil and China to convene an International Conference of members of the United Nations with a view to establishing a new, autonomous, international health organisation.

The ensuing International Health Conference that was held in New York in the summer of 1946 approved, on its final day, the constitution of the new World Health Organization, replacing the pre-existing international health organisations. On 7 April 1948, a date that is now marked as the World Health Day, the WHO's Constitution came into force.

As will be described below WHO has largely focused on reducing the global burden of diseases with a focus on the poorer countries. The traditional reasons for health co-operation across borders, such as containment of infectious diseases and functions to make international comparisons such as a unified disease classification, are still valid. But the global environment is changing faster than ever before, providing new opportunities as well as posing new threats that require new forms of collaboration. As this chapter shows there is a growing number of international health organisations and initiatives.

Many nations now face the double burden of both tackling the largely preventable and curable health problems affecting their poor, while, at the same time facing the new disease burden associated with ageing populations. In addition, the health problems of development, such as pollution and altered lifestyles, entail new health threats.

Globalisation and increased international trade expose people to health risks that stem

[1]   www.ph.ucla.edu/epi/snow/snowbook

from causes that are trans-national in nature, such trade in food and hazardous products, and environmental changes in climate, as well as air and water quality. Trade is important for health not only due to trade in health-related goods but also with regard to trade in health services and migration of trained health staff. The consequences of IT and the Internet have only begun to emerge. There are health risks from unregulated sales of pharmaceuticals and other products over the Internet, as well as untapped opportunities for health systems to become more responsive and effective and for health education to have greater impact.

The future is characterised by increasingly complex health challenges, globalisation and increasing interdependence, a dramatic increase in ease of communications, a vastly expanded traffic in goods, services and persons across borders, and the emergence of new players in the international health arena.

12.1.2 A classification of organisations

A whole new range of 'players' are entering the international health arena, on top of the proliferation of UN organs, multilateral development banks (MDBs) and national agencies for international development cooperation. Although not semantically correct the latter are often known as 'bilateral agencies'. Though USAID in the US, DFID in U.K., Norad in Norway and Sida in Sweden may have bilateral agreements with other countries they are definitely national agencies that are responsible to their respective governments.

Regional international organisations such as the EU are becoming more important as are the philanthropic foundations based largely in the US. The result is a complex web of players and public-private partnerships, with sometimes confusing and overlapping mandates and functions. These organisations come in many shapes and forms. For clarity it may be useful to structure them in categories as show in box 12.1.

In reality, the situation is not as clear-cut as indicated above. There may be combinations, for example, an NGO working on a regional or international basis. An ongoing 'globalisation' of NGOs has yielded the term INGOs, for International Non- Governmen-

---

Box 12.1

Categories of organisations with international health activities

International
Organisations based on several governments, such as those belonging to the UN family. Can be sub-divided into UN programmes and funds, and UN specialised agencies. The programmes and funds are not member organisations with assessed contributions from member states. Used to be called multilateral organisations.

Regional
Organisations based on collaboration between governments in one geographical area.

National
Government agencies in one country that deal directly (one-to-one) with other governments in bilateral co-operation agreements.

Non-governmental
Private, not-for-profit and non-governmental organisations (NGOs) that may be national or international. They may either be member organisations (with individuals as members) or umbrella organisations (with other organisations as members).

Philanthropic foundations
Expression used mainly in the US for institutions handling considerable private donations for international development.

Industry & corporations
For-profit entities.

---

tal Organisations. National governments have no control of the INGOs that mostly also stand independent and outside democratic control. They are most often registered as a charity foundation in each country and operate under the leadership of self-nominated boards.

Industry is usually taken to be private, but there are also companies with a greater or lesser degree of government ownership. Many national agencies also commission the implementation of their bilateral collaboration with low and middle-income countries to private consulting companies. NGOs may be organised in different ways and classified according to the laws of different countries. There are also institutes and organisations that are semi- or partly owned or influenced by governments, although appearing as NGOs. The term 'civil society organisations' (CSOs) is sometimes used in a broad sense to include NGOs as well as looser networks and other types of non-state collaboration.

12.2 International organisations

12.2.1 World Health Organization, WHO (UN specialised agency)

Established 1948
192 member states
Annual budget: Regular budget USD 428 million, extra-budgetary resources USD 690 million (annual average of biannual budget 2002 to 2003)
Staff: 3,800
Web site: www.who.int
World Health Report available on-line at: http://www.who.int/whr

WHO is the truly global health organisation for the world's nations. It is the specialised agency within the UN system that is entrusted to handle health and medical issues. It has, according to its Constitution, the function to act as the directing and co-ordinating authority on international health

work. It is also one of the largest specialised agencies in the United Nations family.

WHO's role as a specialised agency is based on the United Nations Charter and its objectives, as expressed in Article 55 as a pledge to promote solutions of international, economic, social, health, and related problems.

WHO's founding fathers—and it was, indeed, an exclusively male club at the time—provided the organisation with a Constitution which defined health more broadly than ever before, in the now famous words:

> "Health is a state of complete physical, mental and social well-being, not merely the absence of disease or infirmity."

The organisation that was set up was provided with a headquarters in Geneva and six regional offices: in Alexandria (recently moved to Cairo), Brazzaville, Copenhagen, Manila, New Delhi and Washington. Its highest policy-making body was determined to be the World Health Assembly, WHA, which consists of representatives of all the member states and which usually meets in Geneva in May every year. The Assembly elects an Executive Board with 32 members, representing the various regional groupings. The day-to-day affairs of the WHO are handled by the Secretariat and tasks are distributed between the headquarters, the regional offices and country offices in low-income countries, which are headed by the World Health Organization representatives, known as WRs.

In 1998, WHO celebrated its 50th anniversary. The organisation could then look back upon a period of unprecedented health gains in the countries of the world, including the first ever eradication of a disease pathogen from the earth (the smallpox virus). However, it was also a period of major setbacks, such as the failed attempt to eradicate malaria, and even more importantly, a period that saw an increasing disparity in health between the richest and the poorest countries.

The backbone of WHO's finances are the assessed contributions which could be seen as the 'membership' fees from the member states. Applying the UN scale of assessment, each country has to pay an amount in proportion to its gross national product. These contributions make up the regular budget, which finances the basic structure and work of WHO.

The regular budget is allocated with roughly one-third to global and interregional work, including the cost of the headquarters with the remainder divided among the regions. On top of that come the extrabudgetary funds, which are voluntary contributions for specific purposes from member states and, for that matter, from organisations or even private individuals. The vast majority of these contributions originate from the development co-operation budgets of the rich countries. A problem has been the policy of zero growth of the regular budget that was established by the World Health Assembly in the early 1980s (Vaughan et al., 1996). Therefore, the organisation has had to rely increasingly on extrabudgetary contributions. These extra-budgetary resources have in recent years come to exceed the regular budget and now constitute well over 60 % of the funds made available for WHO.

Together with the United States, the Nordic countries were for many years the major contributors of extra-budgetary funds, which were channelled to some of the major programmes of WHO, such as the programmes for research on human reproduction and on tropical diseases. Today, other countries, such as Japan and Italy, have also become important donors to WHO. Extrabudgetary funds have been channelled predominantly to large and vertically managed programmes in the areas of disease control, health promotion and human reproduction. By contrast, about 70 % of the regular budget expenditure has been for organisational expenses and for the support of programmes in the area of health systems.

It should be remembered that WHO is not primarily a donor or technical assistance agency for the poorest countries. Its main role is to direct international health work and to set global standards for health actions. These functions are generally referred to as the normative functions. WHO also has an important role, as foreseen in the Constitution, to co-operate with governments to reinforce national health programmes and to develop and transfer appropriate health technology and information.

Among today's priority programmes, the Roll Back Malaria Initiative (RBM) and the Tobacco Free Initiative (TFI) are prominent among continued efforts in areas such as tropical diseases and tuberculosis, injury prevention, non-communicable diseases and immunisation, including polio eradication, for which WHO is the lead agency.

The World Health Assembly in May 2003 unanimously adopted the Framework Convention on Tobacco Control which is the first of its kind, further strengthening WHO's role in global health development. The International Agency for Research on Cancer in Lyon is closely affiliated with WHO.

It should also be mentioned that WHO has strengthened its capacity to analyse and work with health policies in a broad sense, including economic aspects—which became dominated by the World Bank in the last decade. There is also an effort to connect WHO's work to an analysis of the relationship between poverty and health, and between health and poverty.

A new step in this direction was taken in 2001, through the work of the Commission on Macroeconomics and Health, chaired by Jeffrey Sachs. The commission has come far from the ideological vision of WHO's Primary Health Care Strategy in 1978, although it basically discusses the same issues. The argument for health is no longer only that health is a goal in itself but also that health is an important factor for economic growth. The commission calculated the overall additional resource needs for the low and middle-income countries to reach the millennium development goals (MDGs). This was estimated to be possible with an increase of their budgetary outlays for health with 1 % of GNP by 2007, and 2 % of GNP by 2015 relative to current levels, and to increase donor spending for health to USD 27 billion in 2007 and USD 38 billion in 2015. These calculations were based on a cost for a package of essential health interventions of USD 34 per capita, a modest sum compared to the more than USD 2 000 per capita expenditures in the high-income countries. The additional sum needed from abroad constitute only about 0.1 % of the GNP of the high-income countries. It would, however, constitute a considerable increase in relation to what is today spent in the least developed countries. From a present total of USD 13 per capita, of which public spending is USD 7 to a minimum of 34 USD per capita (Sachs 2001). In its 2003 annual report WHO connects this analysis with a revival of the principles of the primary health care strategy (WHO 2003).

It is inherently difficult for an organisation such as WHO to set clear priorities. Member states have different interests and biases for different types of activities. The United States has always been a strong supporter of technological interventions such as immunisation and eradication programmes. Russia has a particular interest in chronic diseases. The Nordic countries have often advocated stronger action by WHO in areas such as pharmaceuticals, alcohol and tobacco, while countries with strong industrial interests in these areas have tended to resist such actions. Thus, the Nordic countries were instrumental in the development of the Code of Marketing of Breastmilk Substitutes in the early 1980s, while the only country to vote against this resolution to protect breastfeeding was the United States.

In spite of its broad definition of health, WHO has in the past tended to view health from a predominantly medical perspective. This could possibly be traced to the almost total dominance of medical doctors among the professional staff. Under the Brundtland administration (1998 to 2003), a change began to appear. It is still too early to say to what extent the new directions will bear fruit. Clearly the organisation is moving into areas that are more or less new to it. But if health is accepted as a concept that stretches beyond the biomedical sphere, then these changes are necessary, and indeed overdue.

In July 2003 Dr. Jong-wok Lee from South Korea succeeded Dr. Gro Harlem Brundtland as Director General of WHO. He has particularly committed himself to increasing the country focus of the organisation, to integrate specific disease programmes into a comprehensive effort to strengthen health systems and to work towards the achievement of the Millennium Development Goals. However, the major new initiative, launched in December 2003, has been the very medically oriented so-called three by five initiative; an effort to ensure drug treatment for three million AIDS victims in the developing world by 2005 (WHO 2003).

12.2.2 United Nations Children's Fund, UNICEF (UN fund)

Founded in 1946
Fund under UNDP, no members.
Executive board with 41 members representing governments, elected by ECOSOC
Annual budget: USD 1,218 million (2001), of which USD 336 million for direct health activities
Staff: around 6 000, 85 % of which located in the field offices
Web site: www.unicef.org

With its special mandate to work with children, UNICEF is a unique organisation. In the very beginning, the mandate was specifically to help children in war-torn Europe during the bitter winter of 1946/7. Its original acronym was ICEF, for the International Children's Emergency Fund. When it was due to close down in 1950, nations from the developing world mounted an effort to save it, and succeeded. It then became the United Nation's Children's Fund, but was given the acronym UNICEF.

There is little doubt that UNICEF is the best-known member of the UN family. This is because it has a high media profile, with a well-developed 'marketing' function. UNICEF has an organisation that reaches out to all countries through its national committees, and it has consistently worked with problems where its impact can be measured and demonstrated. The organisation was awarded the Nobel Peace Price in 1965.

With James Grant as its Executive Director between 1983 and 1995, UNICEF made a strong investment in health relative to its two other main sector activities, education and water/sanitation. In its promotion of the Child Survival Revolution in the 1980s and early 1990s, UNICEF's health activities focused strongly on two particular technical interventions: oral rehydration (ORS) to treat diarrhoea, and immunisation.

UNICEF is organised with headquarters in New York and eight regional offices, which have a more technical role, relative to the WHO regional offices. UNICEF's presence is particularly strong in low and middle-income countries, with representation in over 125 countries, with both international and national employees. The supply division of UNICEF, located in the Freeport of Copenhagen, effectively procures a variety of products for developing countries, especially drugs and vaccines. From a very small and modest office in this major Danish port UNICEF procures 40 per cent of the world's doses of vaccine for children.

A special feature of UNICEF is the existence of national committees for the organisation. The main role of these committees is to inform the general public about UNICEF and its work, to raise awareness and interest in children's issues, and to collect money for the organisation. As a UN fund, UNICEF relies wholly on voluntary contributions. The United States has always been a strong supporter of UNICEF and is the largest contributor in financial terms. The Nordic countries are also important contributors on a per capita basis. Out of UNICEF's total income, close to 64 % originates from governments, and the remainder from private contributions, mainly through the national committees and the sale of UNICEF greeting cards and other products.

In the early 1980s, a few years after the primary health care concept was launched, the competing concept of selective health interventions was developed. The essence of this strategy was to focus on a few essential health interventions in situations where a more comprehensive solution might not be within reach. UNICEF immediately grasped this idea and began a strong push for what it termed GOBI, an acronym standing for growth monitoring, oral rehydration, breastfeeding and immunisation.

After an immediate clash with WHO, which was promoting a broader vision of primary health care, both parties reached an agreement. This agreement included that UNICEF broadened its initially narrow GOBI approach to include three F's: female education, food supplements and family planning. WHO made adjustments and gave its wholehearted support to the interventions advocated by UNICEF that eventually became quite successful during the 1980s.

The explicit link made by UNICEF between operations and advocacy for children has probably been a contributing factor behind its successes. It seems clear that UNICEF's critique has helped to mediate the Structural Adjustment Programmes of the International Monetary Fund in the direction of more protection of the social sectors, a policy called 'Adjustment with a Human Face'. In recent years the advocacy function has developed in the direction of children's rights. Children in war situations have been of particular concern to UNICEF, including those affected by landmines or psychologically traumatised by experiences of armed conflicts.

UNICEF's publications contain a wealth of information about children, as well as annually updated statistics. The State of the World's Children, which is published annually on 8 December, is a particularly useful publication that 20 years ago initiated a systematic monitoring of health and social development in all the countries of the world.

12.2.3   United Nations Population Fund, UNFPA (UN fund)

Established 1969
Annual budget: USD 396 million (2001)
Staff: About 1 000
Web site: www.unfpa.org

Demographic statistics have always been part of the work of the United Nations, which has a specialised population division in its New York headquarters for that purpose. However, the concern of the rapidly growing world population that started to emerge in the 1950s, and the consequent interest in family planning activities was for a long time too politically sensitive an issue for the United Nations. Thus, it was not until 1969 that the United Nations Fund for Population Activities, UNFPA (today United Nations Population Fund), was created. UNFPA is a fund comprised solely of voluntary contributions, working under the auspices of the UNDP. UNFPA's mandate is fourfold:

1   to build knowledge and capacity to respond to needs in population and family planning;
2   to promote awareness of population problems;
3   to assist developing countries, on request, to deal with their population problems;
4   to play a leading role in the UN system to co-ordinate projects in population.

In its early years, UNFPA focused strongly on support for family planning programmes, in addition to its population statistics work. Some of its activities, especially its large-scale support for the population programme in China that had coercive aspects, have been heavily criticised. Among other things, this resulted in the total withdrawal of US funding in 1985, the US having previously been the largest contributor to UNFPA.

In later years, and especially after the International Conference on Population and Development (ICPD) in Cairo in 1994, which was organised by UNFPA, the organisation has become active in a broad range of Sexual and Reproductive Health issues.

12.2.4   United Nations Development Programme, UNDP (UN programme)

The major technical co-operation programme of the United Nations
Open to all members of the specialised agencies and commissions
Founded in 1965
Annual budget: USD 283 million (average of 2002–2003)
Staff: 5 300
Web site: www.undp.org

United Nations Development Programme is the major organisation dealing with development issues in the UN system. It works under the auspices of the Economic and Social Council, ECOSOC, of the central UN administration. UNDP is the world's largest voluntarily funded international technical assistance organisation.

UNDP's overriding priority is poverty eradication. The main activities today are human resources and institutional development. The organisation does not generally deal with specific health issues, although it is an active partner in some of WHO's special programmes, especially in the programme for Research and Training in Tropical Diseases (TDR). It is also a major partner in UNAIDS (see below).

UNDP's history has been marked by criticism for weak performance and by recurrent funding crises. However, with offices in 132 countries, it does have a special role in co-ordinating UN activities. This role may become more important with the new mechanisms for UN agency collaboration, such as

UNDAF (United Nations Development Assistance Framework).

UNDP annually produces the Human Development Report[1], which in recent years has featured ranking lists of countries according to their general development status and not just their economic power. This Human Development Index has become well known in large parts of the world. UNDP has been given a special role to co-ordinate the UN effort to monitor progress towards the Millennium Development Goals and to assist member countries to set and monitor their own development goals.

12.2.5 World Bank, including IDA

Usually known as the World Bank, WB
Established: 1945
Owned by its member countries, which have voting rights according to the size of their contributions.
Annual budget: Disbursements of USD 1 046 million for health (1997)
Web site: www.worldbank.org

The World Bank group, or as it also is called, the Bretton Wood institutions, originated in 1944, and developed in the aftermath of the Second World War. Today, this group consists of five associated institutions with the International Bank for Reconstruction and Development (IBRD) and the International Development Association (IDA) being the major ones. The term 'the World Bank' is often loosely used to include the IDA.

IBRD's aims are to promote sustainable economic development and to reduce poverty, primarily by providing loans at basically commercial interest rates. Borrowing on the ordinary financial markets finances IBRD. Obviously, the bank's activities have to be focused on infrastructure and on economically viable projects. IBRD only lends money to countries that are considered to be creditworthy, i.e. able to pay back their loans. This principle excludes the poorest countries, as

well as some others. IBRD's cumulative lending as of mid-1999 had reached USD 454 billion.

IDA's goal is to reduce poverty in low-income countries. IDA is different from the WB, as it is financed by grants from donor countries, which are replenished every three years. IDA lends money at heavily subsidised rates, through what are known as 'soft loans'. The real value of an IDA loan approaches an outright grant.

The focus of IDA operations is on the poorest countries—those with a per capita income of less than USD 1,500 and not considered creditworthy for commercial loans. In practice, the limit is lower, around USD 930. Above that limit there are a number of countries that are eligible both for IDA and IBRD loans and above that category there are countries that are eligible only for IBRD loans. Countries with a per capita income above USD 5,445 will not receive any support from the World Bank group. Countries may 'graduate' from one category to another. Thus, China was removed from the list of eligible countries for both IBRD and IDA loans and moved into the category of 'only IBRD loans' on 30 June 1999.

With the exception of 'population projects', which emphasised family planning activities, the World Bank did not enter the health field for a long time. Many countries have also thought that it would be wrong to borrow money for health care purposes. However, this has now changed. Since the early 1980s, the Bank has become more and more involved in the health and social sectors. Today, it is the most important player in the international financing of health services in low and middle-income countries.

The Bank has also become more active in health policy issues, as marked by the publication in 1993 of its annual World Development Report under the theme: 'Investing in Health'. This publication has been hailed as a landmark report. For the first time it employed a combination of burden-of-disease and cost-effectiveness arguments to propose

---

[1] www.undp.org/hdr2003

a health policy agenda for countries in varying circumstances.

The World Bank has been heavily criticised for its support of the Structural Adjustment Programmes (SAPs) that the International Monetary Fund (IMF) imposed on countries as a condition for lending money to support or save their macroeconomic stability. The SAPs involved a requirement to cut down on government expenditures, often in the social sector, thereby hurting the poor most. Such criticism has also been levelled by other UN agencies. UNICEF produced a report entitled 'Adjustment with a Human Face', advocating structural reforms which would not have such a negative effect on the poor.

Gradually the Bank has listened to the critique, and the adjustment programmes have been modified in order to better protect the poor. At the end of the 1990s the term 'heavily indebted poor countries', HIPC, was coined in connection with the emerging discussions on debt relief. The idea of this is that, instead of having to repay excessive debts, countries will instead finance essential social services, as agreed with the creditors through what are known as Poverty Reduction Strategy Papers, PRSP. This process is still in an early stage, but in some countries, such as Tanzania, considerable amounts of local funds have been injected into the health sector through the debt relief process.

12.2.6 UNAIDS (UN co-sponsored programme)

> *Established 1996*
> *Headquarters in Geneva*
> *Annual budget: around USD 30 million*
> *Staff: over 250*
> *Web site: www.unaids.org*

When the threat of HIV/AIDS became a reality in the mid 1980s, WHO established a unit to deal with the pandemic, the Global Programme on AIDS (GPA), and launched a Global AIDS Strategy. Other UN organisations started their own AIDS initiatives, although, as commonly occurs, the co-ordination of policies, strategies and support activities rapidly became a problem. With time it was found that HIV/AIDS, as a threat to health, concerned many sectors in society outside the health sector, which so far has not been in a position to provide a cure for the disease. Thus, it was thought that HIV/AIDS, rather than remaining the responsibility of the health sector, as a WHO programme, it should be a joint responsibility within the UN system.

After a lengthy investigation, it was finally agreed in 1996 to dismantle the old structures and establish a new, joint, co-sponsored UN programme, the Joint United Nations Programme on HIV/AIDS, bringing together six agencies: WHO, UNDP, UNICEF, UNFPA, UNESCO and the World Bank, today expanded by two more UN organisations.

The aim of this programme, entitled UN-AIDS, is to lead, strengthen and support an expanded response aimed at preventing HIV transmission and alleviating the impact of the epidemic. Four objectives have been set to fulfil its role:

- to foster an expanded national response, particularly in developing countries;
- to promote strong commitment by governments to an expanded response to HIV/AIDS;
- to strengthen and co-ordinate UN action on HIV/AIDS at the global and national levels;
- to identify, develop, and advocate international best practice.

UNAIDS has been successful in lowering the prices on antiretroviral drugs and on improving the monitoring of the HIV pandemic. Regarding the main task to curb the epidemic through preventive measures the challenge remains.

12.2.7   World Trade Organisation, WTO

Established 1995 as a successor to GATT
Main objective: to help international trade to
flow smoothly, freely, fairly and predictably.
More than 130 member countries
Annual budget: USD 80 million
Secretariat based in Geneva with 500 staff.
Web site: www.wto.org

Outside the UN family, the World Trade Organisation, WTO, in its aim to reduce barriers to trade, is becoming increasingly important in dealing with trade in health-related
goods and in products that can influence
health. In the Doha agreement of 2001, it
was agreed that developing countries might
obtain patented drugs of particular public
health importance (especially for HAART
treatment of HIV/AIDS) on special conditions, through what is known as parallel import or compulsory licensing. This is to off-
set the effects of the current rules on intellectual property rights in the world trading
system, knows as TRIPS (trade-related aspects of intellectual property rights) that
makes patented drug inaccessible to the
poor in the world.

12.2.8   Other international organisations

To deal in detail with all the principal organisations in international health lies beyond
the scope of this book. However, it should
be mentioned that a large number of other
organisations besides those mentioned
above carry out activities with a direct or indirect impact on health. Within the UN system, the Food and Agriculture Organisation,
FAO, is concerned with food supply and
food safety aspects, and with improving the
conditions of rural people, and the International Labour Organisation, ILO, is concerned with workers' issues and safety at
work. A substantial number of the existing
182 ILO conventions and 190 recommendations have dealt with issues related to
health. The International Atomic Energy
Agency, IAEA, has developed a number of

conventions and codes dealing with nuclear
safety, with particular relevance to the protection of public health.

The United Nations Environmental Programme, UNEP, deals with environmental
matters of obvious concern to health, while
the United Nations High Commissioner for
Refugees has a mandate that encompasses
health for refugees. The UN Commissioner
for Human Rights is becoming increasingly
important as rights issues gain prominence
on the health agenda. The United Nations
Educational, Scientific and Cultural Organisation, UNESCO, deals with the area of research and science, with a particular emphasis on biomedical science.

12.3 Regional organisations

Examples of regional organisations involved
in health co-operation include the regional
development banks (MDBs), which have increased their lending for health projects
with a method of operation that resembles
the World Bank group.

The UN regional economic commissions,
one for each continent, also have a role to
play, albeit a minor one in health.

One of the particular aims of The European Union is the protection of public
health within the Community. It encourages co-operation between the Member
States in the field of health. It comprises one
of the larger development co-operation
agencies under its Development Directo-
rate-General, although it is heavily criticised
for inefficiency and bureaucratic procedures. This has provided an average of USD
400 million in health aid per year to low-income countries.

The member states of the Organisation of
African Unity, established in 1963, and the
African Economic Union, established under
the auspices of OAU, have an agreement to
promote and increase co-operation in the
field of health.

12.4 National agencies

Most high-income countries are involved in development co-operation with low and middle-income countries through bilateral, country-to-country relationships. For this purpose national development co-operation agencies have been set up, and some of these are listed below.

The greater part of official development assistance, ODA, originates from the European and North American member states of the Organisation of Economic Co-operation and Development, OECD. Its Development Assistance Committee, DAC, has a particular role to produce statistics on development co-operation. DAC collects data and publishes annual reports on aid flows.[1]

The share of the bilateral aid allocated to the social sectors increased during the 1990s to some 29 % in 1997. In real terms, bilateral health assistance had reached USD 2.7 billion in 1997. Some few examples of bilateral development co-operation agencies are mentioned below.

12.4.1   United States Agency for International Development, USAID

USAID is the main official US development co-operation agency. It is an offshoot of the Marshall Plan for Europe after the Second World War and the Act for International Development passed by Congress in 1949. The US assistance programme has often been closely connected with commercial, political and military interests, and it is exposed to a detailed regulation by the US Congress, which occasionally decides on specific conditions for the provision of assistance. USAID also supports some very important initiatives. One outstanding example is the Demographic Health Surveys that provide much of the information about the health status of children in low-income countries. These surveys are commissioned to a private company

called Macro International Inc., which in a highly professional way implements these studies in conjunction with national agencies. All data obtained is freely available on the Internet.[2]

USAID is, in financial terms, by far the most important bilateral player in global health, with a commitment of USD 917 million in the fiscal year 2001. Its main areas have been family planning, reproductive health, child survival, maternal health, HIV/AIDS and infectious diseases.[3] However, USAID has significantly reduced its support to reproductive health issues such as abortion and contraceptives due to the conservative influence within the current US administration.

12.4.2   Department for International Development, DFID (U.K.)

Under previous governments, the DFID and its predecessor, ODA, emphasised economic and financial issues and accountability, expressed as 'value for money'. Under the Blair government, the focus has shifted to the alleviation of poverty[4] with a strong increase of the developmental aid budget. DFID possesses considerable professional expertise in the health sector.

12.4.3   Swedish International Development Co-operation Agency (Sida).

Sida was established in 1965 as a successor to an earlier government agency (NIB). In its early phase, Sida had a strong focus on population and family planning issues. From the mid-1970s, this emphasis was gradually replaced by a broad-based primary health care strategy and strong support for multilateral actions. From the late 1990s, the health sector priorities of Sida have been

---

[1]   www.oecd.org/dac

[2]   www.measuredhs.com
[3]   www.usaid.gov
[4]   www.dfid.gov.uk

health planning and management and sexual and reproductive health. Sweden is today among those donor countries which provide the smallest amount of health aid, in relative terms (only 2.2 % of total bilateral aid in 2001) but with a sharp increase in overall development aid to reach the one percent of GNP target.[1]

12.5 Non-governmental organisations (NGOs)

The demarcation line between public, i.e. governmental organisations and the private sector is not always clear-cut. Institutes such as the Pasteur institutes in many countries often occupy a semi-governmental position. In other countries, especially the former socialist countries, NGOs were often regarded with mistrust and not permitted to operate except in close alliance with governments. For example the Red Cross association in some countries can still be seen as a semi-governmental entity.

By and large the organisations below are international non-governmental organisations (INGOs), with a global scope. However, purely national NGOs are playing an increasingly important role in many countries, sometimes in collaboration with international organisations or as member organisations of global federations.

Long before any official development co-operation was even considered, NGOs were active in health activities in different countries. Since the late 19th century, especially in Africa, a variety of churches and missionary societies have been heavily involved in health and education projects, in addition to their main religious objectives. As the colonial powers tended to neglect the health of the indigenous peoples in their colonies, the health care provided by missions was often the only form of western health care

available. Other organisations, such as the International Committee of the Red Cross, were also active in health activities.

In the early post-colonial era, health was placed high on the agenda of official development co-operation. The expectation that the governments of the newly independent states would quickly become capable of running their own—at that time mostly free—health services was strong. The role of NGOs was seen as complementary, at most.

At the same time many NGOs did receive support from their home countries in order to provide more and better services for groups that were not easily reached by governments. The importance of the NGOs in health was vastly different between regions and countries. In most Asian countries, they were insignificant in terms of funding and activities, while in some African countries they actually ran, and still run, a considerable part of the health services, sometimes more than half.

Today, the NGOs constitute a varied group. The traditional NGOs, such as churches and missions, are still active, although now more often through their local partner churches or through special disaster relief organisations, such as Caritas International Medical Mission Board (Catholic) or the Church World Service (Protestant and Orthodox). Among the best-known humanitarian organisations, we find the Red Cross (considered to be the world's largest NGO), the Save the Children associations in many countries, Médecins Sans Frontières, World Vision, Oxfam, PATH, Rotary International, and CARE.

In specific areas NGOs are prominent at a global level; for example, the International Planned Parenthood Federation, IPPF, promotes responsible parenthood, family planning and nowadays also broader reproductive health action. In some countries NGOs constitute a special form for recognised activities, for instance in Nepal, where more than 10 000 NGOs are reported to exist.

---

[1]   www.sida.se

Examples of NGOs which are important in global health (out of hundreds of thousands of NGOs) are:

12.5.1 International Committee of the Red Cross, ICRC

Founded in 1863 as a Swiss organisation, governed by a committee of 15 to 25 Swiss nationals, with headquarters in Geneva.
Active in war and disaster situations, and increasingly in conflict prevention.
Annual budget (2000): USD 700 million
Expatriate field staff: 1 000 to 1 200
Web site: www.icrc.org

12.5.2 International Federation of Red Cross & Red Crescent Societies (IFRC)

(Previously the League of Red Cross and Red Crescent Societies)
Federation of 177 national Red Cross and Red Crescent societies, founded in 1919 with headquarters in Geneva. Total of 97 million members and volunteers, and 300 000 employees.
Main tasks are to co-ordinate international assistance from national societies to disaster victims, promote the establishment of national societies and act as a body for liaison, co-ordination and study for national societies.
Web site: www.ifrc.org

12.5.3 International Planned Parenthood Federation, IPPF

Established in 1952,
Federation of national family planning or sex education organisations
Around 180 member organisations
Annual turnover of the whole system around USD 850 million, central organisation around USD 80 million
Staff (volunteers): Several million
Web site: www.ippf.org

12.5.4 Médecins Sans Frontières, MSF ('Doctors Without Borders')

Established in 1971 in France as a medical humanitarian organisation
Now with 5 operational branches (France, Belgium, Holland, Switzerland, Spain) and supporting organisations in 13 other countries
Annual budget: 300 million US
Staff: 3 000 international volunteers, 15 000 national staff, working in more than 80 countries
Web site: www.msf.org

12.5.5 World Council of Churches (WCC)

Established 1948
WCC is a fellowship of 348 churches in more than 120 countries in all continents mainly from the Orthodox, Anglican, Reformed, Methodist and Lutheran traditions.
Its headquarter in Geneva supports member-churches as well as other churches and faith-based organisations in their health service projects around the world, mainly through studies, training and advice.
Web site: www.wcc-coe.org

12.5.6 Caritas Internationalis

Founded in 1951
Caritas is a network of Catholic relief, development and social service organisations supporting and running health service and development projects over 200 countries.
Caritas works without regard to creed, race, gender, or ethnicity, and is one of the world's largest humanitarian networks.
Web site: www.caritas.org

12.6 Philanthropic foundations

The philanthropic foundations constitute a particular form of work, particularly prominent in the United States. Some of them have long been active in international health work, e.g. the Rockefeller Foundation (established in 1913) and the Ford Foundation, both of which have been and are heavily involved in health work at different levels, e.g. research, training and epidemiological work. The Aga Khan Foundation is well known for its support to promote social development in low-income countries, and for its educational institutions.

12.6.1   The Rockefeller Foundation

Established: 1913
Assets: USD 3.5 billion
Grants for health 2000: USD 197 million
Web site: www.rockfound.org

12.6.2   The Bill and Melinda Gates Foundation

Established 1999
Assets: over USD 30 billion
Grants for global health 2001: USD 856 million
Health, especially immunisation, HIV/AIDS, and reproductive and child health with a special focus on innovation.
Financing of the Children's Vaccine Program
Web site: www.gatesfoundation.org

The Gates' Foundation has in only a few years become one of the major actors in global health collaboration. It can be expected that this and other similar philanthropic organisations will play an increasingly important role in world health co-operation in the future.

12.7 Industry & corporations

Industry's role in health care is complex and not easy to interpret. It has an obvious role to play on the supply side for clinical services (increasingly an area for private enterprise in many areas of the world), pharmaceutical products and equipment. For example, private industry is today the only sector that can translate basic research into product development for new pharmaceuticals.

The provision of health services for employees is a traditional area of activity. A new trend is towards greater involvement in society through contributions to health and welfare activities, possibly as an aspect of what is considered good business practice.

12.8 The future of global health collaboration

As the mechanisms for international health collaboration have appeared to be insufficient to meet the new—and the old—threats to health, new entities have emerged, replacing or complementing the old institutions. There are already about 70 health initiatives in which WHO is participating.

The prime example of this is UNAIDS (see section 12.2.6 above). More recently, the Global Forum for Health Research has been formed as a focal point for new efforts to intensify health research. Another example of such collaboration is the Global Alliance for Vaccines and Immunisation (GAVI).[1] This alliance was created in 1999 as a partnership between WHO, UNICEF, the World Bank, bilateral agencies, countries, Bill & Melinda Gates foundations and the pharmaceutical industry, in order to promote immunisation of children in a rights perspective (the right of every child to be protected against immunisation-preventable diseases). With a Vaccine Fund of over USD 1.3 billion at its disposal through grants from the Gates Foundation and countries such as Norway, Netherlands, Sweden, the UK and the US, GAVI has in less than five years committed over USD 1.2 billion in support to 70 of the world's poorest countries.

Most recently, the Global Fund to Fight AIDS, Tuberculosis and Malaria (GFATM) started to provide its first support to countries in 2002, with the goal of mobilising up to USD 10 billion per year for its activities.[2] In the start the fund has mobilised about 1

---

[1]   www.vaccinealliance.org
[2]   www.globalfundatm.org

billion USD per year, and it has created a seemingly efficient and transparent mechanism for assessing applications and disbursements of funds. In the honourable attempt to raise new money for health improvements for those in greatest need the Global Fund is facing a dilemma, which it shares with similar initiatives. In order to mobilise substantial amounts of new funds the Fund must focus on issues and actions that coincide with the perceptions of the potential contributors. However, contributors' conceptions may not coincide with the cost-effective and evidence-based actions that are first needed in low-income countries. One such example is the provision of free anti-retroviral drugs. With a scientifically highly qualified leader for the Global fund and a transparent mechanism for assessing applications one can hope that this new institution will manage to strike the best balance between what is most needed and what is easiest to find money for. It seems that it remains easier to raise money for drugs to treat the sick rather than to prevent diseases to occur.

Another large-scale initiative that was launched in July 2003 is the Health Metrics Network as a collaborative effort between WHO, the Gates' Foundation and others to improve health measurements.

UNAIDS, GAVI and the global fund are probably only the start. There is a growing awareness that previous competition and turf wars between international agencies must be replaced by collaborative efforts and, whenever possible, joint programming. New linkages, networks and joint programmes can be expected to emerge from this insight, complementing or replacing existing structures.

In addition to these new organisational forms, reform efforts are under way within the UN system to make collaboration between the agencies more effective. The United Nations Development Groups, UNDG, is working in a number of pilot countries to develop what are known as United Nations Development Assistance Frameworks, UNDAFs, as a means of joint programming. The World Bank, for its part, is establishing Comprehensive Development Frameworks (CDFs), which aim to integrate WB loans and support from other external partners in different sectors. A variety of working groups and committees strengthen the multilateral work in many sub-sectors of health. One example is the Interagency Pharmaceutical Co-ordination Group (IPC), consisting of senior pharmaceutical advisers of WHO, WB, UNAIDS, UNFPA and UNICEF who meet regularly to co-ordinate pharmaceutical policies and prepare interagency statements and technical documents.

A more crucial issue will be how international contributions to the health sector should match the national health budgets. There are governments such as the one in Uganda that has considered the international contributions to their health sector to be so big that the countries have to cut down their own health budget to secure the macroeconomic stability. Many assumed that this was due to foreign pressure from IMF, but it has to be realised that all serious governments will adjust their budgets in relation to the size of foreign contributions in different sectors. The main issue regarding future international support to the health sector in low-income countries may be how the national government assesses the investment need in health in relation to the needs in the other social sectors.

Another emerging aspect of the globalisation of health with the focus on middle-income countries is that international companies start to operate curative hospital service around the world. Other trans-actional companies also start to offer health insurance at an international level. It is noteworthy that the governments in China and Vietnam have embarked on a very market oriented policy for hospital services that may open for international trade both in operating hospitals and providing hospital services to patients. Hospitals services are very labour intensive and middle-income countries with high medical qualifications among their staff may start to provide curative services in a much larger scale than today. A number of new examples are emerging every year. These types of trans-national curative services will need regulations and policy decisions both in the country of the patient and the country of the hospital. Countries in the former Soviet Union and South Africa are already providing cosmetic surgery to patients from West Europe on a regular basis. It is not surprising that Cuba is one of the countries that is leading the process of commercial international provision of curative services as the country has an abundance of highly qualified medical practitioners that work on low salaries.

The number of international contacts in what we might call international health co-operation is increasing in all fields. The multilateral system centred on the United Nations continues to be of significance, civil society and a variety of organisations are meeting, combining or working together, and research contacts are multiplying. Training and work by young people across national borders is rapidly becoming a necessary part of their careers, rather than an exotic adventure.

Some of the developments of the last few years deserve further discussion and action. The multi-sectoral nature of emerging health problems so clearly demonstrated by the HIV/AIDS pandemic is one of them. Whether the solution to that is specialised organisations outside the traditional ones is another matter. It may be that the existing organisations will have to broaden the scope of their work to cater for new needs for co-operation.

It seems now rather clear that the Millennium Development Goals that were set by the global community will not be reached by 2015. In fact if developments continue as now it will take many decades before some of the goals will be met.

A number of ideas to increase overall development aid have been presented in recent years, the Tobin tax (taxation on international capital transactions), environmental taxes, global lotteries etc. For the moment the most realistic of these appears to be an idea rasied by the British Chancellor of the Exchequer, Gordon Brown, about the creation of a so called International Finance Facility (IFF). This idea implies the sale of bonds in the capital markets backed up by donor pledges to provide funding over a 15 or 20 year period. This is a simple idea although technically complex; the goal being to double international development aid from currently about USD 50 billion annually, thereby being able to invest more to help the world attain the MDGs.

As a pilot of this large scale IFF it has been proposed to raise USD 4 billion for a specific immunization project, to be handled by GAVI. Strongly backed by Britain and France this initiative may actually be realized early in 2005.

The recent reorganisation of WHO shows, if nothing else, a growing sense that the multilateral organisations must be more responsive to their constituencies, their member states. They cannot continue to work according to old prescriptions. They will have to compete with other possible solutions, such as regional organisations or private sector activities.

Clearly, these developments do not replace the original purpose of international health collaboration: to prevent the spread of communicable diseases across national borders. A few years ago, a man that lived in the neighbourhood of Geneva Airport died of malaria caused by a mosquito that had apparently been brought there by a plane from an endemic area. This was not a public health problem, but it shows that, as diseases know no national borders, international health co-operation will continue to have to deal with trans-national health issues.

If present trends continue, civil society and private players are bound to become more prominent. It is not just the fact that wealthy individuals are likely to continue donating large amounts of money to health programmes. There also seems to be a growing sense of corporate social responsibility from companies, including possible involvement in health programmes outside their own work sector. It is difficult to predict the final outcome of the directions of international health collaboration as described above. One may see the diversification of global health initiatives as a sad weakening of the UN system leading towards a commercial globalisation of the health sector; or as an evidence based move towards a more effective enlightened self-interest that will benefit the health of all in this world. It is partly up to the readers of this book to make sure that collaboration for better global health goes the right way.

References and suggested further reading

Basch PF. A Historical Perspective on International Health. Infectious Disease Clinics of North America, 1991;5:183–96.

Development Assistance Committee, Development Co-operation Report. Paris: OECD; 2002.

WHO. Facts about WHO. Geneva: World Health Organization; 1990.

Lucas A, Mögedal S, Walt G, Hodne SS, Kruse SE, Lee K, Hawken L. Co-operation for Health Development. WHO's support to programmes at country level. WHO: 1997.

Sachs JD. Macroeconomics and Health: Investing in Health for Economic Development. Report of the Commission on Macroeconomics and Health (CMH) to WHO: 2001. www.cmhealth.org

Musgrove P, Zeramdini. A. Summary Description of Health Financing in WHO Member States. CMH Working Paper Series, Paper No. WG3:3. www.cmhealth.org

Pouiller JP, Hernandez P, Kawabata K, Savedoff WD. Patterns of Global Health Expenditures: Results for 191 Countries. EIP/HFS/FAR Discussion Paper No. 51. WHO, 2002 (mimeo).

Reich MR, Marui E. International Co-operation for Health. Problems, Prospects and Priorities. Auburn House Publishing Company; 1989.

Vaughan JP, Mogedal S, Kruse S-E, Lee K, Walt G, de Wilde K. Financing the World Health Organisation: global importance of extra budgetary funds. Health Policy 1996;35:229–245.

WHO. The World Health Report 2000. Health Systems: Improving Performance. WHO; 2000.

WHO. The World Health Report 2003.

World Development Report 1993. Investing in Health. Published for the World Bank. Oxford: Oxford University Press; 1993.

Abbreviations

AIDS	Acquired Immune Deficiency Syndrome	MDG	Millennium Development Goals
ARV	Anti Retro-Viral drugs	MGM	Male Genital Mutilation
BCG	Bacille Calmette-Guérin (Tuberculosis vaccine)	MMR	Maternal Mortality Ratio
		NAIDS	Nutritionally Acquired Immune Deficiency Syndrome
BMI	Body Mass Index	NGO	Non-Governmental Organization
CBR	Crude Birth Rate	PHC	Primary Health Care
CDR	Crude Death Rate	PPP	Purchasing Power Parity
CMH	Commission on Macroeconomics and Health	PVO	Private Voluntary Organizations
		OAU	Organization for African Unity
CVD	Cardiovascular Disease	ODA	Official Development Assistance
DAC	Development Assistance Committee (of OECD)	OECD	Organization for Economic Co-operation and Development
DALY	Disability Adjusted Life Years	OPV	Oral Polio Vaccine
DHS	Demographic and Health Survey	ORT	Oral Rehydration Therapy
DTP	Diphteria-Tetanus-Pertussis	SAP	Structural Adjustment Program
EPI	Expanded Program on Immunization	SARS	Severe acute respiratory syndrome
		SF	Symphysis Fundus distance
FGM	Female Genital Mutilation	STI	Sexually Transmitted Infection
GAVI	Global Alliance for Vaccines and Immunization	SWAps	Sector Wide Approach
		TFR	Total Fertility Rate
GDP	Gross Domestic Product	TRIPS	Trade Related Aspects of Intellectual Property Rights
GFATM	Global Fund to fight AIDS, Tuberculosis and Malaria		
		U5MR	Under Five Mortality Rate
GNP	Gross National Product	UNAIDS	Joint United Nations Program on HIV/AIDS
HALE	Health Adjusted Life Expectancy		
HFA	Height For Age	UNDP	United Nations Development Program
HIV	Human Immunodeficiency Virus		
HPV	Human Papilloma Virus	UNFPA	United Nations Population Fund
IBRD	International Bank of Reconstruction and Development	UNICEF	United Nations Children's Fund
		USD	US dollars
ICD	International Classification of Disease	YLL	Years of Life Lost
		VAD	Vitamin A Deficiency
IDA	International Development Association (part of WB group)	WB	World Bank
		WDR	World Development Report (World Bank)
IDA	Iron Deficiency Anemia		
IDD	Iodine Deficiency Disorders	WFA	Weight For Age
IEC	Information Education Communication	WFH	Weight For Height
		WHA	World Health Assembly (WHO's annual meeting of member states)
IMF	International Monetary Fund		
IUD	Intrauterine device	WHO	World Health Organization
IMR	Infant Mortality Rate	WDR	World Development Report (by WB)
IPV	Inactivated (killed) polio vaccine	WHR	World Health Report (by WHO)
LBW	Low Birth Weight	WTO	World Trade Organization
LE	Life Expectancy (at birth)		

Appendix 1

Regional summaries in all Unicef statistics referred to in this book

Regional averages given at the end of each table are calculated using data from the countries and territories as grouped below.

Sub-Saharan Africa
Angola; Benin; Botswana; Burkina Faso; Burundi; Cameroon; Cape Verde; Central African Republic; Chad; Comoros; Congo; Congo, Democratic Republic of the; Côte d'Ivoire; Equatorial Guinea; Eritrea; Ethiopia; Gabon; Gambia; Ghana; Guinea; Guinea-Bissau; Kenya; Lesotho; Liberia; Madagascar; Malawi; Mali; Mauritania; Mauritius; Mozambique; Namibia; Niger; Nigeria; Rwanda; Sao Tome and Principe; Senegal; Seychelles; Sierra Leone; Somalia; South Africa; Swaziland; Tanzania; United Republic of; Togo; Uganda; Zambia; Zimbabwe.

Middle East and North Africa
Algeria; Bahrain; Cyprus; Djibouti; Egypt; Iran, Islamic Republic of; Iraq; Jordan; Kuwait; Lebanon; Libyan Arab Jamahiriya; Morocco; Occupied Palestinian Territory; Oman; Qatar; Saudi Arabia; Sudan; Syrian Arab Republic; Tunisia; United Arab Emirates; Yemen.

South Asia
Afghanistan; Bangladesh; Bhutan; India; Maldives; Nepal; Pakistan; Sri Lanka.

East Asia and Pacific
Brunei Darussalam; Cambodia; China; Cook Islands; East Timor; Fiji; Indonesia; Kiribati; Korea, Democratic People's Republic of; Korea, Republic of; Lao People's Democratic Republic; Malaysia; Marshall Islands; Micronesia, Federated States of; Mongolia; Myanmar; Nauru; Niue; Palau; Papua New Guinea; Philippines; Samoa; Singapore; Solomon Islands; Thailand; Tonga; Tuvalu; Vanuatu; Viet Nam.

Latin America and Caribbean
Antigua and Barbuda; Argentina; Bahamas; Barbados; Belize; Bolivia; Brazil; Chile; Colombia; Costa Rica; Cuba; Dominica; Dominican Republic; Ecuador; El Salvador; Grenada; Guatemala; Guyana; Haiti; Honduras; Jamaica; Mexico; Nicaragua; Panama; Paraguay; Peru; Saint Kitts and Nevis; Saint Lucia; Saint Vincent and the Grenadines; Suriname; Trinidad and Tobago; Uruguay; Venezuela.

CEE/CIS and Baltic States
Albania; Armenia; Azerbaijan; Belarus; Bosnia and Herzegovina; Bulgaria; Croatia; Czech Republic; Estonia; Georgia; Hungary; Kazakhstan; Kyrgyzstan; Latvia; Lithuania; Moldova, Republic of; Poland; Romania; Russian Federation; Slovakia; Tajikistan; the former Yugoslav Republic of Macedonia; Turkey; Turkmenistan; Ukraine; Uzbekistan; Yugoslavia.

High-income countries
Andorra; Australia; Austria; Belgium; Canada; Denmark; Finland; France; Germany; Greece; Holy See; Iceland; Ireland; Israel; Italy; Japan; Liechtenstein; Luxembourg; Malta; Monaco; Netherlands; New Zealand; Norway; Portugal; San Marino; Slovenia; Spain; Sweden; Switzerland; United Kingdom; United States.

Low- and middle-income countries

Afghanistan; Algeria; Angola; Antigua and Barbuda; Argentina; Armenia; Azerbaijan; Bahamas; Bahrain; Bangladesh; Barbados; Belize; Benin; Bhutan; Bolivia; Botswana; Brazil; Brunei Darussalam; Burkina Faso; Burundi; Cambodia; Cameroon; Cape Verde; Central African Republic; Chad; Chile; China; Colombia; Comoros; Congo; Congo, Democratic Republic of the; Cook Islands; Costa Rica; Côte d'Ivoire; Cuba; Cyprus; Djibouti; Dominica; Dominican Republic; East Timor; Ecuador; Egypt; El Salvador; Equatorial Guinea; Eritrea; Ethiopia; Fiji; Gabon; Gambia; Georgia; Ghana; Grenada; Guatemala; Guinea; Guinea-Bissau; Guyana; Haiti; Honduras; India; Indonesia; Iran, Islamic Republic of; Iraq; Israel; Jamaica; Jordan; Kazakhstan; Kenya; Kiribati; Korea, Democratic People's Republic of; Korea, Republic of; Kuwait; Kyrgyzstan; Lao People's Democratic Republic; Lebanon; Lesotho; Liberia; Libyan Arab Jamahiriya; Madagascar; Malawi; Malaysia; Maldives; Mali; Marshall Islands; Mauritania; Mauritius; Mexico; Micronesia, Federated States of; Mongolia; Morocco; Mozambique; Myanmar; Namibia; Nauru; Nepal; Nicaragua; Niger; Nigeria; Niue; Occupied Palestinian Territory; Oman; Pakistan; Palau; Panama; Papua New Guinea; Paraguay; Peru; Philippines; Qatar; Rwanda; Saint Kitts and Nevis; Saint Lucia; Saint Vincent/Grenadines; Samoa; Sao Tome and Principe; Saudi Arabia; Senegal; Seychelles; Sierra Leone; Singapore; Solomon Islands; Somalia; South Africa; Sri Lanka; Sudan; Suriname; Swaziland; Syrian Arab Republic; Tajikistan; Tanzania, United Republic of; Thailand; Togo; Tonga; Trinidad and Tobago; Tunisia; Turkey; Turkmenistan; Tuvalu; Uganda; United Arab Emirates; Uruguay; Uzbekistan; Vanuatu; Venezuela; Viet Nam; Yemen; Zambia; Zimbabwe.

Least developed countries

Afghanistan; Angola; Bangladesh; Benin; Bhutan; Burkina Faso; Burundi; Cambodia; Cape Verde; Central African Republic; Chad; Comoros; Congo, Democratic Republic of; Djibouti; Equatorial Guinea; Eritrea; Ethiopia; Gambia; Guinea; Guinea-Bissau; Haiti; Kiribati; Lao People's Democratic Republic; Lesotho; Liberia; Madagascar; Malawi; Maldives; Mali; Mauritania; Mozambique; Myanmar; Nepal; Niger; Rwanda; Samoa; Sao Tome and Principe; Senegal; Sierra Leone; Solomon Islands; Somalia; Sudan; Tanzania, United Republic of; Togo; Tuvalu; Uganda; Vanuatu; Yemen; Zambia.

Appendix 2

Regional summaries of World Health Organization statistics referred to in this book

Below are the regions of the world listed by country used for WHO statistics in this book. WHO also divides some of its health data into high-income and Low- and middle-income countries. Sometimes China and India are referred to separately because of their large population.

African region (AFR)
Algeria, Angola, Benin, Botswana, Burkina Faso, Burundi, Cameroon, Cape Verde, Central African Republic, Chad, Comoros, Congo, Côte d'Ivoire, Democratic republic of Congo, Equatorial Guinea, Eritrea, Ethiopia, Gabon, Gambia, Ghana, Guinea, Guinea-Bissau, Kenya, Lesotho, Liberia, Madagascar, Malawi, Mali, Mauritania, Mauritius, Mozambique, Namibia, Niger, Nigeria, Rwanda, Sao Tome et Principe, Senegal, Seychelles, Sierra Leone, South Africa, Swaziland, Togo, Uganda, United Republic of Tanzania, Zambia, Zimbabwe.

Region of the Americas (AMR)
Antigua and Barbuda, Argentina, Bahamas, Barbados, Belize, Bolivia, Brazil, Canada, Chile, Colombia, Costa Rica, Cuba, Dominica, Dominican republic, Ecuador, El Salvador, Grenada, Guatemala, Guyana, Haiti, Honduras, Jamaica, Mexico, Nicaragua, Panama, Paraguay, Peru, Saint Kitts and Nevis, Saint Lucia, Saint Vincent and the Grenadines, Suriname, Trinidad and Tobago, United States of America, Uruguay, Venezuela.

Eastern Mediterranean Region (EMR)
Afghanistan, Bahrain, Cyprus, Djibouti, Egypt, Islamic Republic of Iran, Iraq, Jordan, Kuwait, Lebanon, Libyan Arab Jamahiriya, Morocco, Oman, Pakistan, Qatar, Saudi Arabia, Somalia, Sudan, Syrian Arab Republic, Tunisia, United Arab Emirate, Yemen.

European Region (EUR)
Albania, Andorra, Armenia, Austria, Azerbaijan, Belarus, Belgium, Bosnia and Herzegovina, Bulgaria, Croatia, Czech republic, Denmark, Estonia, Finland, France, Georgia, Germany, Greece, Hungary, Iceland, Ireland, Israel, Italy, Kazakhstan, Kyrgyzstan, Latvia, Lithuania, Luxembourg, Malta, Monaco, Netherlands, Norway, Poland, Portugal, Republic of Moldova, Romania, Russian Republic, San Marino, Slovakia, Slovenia, Spain, Sweden, Switzerland, Tajikistan, The former Yugoslav Republic of Macedonia, Turkey, Turkmenistan, Ukraine, United Kingdom, Uzbekistan, Yugoslavia.

South East Asia Region (SEAR)
Bangladesh, Bhutan, Democratic People's Republic of Korea, India, Indonesia, Maldives, Myanmar, Nepal, Sri Lanka, Thailand.

Western Pacific Region (WPR)
Australia, Brunei Darussalam, Cambodia, China, Cook Islands, Fiji, Japan, Kiribati, Lao People's Democratic Republic, Malaysia, Marshall Islands, Federated States of Micronesia, Mongolia, Nauru, New Zealand, Niue, Palau, Papua New Guinea, Philippines, Republic of Korea, Samoa, Singapore, Solomon Islands, Tonga, Tuvalu, Vanuatu, Viet Nam.

Appendix 3

Regional summaries of the world according to the World Bank

East Asia and Pacific
American Samoa, Cambodia, China, Fiji, Indonesia, Kiribati, Dem. Rep. Korea, Rep. Korea, PDR Laos, Malaysia, Marshall islands, Fed. Sts. Micronesia, Mongolia, Myanmar, Palau, Papua New Guinea, Philippines, Samoa, Solomon Islands, Thailand, Tonga, Vanuatu, Vietnam.

Europe and Central Asia
Albania, Armenia, Azerbaijan, Belarus, Bosnia and Herzegovina, Bulgaria, Croatia, Czech Republic, Estonia, Georgia, Hungary, Isle of Man, Kazakhstan, Kyrgyz Republic, Latvia, Lithuania, FYR Macedonia, Moldova, Poland, Romania, Russian Republic, Slovak Republic, Tajikistan, Turkey, Turkmenistan, Ukraine, Uzbekistan, FR Yugoslavia.

Latin America and the Caribbean
Antigua and Barbuda, Argentina, Belize, Bolivia, Brazil, Chile, Colombia, Costa Rica, Cuba, Dominica, Dominica Republic, Ecuador, El Salvador, Grenada, Guatemala, Guyana, Haiti, Honduras, Jamaica, Mexico, Nicaragua, Panama, Paraguay, Peru, Puerto Rica, St. Kitts and Nevis, St. Lucia, St.Vincent and the Grenadines, Suriname, Trinidad and Tobago, Uruguay, Venezuela.

Middle East and North Africa
Algeria, Bahrain, Djibouti, Egypt Arab Rep., Islamic Rep. Iran, Iraq, Jordan, Lebanon, Libya, Malta, Morocco, Oman, Saudi Arabia, Syrian Arab Republic, Tunisia, West Bank and Gaza, Rep Yemen.

South Asia
Afghanistan, Bangladesh, Bhutan, India, Maldives, Nepal, Pakistan, Sri Lanka.

Sub-Saharan Africa
Angola, Benin, Botswana, Burkina Faso, Burundi, Cameroon, Cape Verde, Central African Republic, Chad, Comoros, Dem.Rep. Congo, Rep Congo, Côte d'Ivoire, Equatorial Guinea, Eritrea, Ethiopia, Gabon, Gambia, Ghana, Guinea, Guinea-Bissau, Kenya, Lesotho, Liberia, Madagascar, Malawi, Mali, Mauritania, Mauritius Mayotte, Mozambique, Namibia, Niger, Nigeria, Rwanda, Sao Tome and Principe, Senegal, Seychelles, Sierra Leone, Somalia, South Africa, Sudan, Swaziland, Tanzania, Togo, Uganda, Zambia, Zimbabwe.

High income OECD
Australia, Austria, Belgium, Canada, Denmark, Finland, France, Germany, Greece, Iceland, Ireland, Italy, Japan, Luxembourg, Netherlands, New Zealand, Norway, Switzerland, Portugal, Spain, Sweden, Switzerland, United Kingdom, United States.

Other High Income
Andorra, Aruba, Bahamas, Bermuda, Brunei, Cayman Islands, Channel Islands, Cyprus, Faeroe Islands, French Polynesia, Greenland, Guam, Hong Kong China, Israel, Kuwait, Liechtenstein, Macao China, Monaco, Netherlands Antilles, New Caledonia, Northern Mariana Islands, Qatar, San Marino, Singapore, Slovenia, United Arab Emirate, Virgin Islands.

Appendix 4
Websites

Website	Organisations	Contents
Medical journals:		
www.ajph.org/cgi/etoc	American Journal of Public Health	
http://bmj.com/	Brittish Medical Journal	
www.who.int/bulletin/ tableofcontents.htm	Bulletin of the World Health Organization	
www.thelancet.com	Lancet Homepage	Many free articles accessible, some require subscription
www.nlm.nih.gov	National Library of Medicine	Home of Medline
www.ncbi.nlm.nih.gov/PubMed/ medline.html	PubMed	Search medical articles
www.elsevier.com/locate/ ContentsDirect	Elsevier Science	ContentsDirect, where you can subscribe for free to emails with Tables of Content for several journal
Health topics:		
www.aidsinfo.nih.gov	National Institute of Health, US	HIV/AIDS
www.aidsmap.com		HIV/AIDS
www.ctu.mrc.ac.uk/penta/	Paediatric European Network for the Treatment of AIDS	AIDS treatment
www.comminit.com		Health communication
www.cdc.gov/nccdphp	The Centers for Disease Control and Prevention in the US	Nutrition and physical activity
www.fao.org	FAO, Division of Nutrition	Nutrition
	WHO/PAHO	Health Library for disasters
www.hsph.harvard.edu/hcpds/ workingpapers. html	Harvard School of Public Health	Gender issues
www.hsph.harvard.edu/ Organizations/healthnet/	Global Reproductive Health Forum, Harvard School of Public Health	Reproductive Health issues
www.iapac.org	(International Association of Physicians in AIDS Care) ARV treatment guidelines	ARV treatment
www.idf.org	International diabetes federation	Diabetes
www.ids.ac.uk/bridge/	Bridge	Gender and Health
www.ifpri.org	International Food Policy Research Institute	Obesity
www.inacg.ilsi.org	International Nutritional Anemia Consultative Group (INACG)	Iron deficiency anaemia
www.iotf.org	International Obesity Task Force	Obesity

Website	Organisations	Contents
www.izincg.ucdavis.edu	International Zinc Nutrition Consultative Group (IZINCG)	Zinc deficiency
www.ivacg.ilsi.org	International Vitamin A Consultative Group (IVACG)	Vitamin A issues
www.measuredhs.com	Demographic and Health Survey	Demography and health
www.paho.org/genderandhealth/#Gender Equity	PAHO	Gender issues
www.people.virginia.edu/~jtd/iccidd	International Council for the Control of Iodine Deficiency Disorders (ICCIDD)	Iodine deficiency
www.pitt.edu/~super1/		The "Supercourse" – lectures on health topics for self learning
www.qweb.kvinnoforum.se	Kvinnoforum in Stockholm.	Women's health and gender issues.
www.reproductiverights.org.	'Center for Reproductive Rights'.	Legal aspects of the implementation of reproductive rights and its Violations.
www.unesco.org		Education
www.unsystem.org/scn	United Nations System Standing Committee on Nutrition	Nutrition
www.unaids.org (epidemiology)		
www.und.ac.za/und/heard/	The Health Economics & HIV/AIDS Research Division (HEARD) South Africa	AIDS info
www.who.int/child-adolescent-health	WHO	Integrated management of childhood illnesses
www.who.int/nutgrowthdb	WHO	Global Database on Child Growth
www.who.int/nut	WHO	Nutrition
Organisations:		
www.usaid.gov	The United States Agency for International Development	US governmental aid agency
www.arrow.org.my	'ARROW', an NGO based in Kuala Lumpur, Malaysia	Reproductive health.
www.gatesfoundation.org	The Bill and Melinda Gates Foundation	
www.ifrc.org	The International Federation of Red Cross and Red Crescent Societies (IFRC)	
www.vaccinealliance.org/home/index.php	Global Alliance for Vaccines and Immunization	
www.globalforumhealth.org/pages/index.asp	Global Forum for Health Research	Health research
www.icrc.org	International Committee of the Red Cross	
www.msf.org/	Medécins Sans Frontières	International Humanitarian Organisation
www.oecd.org/~dac	OECD	

Website	Organisations	Contents
www.ippf.org	International Planned Parenthood Federation	
www.rockfound.org	The Rockefeller Foundation	
www.sida.se	Swedish International Development Cooperation Agency	Swedish governmental aid agency
www.unaids.org	The Joint United Nations Programme on HIV/AIDS	
www.undp.org	United Nations Development Programme	
www.unicef.org/	The United Nations Childrens Fund	
www.dfid.gov.uk	The (British) Department for International Development, DFID	Brittish governmental aid agency
www.unfpa.org	United Nations Population Fund	
www.wcc-coe.org	World Council of Churches	
www.caritas.org	Caritas	Catholic relief network
www.wto.org	World Trade Organisation	
www.wfp.org/index2.html	World Food Program	
www.who.int	WHO- World Health Organization	
www.worldbank.org	The World Bank	
Universities:		
www.phs.ki.se/ihcar/	Karolinska Institute Department of Public Health, Division of International Health	
www.jhsph.edu/	John Hopkins School of Public Health	
www.hsph.harvard.edu	Harvard School of Public Health	
www.lshtm.ac.uk/	London School of Hygiene and Tropical Medicine	
www.dcp2.org	Disease Control Priorities Project World Bank, WHO and others	Update for cost effective actions for global health

Index